THE POPULARIZATION OF MEDICINE
1650–1850

THE WELLCOME INSTITUTE SERIES IN THE HISTORY OF MEDICINE

Edited by W.F. Bynum and Roy Porter
The Wellcome Institute

THE POPULARIZATION
OF MEDICINE
1650–1850

Edited by
ROY PORTER

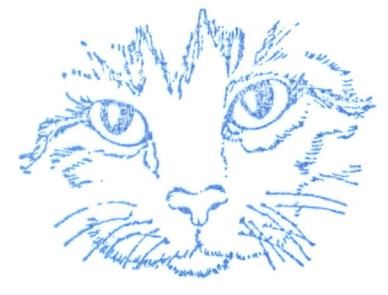

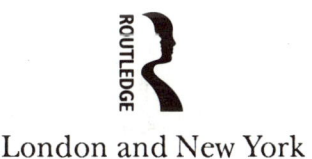

London and New York

First published in 1992
by Routledge
11 New Fetter Lane, London EC4P 4EE

Simultaneously published in the USA and Canada
by Routledge
a division of Routledge, Chapman and Hall Inc.
29 West 35th Street, New York, NY 10001

Typeset in Baskerville by LaserScript, Mitcham, Surrey
Printed and bound in Great Britain
by Biddles Ltd, Guildford and King's Lynn

British Library Cataloguing in Publication Data
The popularization of medicine, 1650–1850. –
(The Wellcome Institute series in the history of medicine)
I. Porter, Roy, *1946*– II. Series
362.10941

Library of Congress Cataloging in Publication Data
The popularization of medicine. 1650–1850/edited by Roy Porter.
p. cm. – (The Wellcome Institute series in the history of medicine)
Includes bibliographical references and index.
1. Medicine, Popular – History – 17th century. 2. Medicine,
Popular – History – 18th century. 3. Medicine, Popular – History –
19th century. I. Porter, Roy, 1946– . II. Series.
[DNLM: 1. History of Medicine, 17th Cent. 2. History of Medicine,
18th Cent. 3. History of Medicine, 19th Cent. WZ 56 P831]
RC81.P83   1991
610'.9'03 – dc20
DNLM/DLC
for Library of Congress   91-32849
CIP

ISBN 0–415–07217–4

Contents

Contents

Illustrations

·Contributors

Antoinette Emch-Dériaz holds degrees in Sciences from the College and the University of Geneva, and a PhD in Intellectual History from the University of Rochester, NY. She has a record of publications in the field of eighteenth-century studies and teaches at the University of Mississippi.

Mary E. Fissell is currently Research Associate in the Wellcome Unit for the History of Medicine at Manchester University. She is the author of *Patients, Power, and the Poor in Eighteenth Century Bristol* (1991) and is embarking on a study of early modern vernacular health texts.

Norman Gevitz is Associate Professor of the History of Medicine at the University of Illinois College of Medicine, Chicago. He is the author of *The D.O.'s Osteopathic Medicine in America* and editor of *Other Healers: Unorthodox Medicine in America.* He is currently working on a history of domestic medicine in the United States.

Stephen Jacyna is Research Officer in the History of Medicine Unit at Manchester University. He is currently completing a monograph on the Edinburgh Medical School in the nineteenth century.

Enrique Perdiguero is Associate Professor in the History of Medicine at the University of Alicante. After studying medicine he did four years of research on the popularization of medicine in the Spanish Enlightenment, the topic of his doctoral thesis completed in 1989. He is currently working on fringe medicine and popular works on medicine of nineteenth-century Spain.

Roy Porter is Senior Lecturer in the Social History of Medicine at the Wellcome Institute for the History of Medicine. Recent books include *Patient's Progress* (co-authored with Dorothy Porter, 1989), *Health for Sale: Quackery in Georgian England, 1660–1850* (1990) and *Doctor of Society: Thomas Beddoes and the Sick Trade in Late-Enlightenment England* (1992).

Matthew Ramsey teaches history at Vanderbilt University in Nashville, Tennessee. He is the author of articles on the social history of medicine in the eighteenth and nineteenth centuries and of *Professional and Popular Medicine in France, 1770–1830: The Social World of Medical Practice* (1988). He is now completing a companion volume on the development of professional monopoly in French medicine.

Maria Szlatky, PhD, Research Fellow and historian. She has been working for the Semmelweis Medical Historical Museum, Library and Archives in Budapest. She has published two books (in Hungarian) on sixteenth to eighteenth century Hungarian medical literature (1983, 1989). She has also published several articles on the history of medicine in Hungarian periodicals. Her recent field of research is European medical literature as the source and origin of Hungarian medical texts.

Andrew Wear lectures in the history of medicine at University College London and the Wellcome Institute for the History of Medicine. He has research interests in Renaissance anatomy and in the social history of early modern England.

Philip K. Wilson received an MA in Medical History from Johns Hopkins University, and lectured for two years in Kansas City. Receiving a Wellcome Trust Studentship enabled him to continue historical research at the Wellcome Institute for the History of Medicine in London, where he is currently writing his doctoral thesis on the career and writings of London surgeon/physician Daniel Turner. He is delineating the organizational structure of early eighteenth-century surgery in London together with reconstructing aspects of the surgical art and practice as relayed through Turner's case histories.

Acknowledgements

This book arose from a conference held at the Wellcome Institute for the History of Medicine in London in January 1991. I am most grateful, as always, to the Wellcome Trust for its generous provision of funds to enable scholars to travel from many different countries to attend such events. I would also like to thank Frieda Houser whose organizing abilities once more helped to make holding the symposium a genuine pleasure. The contributors to the conference have produced versions of their papers for publication in double-quick time: their co-operation has been exemplary. And I am further grateful to Stephen Jacyna for allowing a paper of his, not given at the symposium but precisely on its themes, to be printed in this volume. Kate Legon has compiled a superb index.

Roy Porter
Wellcome Institute for the History of Medicine

Introduction

Roy Porter

Scholars have been recognizing more clearly since the early 1980s that what they study is not so much the history of medicine as histories of the medicines. For there has never been a single, homogeneous body of theory and practice answering to the name 'medicine'; the terrain of healing has always been characterized by great diversity. Academics have traditionally made 'learned medicine' or 'scientific medicine' their study. In recent years, greater attention has been given to 'popular medicine' and the folk tradition.[1] There is active research interest today in quack, irregular, and alternative medicine, too.[2] But, in all this, one important aspect seems largely to have remained in the shadows: the development of medical popularization, the process by which regular medicine is diffused to the wider lay public.

Today, doctors, their spokesmen, and media programmes bombard the public with medical information and education; ordinary people are avid consumers of advice and instruction from the professionals. All parents have invested in their *Dr Spock* or its successors; many families own their *B.M.A. Medical Handbook* or some equivalent; women buy *Our Bodies, Our Selves* (historically speaking, a not unusual instance of an essentially 'regular' text, spiced with a pinch of alternative ideology); newspapers and magazines all carry 'Dr X Answers Your Problems' columns, BBC radio runs 'Medicine Now', and endless television programmes explain the latest in medical science and clinical practice.[3]

Clearly, the phenomenon of diffusion is not unique to the late twentieth century culture of mass communications and electric media. For, as Paul Slack has emphasized, as long as there have been printed books, there have been printed books

1

purveying medical advice, 'secrets' and recipes from the experts or pseudo-experts (often, though not always, medical practitioners) to the public.[4] Before Gutenberg, instruction filtered down in manuscript and by word of mouth; nor did these less formal channels of exchange, of course, dwindle with the advent of printing, though the selective accidents of the preservation of evidence may occasionally convey that impression.

In fact, at least from the sixteenth century, it was common for gentry families to keep personal manuscript recipe books, where, cheek by jowl with cooking tips ('receipts') and household hints, there could be found medical remedies, many of them culled from learned sources.[5] From the mid-seventeenth century, Culpeper's *Herbal* began to assume exemplary status as a household name. In the eighteenth century, the writings of S.-A.-A.-D. Tissot achieved great popularity, especially in French-speaking nations, as did those of William Buchan, particularly in the English-speaking world, though not exclusively so, as is shown below by Enrique Perdiguero's discussion of Spain and Maria Szlatky's account of Hungary. And then, in North America, John Gunn's *Domestic Medicine, or the Poor Man's Friend* (1830) attained classic status. All were proofs of the vitality of, and demand for, a type of medicine that won a measure of approval from the faculty while simultaneously gaining the custom of an avid book-buying public. Tissot's *Avis au peuple* (1761) and Buchan's *Domestic Medicine* (1769) were widely translated, and went through scores of editions; Gunn's text may well have enjoyed over a couple of hundred reprintings: it certainly made Gunn one of the first doctors to make a living basically out of medical publishing. In the present century, such doctors as Truby King and Benjamin Spock have won international fame thanks to their popularizing skills.

Popularization is a historically significant part of the medical enterprise. But – although a couple of its chapters and a fair number of its footnotes have been written – its full history remains to be charted. This volume lays some of the ground, and points the way towards a more comprehensive history. It spans the period from the sixteenth century to the earlier years of the twentieth. It embraces a wide compass, dealing substantially with Britain, France, Spain, Hungary and North America and touching upon other nations. It combines close studies of the outstanding protagonists, Tissot and Buchan above all, with treatment of other major figures (Elyot,

Parkinson, Raspial, etc.) and more general assessments of the interpretative and historiographical problems posed by the genre. This volume cannot be the last word, but it does provide a connected account of the main figures and features of medical diffusion over the course of four centuries.[6]

Common sense suggests that the elements indispensable to the enterprise of medical popularization are a body of authorized regular medicine; doctors or writers eager to undertake the work of spreading it; a medium of diffusion, be it printed book, flysheet, handbill, pamphlet, or newspaper column; and, finally, a literate audience keen, prepared, or possibly compelled to imbibe such publications. These notions evidently contain difficulties which will be unpicked later; but even from this extremely simplified schema, several things should be clear.

For one thing, the genre is keenly time- and culture-specific. It is the child of societies that have developed certain cultural utilities: the printed book and facilities for its widespread production and distribution; a modicum of education and literacy; sufficient surplus income to permit investment in instruction manuals (and the drugs, apparatus, and treatments they recommend); an ethic inculcating self-help and self-reliance. It is equally a sign of a society beset by epidemic disease or at least perceived health threats,[7] and perhaps lacking adequate medical amenities to counter such threats. Thus, had schemes of universal, publicly organized and publicly funded health care been established, say, in seventeenth century Europe (as many reformers dreamed),[8] there would perhaps have been little reason for writings in this category ever to have been composed; had frontier America in the nineteenth century possessed more professional doctors, fewer would have had to vest their trust in their pocket copy of Buchan or Gunn. Popular medical writing took root in societies capable of supporting quite elaborate schemes of health provision and expertise among the élite but unable or unprepared to extend such facilities right down the social scale. It is possible that dispersing medical knowledge across a wide spectrum of society in a sense stood substitute, so to speak, for the wider public distribution of doctors and health care themselves. Yet this is not to say that the diffusion of popular medical works could not be conterminous with the spread of professional medical care itself.

From elementary remarks such as these, it will be obvious that the study of medical popularization makes little sense unless it fully takes into consideration many other great socio-cultural forces transforming early modern Europe: the deployment of printing as what Elizabeth Eisenstein has called 'an agent of change',[9] and the rise of the book trade;[10] the spread of formal schooling and standardized education;[11] the growth of literacy and the reading habit, with its accompanying conviction in the authority of the book,[12] the development of the family ideal (would *Domestic Medicine* have made such an appeal except where domesticity itself had high cachet?);[13] the rise of authorship as a vocation, a sideline, a religious calling, a bid for fame;[14] the forging, in the new nation-states of Europe, of serviceable vernaculars, shared by learned élites and common people alike, in place of the earlier dependence upon Latin as the language of learning, including medicine.[15] All of these are vast topics, which can be no more than mentioned in this Introduction, though many are taken up in the following essays, in particular in Mary Fissell's analysis of the text–reader relations implied in the genre.

But it is vital to take into account such wider forces for sociocultural change, since, as is shown in the following discussions on specific authors and themes, many of the distinctive preoccupations of popularized medicine – for instance, the common assertion of the superiority of the mother tongue, or the emphasis upon 'experience' – make sense only when contextualized against the wider problems of the relations between high and low cultures: questions of the rival priorities of secrecy and revelation, exclusiveness and openness, the dangers of the multiplication of error, fears that knowledge would fall into the wrong hands, the paradox of knowledge as private property and common patrimony.[16] With the coming of the printed book, there were violent debates as to whether 'a little learning' would automatically prove a dangerous thing.

Such debates raged in many fields, but in theology most fiercely. Given that Protestants, at least, believed that every man should be his own Bible-reader, did that mean that every man was also to be his own Bible-interpreter? All the Protestant churches were initially eager to propagate the Gospel, but most quickly discovered the difficulties and dangers of putting religious dynamite into unskilled hands. The Catholic church had no itch to install a Bible into every cottage; but the Council of Trent was equally insistent upon the need for popularization – if not for spreading the Word, at least for indoctrination through the media of images, ceremonies, sacraments and cate-chising.[17] Beyond religion, there were deep contentions over the safeguarding or scattering of technical expertise. Should guilds and professions keep trade secrets? Were certain forms of wisdom necessarily occult? This was an issue exemplified in the rise of Rosicrucianism and later Freemasonry.[18] The ethic of broad-casting knowledge battled with the fear that popular-ization would lead to profanation.

Above all, early modern society was exercised with the ten-sions between high and low culture, élite and plebeian values.[19] In the eyes of some, only the higher ranks could, and should, possess true knowledge, manners and morals; the masses were irremediably vulgar. For others, genteel codes were nothing more than high and mighty pretensions, whereas truth lay in the grass roots or with force of numbers. Some claimed there was no true wisdom outside books, the older the better. Others saw Ancient tomes as hidebound sources of error, denounced their study as fetishistic, and thought the only valuable books were the Book of God's Word (the Scriptures) and the Book of God's Works (Nature). Some, rather as advocated by Francis Bacon, hoped for a fruitful collaboration between philosophers and craftsmen. Others wanted to ensure that the distinctions between the cultures should be kept rigidly distinct. Even Voltaire, who, as a *philosophe*, had an evangelical commitment to spreading the light, was fearful that, if the poor were disabused of their religious superstitions about sin, one would have to start counting the spoons.[20]

In short, the politics of knowledge dissemination were con-fused and contested. Many were committed to education and instruction. Early Protestants had boundless confidence in the capacity of literacy and print to instil true faith. In later cen-turies, this religious missionary zeal was diluted, or modernized, into a Smilesian faith in self-improvement. For their part, eighteenth-century *philosophes* tended to look upon a well-informed and sturdy people as a progressive force against despotism, obscurantism, feudalism, and (above all) Popish bigotry; spreading the word would further *écraser l'infâme*. By contrast, advocates of the charity school movement, the Society for the Propagation of the Gospel, and the Proclamation Society believed that Christian meekness and obedience could best be imparted through twopenny tracts.[21]

Not only would every species of good be advanced by

5

diffusing knowledge, but evils could be eradicated. Witchcraft, magic, superstition, debauchery, and drunkenness – all such popular errors were believed to result from ignorance that could be dispelled by improving literature.[22] Conduct too could be refined. The early modern peasantry, as historians such as Muchembled have stressed, was widely characterized as feckless, idle, licentious, ever eager for the chaos of carnival.[23] Respectable society hoped that chapbooks and tracts crying down drink and dissipation, and moral tales commending sobriety, order, labour and discipline would tame the beast within. Thus the diffusion of knowledge would serve the cause of moral order, teach true religion, discipline, and acceptance of one's place and obedience to one's betters.

Of course, there is something anachronistic and artificial about dividing modes of popularization into the positive and the negative. It was in the nature of popularizing literature that it aimed to fuse the interests of supplier and consumer alike. From his, by definition, somewhat élite viewpoint, the author would express the hope that his labours would benefit the commonwealth, promote industry, activity, population, good order, public spirit, patriotism and so forth; the consumer would believe that, armed with what the text told him, he would be able to control his affairs and mind his business more effectively, would be esteemed and would rise in the world: self-love and social would be the same. Especially in the Central European tradition of Cameralism, the diffusion of knowledge (if not to everyone, at least to the right people) was believed to be an effective engine of statecraft.[24] And, as Eugene Weber has stressed, the strategies of nineteenth-century nation-builders entertained great expectations of the normalizing role of the school and the carefully crafted and chosen book.[25]

It will be evident how all the ambiguities of popularization just discussed apply to the case of medicine. The religious, personal, and political benefits of enhancing the health of the people through the spreading of better knowledge were self-evident. Ignorance meant illness. All too often, it was believed, the people were prisoners of preposterous medical prejudices, such as the folk-notion that syphilis could be cured by having sex with a virgin. The dissemination of medical truth was expected to undermine white magic, divination, and all the dubious palaver of folk healing. Who could possibly object?

In reality, myriad objections were raised to the genre of

popularizing medical writings, echoing the doubts just discussed regarding the democratization and publication of knowledge in general. Certain religious critics feared that medical knowledge, by concentrating too heavily upon the physical dimensions of life, might encourage materialism and lust; such arguments have remained the staple of attempts this century to curb sex education and VD clinic publicity.[26] Many doctors claimed that, in the wrong hands – lay hands, plebeian hands – knowledge would prove a two-edged sword. Medicine was an art for experts, too dangerous for dabblers. And behind such high-minded and paternalist objections, one may of course discern professionals out to protect their turf, just as behind the high-minded rhetoric of the popularizers, claiming to save the world from ignorance, quackery and oligopoly, one may espy the love of lucre and hope for fame. No one could object to the desire for healthier individuals in a more hygienic commonwealth. Many doubted whether the way to achieve this was to pretend that everyone could be his own doctor.

Yet, for all the doubters and the heated debates, the motors of capitalism irresistibly promoted medical popularization: above all, the growth of surplus wealth,[27] the emergence of a better educated, more assertive populace, the communications revolution,[28] and the disposition of a significant minority of doctors – for reasons idealistic or mercenary – to deploy their knowledge and skills, as it were, wholesale – to heal by the book and not just by the bedside.[29]

And it is such authors, their books, and their impact that this volume traces. Andrew Wear explores the rise of popularizing medical works in England in the first couple of centuries after Caxton.[30] In a discussion of the vexed hermeneutics of these often alien and puzzling texts, Mary Fissell surveys medical tracts produced for the lower classes in the seventeenth and eighteenth centuries.[31] Philip Wilson, taking the same temporal span, examines surgical works targeting a rather better-educated and more sophisticated readership,[32] while Porter goes on to examine the popularizing writings that appeared in England at the close of the eighteenth century, analysing the often violent altercations among doctors themselves divided as to the merits of medical popularization.[33]

Together with Tissot, William Buchan was the most successful eighteenth-century popularizer; and the essays by Matthew Ramsey on France, Enrique Perdiguero on Spain, Maria Szlatky on Hungary, and Norman Gevitz on North America are devoted in part to tracing the reception of the works of this pair in these respective countries and cultures. Each has a distinctive story to tell. In France the course of medical popularization was deeply implicated in the wider politics of knowledge generated by the Enlightenment and the Revolution.[34] In Spain, medical popularization reopened old wounds between the medical profession and the Church.[35] The reception of Tissot in Hungary illuminates the profound rifts between high and low traditions, cosmopolitanism and nativism, and the difficulties of modernizing an *ancien régime* society. In the United States, the tradition of medical popularization finally reached its apogee in a society whose knowledge ethic was aggressively democratic, anticorporatist, and individualistic.[36]

These essays demonstrate the growth of the genre. But they also explore its true complexities. Let us return for a moment to the 'essentials' I listed earlier for the existence of the genre, that is, (1) a body of authorized regular medicine, (2) doctors to spread it, (3) books as a medium of diffusion, (4) a literate audience. It will by now be obvious that these cannot themselves be treated as unproblematic concepts. Their complexities deserve a brief review.

The basic presupposition of 'regular medicine' itself poses problems. What many physicians from the Renaissance to the Enlightenment were pleased to call 'medical truth' was itself a ramshackle edifice of internally inconsistent Classical learning, strengthened, or weakened, by later accretions. The assertion of the existence of some pure, perfect and pristine medical truth-system was itself largely an ideological construct, a myth advanced by a medical profession that was itself not an age-old, adamantine institution but a relatively new body attempting to establish corporate existence and privileges in the epoch of the new monarchs and of Renaissance humanism. Popularization could be part of the tactics of a 'professional medicine', itself but shakily established, attempting to assert its own superiority; or it could serve as a weapon against it. The fortunes of medical popularization may thus tell us as much about the politics of the popularizers as about the lucky beneficiaries of their labours.[37]

Looking closer, it is equally obvious that the individual popularizers warrant attention. Their undertaking wore a somewhat transgressive, equivocal air: they served as go-betweens, linking élite and people, neither fish, flesh, nor fowl. Some, like

Nicholas Culpeper, were marginal to the medical establishment, and radical by disposition; others led chequered careers without great professional success (if you can, do; if you can't, popularize). Others were fired by religious, political, or personal missions. Their ambivalent status raises questions about the public presence of the profession at large, and the medico's perception of his place in the professional pecking order and in wider society – questions which medical historians have barely begun to address.[38]

Third, books are not the pellucid and neutral instruments of information exchange that historians sometimes would like to pretend them to be. Marshall Macluhan and others have demonstrated how the print revolution changed sensibilities and ways of thinking, because the medium itself carried a message.[39] Deconstructionist literary critics (as Mary Fissell emphasizes) have drawn attention to the significance of layout, of language, of implicit messages, of readers' expectations.[40] Cultural historians have examined the very different approaches to the act of reading common in earlier centuries (our own assumptions about reading are not self-evident but are the product of five centuries of print culture, and perhaps also betray the sensibilities of academics).[41] Not least, books were commonly treated as possessing intrinsic healing capacities (at least, by those who didn't regard them, or the reading habit, as contagious diseases).[42] Any agenda of future research on this subject must give high priority to consideration of popular medical literature as a class of physical artifact.

Last – and perhaps most important – who bought these books? Who read them? We remain deplorably ignorant about the actual, as distinct from the imputed, book-owning public[43] in earlier centuries, though study of wills and inventories is gradually lightening the darkness.[44] And how far did owners actually read the books they possessed? Nowadays, millions of cookbooks are bought; a small percentage, it seems, are read, but relatively few dishes are ever made on the basis of their instructions. This was perhaps true of child-care and etiquette manuals in earlier centuries. To own was probably more important than to read.[45] Was there a ceremonial, psychological, almost a talismanic, value to owning Buchan or Tissot, quite independent of any practical use to which their contents were put? Some highly intriguing possibilities in this respect are suggested by Stephen Jacyna's paper which charts the skill with

9

which an early nineteenth-century patient 'shopped around' metropolitan practitioners on the strength of his reading of their published works. In a milieu in which regular medicine (even in its non-popularized mode) was rarely too technical for the educated layman to make at least a stab at understanding, the communication of knowledge from faculty to customer may well have had tangible consequences for the practice, as well as the pretensions, of medicine.

To trace the rise of medical popularization is thus to pose a host of key questions about the history of print culture and of the politics of knowledge, no less than to raise profound issues about the historical relations of medicine and the medical profession to the wider society. It is the hope of the contributors that this book will stimulate the research that will point to answers.

Notes

1. G. Risse, R.L. Numbers and J.W. Leavitt (eds), *Medicine Without Doctors* (New York: Science History Publications, 1977); Doreen Evenden Nagy, *Popular Medicine in Seventeenth-Century England* (Bowling Green, OH: Bowling Green State University Popular Press, 1988); W.O. Hand, 'The Folk-Healer: Calling and Endowment', *Journal of the History of Medicine*, xxvi (1971), 263–75.

2. R. Cooter (ed.), *Studies in the History of Alternative Medicine* (London: Macmillan, 1988); W.F. Bynum and Roy Porter (eds), *Medical Fringe and Medical Orthodoxy 1750–1850* (London: Croom Helm, 1986); Roy Porter, *Health for Sale: Quackery in England 1650–1850* (Manchester: Manchester University Press, 1989); Norman Gevitz (ed.), *Other Healers: Unorthodox Medicine in America* (Baltimore: Johns Hopkins University Press, 1988).

3. See, for instance, Anne Karpf, *Doctoring the Media. The Reporting of Health and Medicine* (London: Routledge, 1988).

4. Paul Slack, 'Mirrors of Health and Treasures of Poor Men: Uses of the Vernacular Medical Literature of Tudor England', in C. Webster (ed.), *Health, Medicine and Mortality in the Sixteenth Century* (Cambridge: Cambridge University Press, 1979), 237–74; see, more generally, John L. Thornton, *Medical Books, Libraries and Collectors: A Study of Bibliography and the Book Trade in Relation to the Medical Sciences*, 2nd edn (London: André Deutsch, 1966).

5. Leonard Guthrie, 'The Lady Sedley's Receipt Book, 1686, and Other Seventeenth-Century Receipt Books', *Proceedings of the Royal Society of Medicine*, vi (1913), 150–70.

6. There has been a certain amount of pioneering work in this area. See notably G. Smith, 'Prescribing the Rules of Health: Self-Help and Advice in the Late Eighteenth Century', in Roy Porter (ed.),

Introduction

Patients and Practitioners: Lay Attitudes to Medicine in Pre-Industrial Society (Cambridge: Cambridge University Press, 1985), 249–82; *idem*, 'Physical Puritanism and Sanitary Science: Material and Immaterial Beliefs in Popular Physiology 1650–1840', in W.F. Bynum and R. Porter (eds), *Medical Fringe and Medical Orthodoxy 1750–1850* (London: Croom Helm, 1986), 174–97; *idem*, 'Cleanliness: the Development of an Idea and Practice in Britain 1770–1850' (University of London, PhD thesis, 1985); A.C. Fellman and M. Fellman, *Making Sense of Self: Medical Advice Literature in Late Nineteenth-Century America* (Philadelphia: University of Pennsylvania Press, 1981). For the German-speaking world, see Mary Lindemann, 'Aufklärung and the Health of the People: Volkschriften and Medical Advice in Braunschweig-Wolfenbüttel', in Rudolf Vierhaus (ed.) *Kultur und Gesellschaft in Nordwestdeutschland zur Zeit der Aufklärung* (forthcoming).

Some aspects of the history of medical popularization and medical advice literature have been studied that will not be further explored in the rest of this book. It is worth briefly documenting these here. See, for instance, on baby and child care: D. Beekman, *The Mechanical Baby: A Popular History of the Theory and Practice of Child-Raising* (London: Dennis Dobson, 1977); C. Hardyment, *Dream Babies: Child Care from Locke to Spock* (London: Jonathan Cape, 1983); on popular psychiatry, Anthony Clare with Sally Thompson, *Now Let's Talk About Me. A Critical Examination of New Psychotherapies* (London: BBC, 1981); Paul A. Robinson, *The Modernisation of Sex: Havelock Ellis, Alfred Kinsey, William Masters, and Virginia Johnson* (Ithaca, NY: Cornell University Press, 1989); on medical advice for women, Barbara Ehrenreich and Deidre English, *For Her Own Good: 150 Years of the Experts' Advice to Women* (London: Pluto Press, 1979); C. Smith-Rosenberg and C.E. Rosenberg, 'The Female Animal: Medical and Biological Views of Woman and Her Role in Nineteenth-Century America', *Journal of American History*, lx (1973), 332–56. For children's advice literature, see Samuel F. Pickering Jr, *John Locke and Children's Books in Eighteenth-Century England* (Knoxville: University of Tennessee Press, 1981); Isaac Kramnick, 'Children's Literature and Bourgeois Ideology: Observations on Culture and Industrial Capitalism in the Later Eighteenth Century', *SECC*, (1983), 11–44; Susan Pederson, 'Hannah More Meets Simple Simon: Tracts, Chapbooks, and Popular Culture in Late Eighteenth-Century England', *Journal of British Studies*, xxv (1986), 84–113; James A. Secord, 'Newton in the Nursery: Tom Telescope and the Philosophy of Tops and Balls', *History of Science*, xxiii (1985), 127–51; Bette O. Goldstone, *Lessons to be Learned: A Study of Eighteenth-Century English Didactic Children's Literature* (New York, Berne, and Frankfurt-am-Main: Peter Lang, 1984). For courtesy literature, see Fenella Childs, 'Prescriptions for Manners in Eighteenth Century Courtesy Literature' (D.Phil. thesis, Oxford University, 1984); L.A. Curtis, 'A Case Study of Defoe's Domestic Conduct Manuals Suggested by *The Family, Sex and Marriage in England 1500–1800*', *Studies in Eighteenth Century Culture*, x (1981), 409–28. A recent investigation is Lamar Riley Murphy, *Enter the Physician. The Transformation of Domestic Medicine 1760–1860* (Tuscaloosa: University of Alabama Press, 1991).

7. L.M. Beier, *Sufferers and Healers: The Experience of Illness in Seventeenth-Century England* (London: Routledge & Kegan Paul, 1987); Dorothy Porter and Roy Porter, *Patient's Progress: Doctors and Doctoring in Eighteenth-Century England* (Cambridge: Polity Press, 1989); Roy Porter and Dorothy Porter, *In Sickness and in Health: The British Experience 1650–1850* (London: Fourth Estate, 1988).

8. J. Bellers, *An Essay Towards the Improvement of Physick* (London: J. Sowle, 1714); Charles Webster, *The Great Instauration: Science, Medicine and Reform, 1626–1669* (London: Duckworth, 1975).

9. On the role of printing see Elizabeth L. Eisenstein, *The Printing Press as an Agent of Change*, 2 vols (Cambridge: Cambridge University Press, 1979). For one dimension of medical printing, see W.F. Bynum, Stephen Lock and Roy Porter (eds), *The History of Medical Journalism* (London: Routledge, 1992).

10. For stimulating recent discussion of the social history of the book trade, see Robert Darnton, *The Business of Enlightenment. A Publishing History of the Encyclopédie, 1775–1800* (Cambridge, Mass: Harvard University Press, 1979); *idem* and Daniel Roche (eds), *Revolution in Print: The Press in France 1775–1800* (California: University of California Press, 1989); J. Feather, *The Provincial Book Trade* (Cambridge: Cambridge University Press, 1986); Marjorie Plant, *The English Book Trade: An Economic History of the Making and Sale of Books* (London: Allen & Unwin, 1965); G.A. Cranfield, *The Development of the Provincial Newspaper 1700–1760* (Oxford: Clarendon Press, 1962).

11. On schooling and education, see V.E. Neuberg, *Popular Education in Eighteenth Century England* (London: Woburn Press, 1971).

12. On literacy, reading, and the book, see David Cressy, *Literacy and the Social Order: Reading and Writing in Tudor and Stuart England* (Cambridge: Cambridge University Press, 1980); Harvey J. Graff (ed.), *Literacy and Social Development in the West: A Reader* (Cambridge: Cambridge University Press, 1981); L. Stone, 'Literacy and Education in England 1640–1900', *Past and Present*, 42 (1969), 42–139; R. Houston, 'The Development of Literacy in Northern England, 1640–1750', *Economic History Review*, xxxv (1982), 199–216; Isabel Rivers (ed.), *Books and Their Readers in Eighteenth Century England* (Leicester: Leicester University Press, 1982; London: St Martin's Press, 1982); Victor Neuburg, *Chapbooks: A Guide to Reference Material in English, Scottish, and American Chapbook Literature of the Eighteenth and Nineteenth Centuries*, 2nd edn (London: Woburn Press, 1972, 1st edn 1964); *idem*, 'The Penny Histories', in *Milestones in Children's Literature* (General Editor, Brian Alderson). New York: Harcourt, Brace and World, 1968); Margaret Spufford, *Small Books and Pleasant Histories: Popular Fiction and its Readership in Seventeenth-Century England* (Athens, Ga: University of Georgia Press, 1981); D. Vincent, *Literacy and Popular Culture. England 1750–1914* (Cambridge: Cambridge University Press, 1989).

For revealing instances of the impact of literacy on individual lives, see C. Ginzburg, *The Cheese and the Worms: the Cosmos of the Sixteenth Century* (London: Routledge & Kegan Paul, 1980); Harriet Blodgett, *Centuries of Female Days: Englishwomen's Private Diaries* (Gloucester: Alan Sutton, 1989); Patricia Crawford, 'Women's Published Writings

1600–1700', in Mary Prior (ed.), *Women in English Society 1500–1800* (London: Methuen, 1985); Paul Seaver, *Wallington's World: A Puritan Artisan in Seventeenth Century London* (London: Methuen, 1985); M. Thale (ed.), *The Autobiography of Francis Place (1771–1854)* (Cambridge: Cambridge University Press, 1972).

13. On domesticity, see W. Rybczynski, *Home: A Short History of an Idea* (London: Heinemann, 1988); R. Chartier (ed.), *A History of Private Life*, vol. 3, *Passions of the Renaissance* (Cambridge, Mass: Belknap Press, 1989); Lawrence Stone, *The Family, Sex and Marriage in England, 1500–1800* (London: Weidenfeld and Nicolson, 1977); R. Trumbach, *The Rise of the Egalitarian Family: Aristocratic Kinship and Domestic Relations in Eighteenth Century England* (New York: Academic Press, 1978); K. Wrightson, *English Society, 1580–1680* (New Brunswick, NJ: Rutgers University Press, 1982).

14. On authorship, see Robert Darnton, *The Literary Underground of the Old Regime* (Cambridge, Mass: Harvard University Press, 1982); Pat Rogers, *Grub Street: Studies in a Subculture* (London: Methuen, 1972), 153–4; J.W. Saunders, *The Profession of English Letters* (London: Routledge & Kegan Paul, 1964).

15. On evolving languages, see Peter Burke and Roy Porter (eds), *The Social History of Language* (Cambridge: Cambridge University Press, 1987); *idem* (eds), *Language, Self and Society: The Social History of Language* (Cambridge: Polity Press, 1991); Andrew E. Benjamin, Geoffrey N. Cantor and John R.R. Christie (eds), *The Figural and the Literal: Problems of Language in the History of Science and Philosophy, 1630–1800* (Manchester: Manchester University Press, 1987).

16. Many of these issues are treated in Simon Schaffer, 'Natural Philosophy and Public Spectacle in the Eighteenth Century', *History of Science*, xxi (1983), 1–43; Steven Shapin and Simon Schaffer, *Leviathan and the Air Pump* (Princeton: Princeton University Press, 1985); Steven Shapin, 'The Audience for Science in Eighteenth-Century Edinburgh', *History of Science*, xii (1974), 95–121.

17. See R.W. Scribner, *Popular Culture and Popular Movements in Reformation Germany* (London: Hambledon, 1987).

18. See William Eamon, 'Arcana Disclosed: The Advent of Printing, the Books of Secrets Tradition and the Development of Experimental Science in the Sixteenth Century', *History of Science*, xxii (1984), 111–50; Frances Yates, *The Rosicrucian Enlightenment* (London: Routledge & Kegan Paul, 1972).

19. The best introductory discussion remains Peter Burke, *Popular Culture in Early Modern Europe* (London: Temple Smith, 1978). See also Mikhail M. Bakhtin, *Rabelais and his World*, trans. by H. Iswolsky (Cambridge, Mass: MIT Press, 1968); E.P. Thompson, 'Patrician Society, Plebeian Culture', *Journal of Social History*, vii (1973–4), 382–405; *idem*, 'Eighteenth Century English Society: Class Struggle Without Class?', *Social History*, iii (1978), 133–65; Robert Darnton, 'The High Enlightenment and the Low Life of Literature in Pre-Revolutionary France', *Past and Present*, li (1971), 81–115; *idem, The Great Cat Massacre and Other Episodes in French Cultural History* (London and New York: Basic Books, 1984); Roger Chartier, *Cultural History. Between Practices and*

Representations (Ithaca: Cornell University Press, 1988); J. Devlin, *The Superstitious Mind: French Peasants and the Supernatural in the Nineteenth Century* (New Haven, Conn: Yale University Press, 1987); David Warren Sabean, *Power in the Blood: Popular Culture and Village Discourse in Early Modern Germany* (Cambridge: Cambridge University Press, 1984); Bob Scribner, 'Is a History of Popular Culture Possible?', *History of European Ideas* x (1989), 175–91.

20. H.C. Payne, *The Philosophes and the People* (New Haven: Yale University Press, 1976).

21. Thomas W. Laqueur, *Religion and Respectability: Sunday Schools and Working Class Culture, 1780–1850* (New Haven and London: Yale University Press, 1976).

22. Keith Thomas, *Religion and the Decline of Magic: Studies in Popular Beliefs in Sixteenth and Seventeenth-Century England* (London: Weidenfeld & Nicolson, 1971; reprinted, Harmondsworth: Penguin, 1978).

23. R. Muchembled, *Popular Culture and Elite Culture in France 1400–1750*, trans. by L. Cochrane (Baton Rouge, La: Louisiana State University Press, 1978; 1985).

24. George Rosen, *From Medical Police to Social Medicine* (New York: Science History Publications, 1974).

25. E. Weber, *Peasants into Frenchman* (London: Chatto and Windus, 1970).

26. Compare Richard Davenport-Hines, *Sex, Death and Punishment. Attitudes to Sex and Sexuality in Britain since the Renaissance* (London: Collins, 1989); J. Stengers and A. Van Neck, *Histoire d'une grande peur: le masturbation* (Brussels: Université de Bruxelles, 1984).

27. On the rise of consumerism, see John Brewer and Roy Porter (eds), *Consumption and the World of Goods* (London: Routledge, 1992).

28. Raymond Williams, *The Long Revolution* (London: Chatto and Windus, 1961; New York: Columbia University Press, 1984).

29. On this market-oriented spirit among the doctors, see G. Holmes, *Augustan England: Professions, State and Society, 1680–1730* (London: George Allen & Unwin, 1982); I.S.L. Loudon, *Medical Care and the General Practitioner 1750–1850* (Oxford: Clarendon Press, 1986); Dorothy Porter and Roy Porter, *Patient's Progress: Doctors and Doctoring in Eighteenth-Century England* (Cambridge: Polity Press, 1989).

30. For background, see also Andrew Wear, 'Puritan Perceptions of Illness in Seventeenth Century England' in Roy Porter (ed.), *Patients and Practitioners* (Cambridge: Cambridge University Press, 1985), 55–99; *idem*, 'Interfaces: Perceptions of Health and Illness in Early Modern England', in Roy Porter and Andrew Wear (eds), *Problems and Methods in the History of Medicine, 1750–1850* (London: Croom Helm, 1987), 230–55; John L. Thornton, *Medical Books, Libraries and Collectors: A Study of Bibliography and the Book Trade in Relation to the Medical Sciences*, 2nd edn (London: André Deutsch, 1966).

31. For one attempt to 'read' similar material, see Bruno Bettelheim, *The Uses of Enchantment: The Meaning and Importance of Fairy Tales* (New York: Vintage Books, Random House, 1977); for another, see Edward A. Bloom, Lilian D. Bloom and Edmund Leites, *Educating the Audience: Addison, Steele, and Eighteenth-Century Culture: Papers Presented*

Introduction

at a Clark Library Seminar 15 November 1980 (Los Angeles: William Andrews Clark Memorial Library, 1984); Jack Zipes, *Breaking the Spell: Radical Theories of Folk and Fairy Tales* (Austin: University of Texas Press, 1979); for discussion of 'readings', see J. Culler, *On Deconstruction* (London: Routledge & Kegan Paul, 1983); see also B. Capp, *Astrology and the Popular Press: English Almanacs, 1500–1800* (London and Boston: Faber & Faber, 1979); Patrick Curry (ed.), *Astrology, Science and Society: Historical Essays* (Woodbridge, Suffolk: Boydell Press, 1987); idem, *Prophecy and Power: Astrology in Early Modern England* (Cambridge: Polity Press, 1989).

32. See also L.M. Beier, *Sufferers and Healers: The Experience of Illness in Seventeenth-Century England* (London: Routledge & Kegan Paul, 1987).

33. For Buchan in England, see C. Lawrence, 'William Buchan: Medicine Laid Open', *Medical History*, xix (1975), 20–35; Charles Rosenberg, 'Medical Text and Medical Context; Explaining William Buchan's *Domestic Medicine*', *Bulletin of the History of Medicine*, lvii (1983), 22–4; for Parkinson, see A.D. Morris, *James Parkinson, his Life and Times* (Boston: Birkhauser, 1989); for Thomas Beddoes and his times, see Roy Porter, *Doctor of Society: Thomas Beddoes and the Sick Trade in Late Enlightenment England* (London: Routledge, 1992).

34. See Jean Pierre Goubert (ed.), *La Médicalisation de la société française, 1770–1830* (Waterloo, Ontario: Historical Reflections Press, 1982); M. Ramsey, *Professional and Popular Medicine in France 1770–1830: The Social World of Medical Practice* (Cambridge: Cambridge University Press, 1988).

35. See Richard Herr, *The Eighteenth Century Revolution in Spain* (Princeton, NJ: Princeton University Press, 1958).

36. For democratic medical culture in the United States, see J.C. Whorton, *Crusaders for Fitness: The History of American Health Reformers* (Princeton: Princeton University Press, 1982).

37. There is valuable discussion on these issues in R. French and A. Wear (eds), *The Medical Revolution of the Seventeenth Century* (Cambridge: Cambridge University Press, 1989).

38. See Roy Porter, *Doctor of Society: Thomas Beddoes and the Sick Trade in Late Enlightenment England* (London: Routledge, 1992); P. Stallybrass and A. White, *The Politics and Poetics of Transgression* (Ithaca, NY: Cornell University Press, 1986).

39. Marshall McLuhan, *Understanding Media: The Extension of Man* (London: A.R.K., 1987); Walter J. Ong, *Orality and Literacy: The Technologizing of the Word* (London: Methuen, 1982); Jack Goody, *The Domestication of the Savage Mind* (Cambridge: Cambridge University Press, 1977).

40. J. Culler, *On Deconstruction* (London: Routledge & Kegan Paul, 1983).

41. Keith Thomas, *Religion and the Decline of Magic: Studies in Popular Beliefs in Sixteenth and Seventeenth-century England* (London: Weidenfeld & Nicolson, 1971; reprinted Harmondsworth: Penguin, 1978); idem, 'Numeracy in Early Modern England', *Transactions of the Royal Historical Society*, xxxvii (1987), 103–32.

42. David Cressy, 'Books as Totems in Seventeenth-Century England and New England', *Journal of Library History*, xxi (1986), 92–106; Roy Porter, '"The Whole Secret of Health": Mind, Body and Medicine in *Tristam Shandy*', in John Christie and Sally Shuttleworth (eds), *Nature Transfigured* (Manchester: Manchester University Press, 1989), 61–84.

43. J. Habermas, *The Structural Transformation of the Public Sphere. An Inquiry into a Category of Bourgeois Society* (Cambridge, Mass: MIT Press, 1989).

44. Lorna Weatherill, 'Consumer Behavior and Social Status in England', *Continuity and Change*, ii (1986), 191–216; *idem*, 'A Possession of One's Own: Women and Consumer Behaviour in England, 1660–1740', *Journal of British Studies*, xxv (1986), 131–56; 60; *idem, Consumer Behaviour and Material Culture, 1660–1760* (London: Routledge, 1988); John Brewer and Roy Porter (eds), *Consumption and the World of Goods* (London: Routledge, 1991).

45. Jay Mechling, 'Advice to Historians on Advice to Mothers', *Journal of Social History*, ix (1975).

1

The popularization of medicine in early modern England

Andrew Wear

Popular medicine in early modern England is not *terra incognita*. In the last few years there have been important studies of the social history of English medicine of this period. From them it is clear that there was a medical marketplace composed of many different types of practitioner, and it was not limited to the physicians, surgeons and apothecaries – the traditional objects of study of medical historians. At the same time, patients' actions and attitudes in relation to illness have been studied.[1] The overall impression produced by the new research is that in early modern England there was a largely unregulated open-market place in which the layperson and the patient had much more choice and power in relation to medical practitioners, and, indeed, that power was shown by the prevalence of lay and of self-treatment.

It would be easy to call this open medicine with its many different kinds of practitioner (and multiplicity of explanations for illness, for instance, religious and magical as well as naturalistic), popular. But popular in relation to what? Our use of the term implies a contrast: élite–popular, high–low culture, written–oral. The new picture of English medicine is one in which people at the time recognized distinctions, for instance, between the learned physician trained in the universities in the classical works of Hippocrates and Galen and the empiric or mountebank with his travelling show and cure-alls. Yet in practice those distinctions were often ignored. People used many different kinds of practitioner without being troubled about the distinctions between them. In this context and at this time, therefore, 'popular' has an ambiguous sense which it had lost by the nineteenth and twentieth centuries; when, in fact, the

17

growth of the academic study of the popular indicates that it was a proper category defined with the aid of its antitheses – by knowledge of what is not popular.

Another difficulty with the idea of popular medicine in the early modern period is that the term 'popular' has been made to do too much. It has encompassed the literate middle class, people like Pepys, as well as illiterate wise men and women. The oral culture of medicine can include Pepys being given word-of-mouth medical advice by friends for an illness as well as what we can reconstruct of the knowledge handed down by a succession of white witches to each other. This problem becomes immediately apparent when discussing popularized medicine, the topic of this chapter. Who was it who could read the books which brought medicine to a 'popular' audience? Clearly not the illiterate, the most 'popular' part of the population. Despite a putative educational revolution between 1558 and the 1640s, the poorest, lowest part of the population still remained illiterate. The higher social groups such as the gentry, yeomen, and merchants and shopkeepers increased their male literacy rates, while husbandmen, poor artisans, labourers and servants still had high illiteracy rates. It is true, as Keith Wrightson and Margaret Spufford have pointed out, that the need to be literate was felt by the poorest and that much of oral culture was in the process of being put into print.[2] Geographically, there was a wide variation in literacy rates; some parishes, especially where there was a school or a teacher, had rates of male illiteracy ranging as low as 28 to 40 per cent in the early 1640s, while other parishes had rates as high as 90 per cent. The distribution of literacy across the country varied enormously. As the testimonies of Richard Lowe and Thomas Tryon indicate, it was possible for the very poor to learn to read and write. Moreover, reading on its own was much more widely practised than reading and writing. Women were often taught only to read. And it is impossible to calculate rates of reading, as reading, unlike writing, leaves behind no record. However, despite the large gains in literacy in early modern England, half the population was probably illiterate in 1750[3] and there were still many whose culture was totally oral, though their numbers were declining. To be able to read popular medical books meant, therefore, that one belonged to a special section of society, the literate. The readership of popular medical books has to be seen in a restricted sense, and the term 'popular' used cautiously.

Despite these caveats is it possible to speak of popularized medicine in early modern England? At first sight, the answer must be yes. Many books were published in England in English (ably discussed by Paul Slack[4]), which digested, popularized, and made accessible the classical works of Hippocrates and Galen. This suggests a model of medical knowledge coming down in a diluted form from the top to the reading public. It also implies the existence of distinctions, for instance, between medical writer and reader, or between learned source and popular author. Another way of putting it is that the popularization of medical knowledge involves the movement or trickle down of that knowledge from high to low culture. As I have indicated there are problems with this view. In practice, distinctions were blurred in an open medical culture in which family members or patients themselves might treat the most serious medical, if not surgical, conditions and in which the patient, the family, neighbours, clergymen and their wives, wise men and women, midwives, uroscopists, herbalists, empirics, astrologers, tooth-drawers, lithotomists, as well as apothecaries, surgeons and physicians, were all able to provide care. The lack of effective regulation of medical practice also helped to blur distinctions and hierarchy among medical practitioners. The College of Physicians controlled medical practice only within London and seven miles around and its powers were whittled away during the seventeenth century.[5] In the rest of the country there was no licensing except for a sporadic form of ecclesiastical licensing. The State and the law, those creators and enforcers of distinctions, were absent from large areas of the medical marketplace.

In this chapter I shall bear in mind the paradox of distinctiveness and openness in early modern English medicine, and I shall be examining how it was expressed by the authors of popularized English medical books. Their perceptions of what they were doing are in terms of contemporary interests and problems and they place their work historically. In the final part of the chapter I shall range more widely to emphasize the point that popular and popularized medicine (the former provides the context for the latter) in this period were *sui generis* and very different from the nineteenth or twentieth centuries.

The popularization of learned medicine

In 1539 Sir Thomas Elyot in the introduction to his *Castell of Health,* one of the most popular and frequently reprinted guides to health, defended his right to publish a work in medicine even though he was not a physician.

> But yet one thing much greveth me, that notwithstand-inge I have ever honoured and specially favoured the revered College of approved Phisitions yet some of them hearing me spoken of, have sayd in dirision, that although I were pretely seene in storyes, yet being not learned in Phisicke, I have put in my books divers errours in presum-ing to write of hearbs and medicines.[6]

In his defence Sir Thomas spelled out how, before he had become twenty years old, a learned physician read to him 'the workes of Galen of temperaments, naturall faculties, the intro-duction of Johannicius with some of the Aphorismes of Hippocrates'.[7]

Clearly Elyot felt he could be as learned as an approved physician of the College. In other words, for an educated person the learning of the physicians was not esoteric and out of reach. The literature of medicine was accessible to those who were not trained in medicine. This is an important point, for the openness of medicine and the ability of laypeople to practise medicine depended partly on the denial of claims that only the medically educated could understand medical books. Indeed, as the main thrust of learned medicine's claim to expertise lay in the scholarly, book-based nature of the discipline, to deny others who were literate entry into this learning might not be credible. Although Galenic medicine was self-consciously based on a mixture of experience and book learning (the union of the empirical and dogmatic schools of Galen's time), it was difficult for the learned physicians to base their claims to a monopoly of expertise upon experience alone, for that pointed in the direc-tion of the empirics and quacks, their hated enemies. There-fore, the best they could do against Sir Thomas Elyot was to point to his errors in transmitting the knowledge he had gained from books – his scholarly errors.

The list of authors that Elyot went on to read for himself comprised the great and the good in medicine:

And afterward by myne owne study I read over in order the more part of the works of Hippocrates, Galen, Oribasius, Paulus, Celius, Alexander Trallianus, Celsus, Plinius the one and the other, wyth Discorides. Nor did I omit to reade the long Canons of Avicenna, the commentaries of Averrois, the practises of Isake, Haliabbas, Rasis, Mesue, and also the more part of them which were their aggregators and followers.[8]

It is worth leaving Sir Thomas for a moment to consider the wider context of the learned medicine that he refers to. Learned medicine, the medicine of Hippocrates and especially of Galen, was undergoing popularization before and during the Renaissance. Printing alone had diffused medical knowledge more widely. Within learned medicine knowledge was also being diluted. In the Renaissance the methodical reduction of knowledge into compendia was in fashion among university medical men. For instance, the *Institutionum Medicinae* (1555) of the German humanist physician Leonard Fuchs gave an orderly, compartmentalized account of medical theory – the elements, qualities, humours, the parts of the body, its actions, then the non-naturals, the causes of illness, account of fevers, brief descriptions from head to toe of the ills of the body, and a discussion of signs and diagnosis. Other works such as the *Medicina Universa* of Giovanni Battista Da Monte (1587) and the *Methodi Vitandorum Errorum* (1603) of Sanctorio Sanctorio structured medical knowledge in more complex ways using models drawn from Galen's medical philosophy.[9] The gist of Greek and Arabic medicine could be read in one volume and the reader was spared having to use the large multi-volume folios of the Junta edition of Galen's work. Andrew Boorde, the sometime suffragan bishop of Chichester who travelled widely in Europe in search of medical education, wrote in his *Breviary of Health* (1547) that 'every man now a dayes is desirous to rede brefe and compediouse matters'[10] as in his own work. It was not only in the Renaissance that the process of abstracting past medical learning had taken place. In the Middle Ages the aggregators whom Elyot mentions produced compilations and abstracts of classical and Arabic medical texts. And before them in Elyot's list of authorities Pliny appealed to a lay popular readership, while others like Oribasius, Alexander of Tralles and Avicenna produced compendia of learned medicine. Galen himself had synthesized previous medical writings. Since Greek times, therefore, popularization in the sense of making medical knowledge available in easier and more accessible forms had been taking place. The difference between lay and medical readerships was not clear-cut. Although much of this was 'popularization' for a medical readership it was not exclusively so. Galen expected his patients to be as learned in medicine as he was and this view of a shared medical culture continued through to the eighteenth century.[11] The sources of medical knowledge could also be lay and popular. Galen showed no professional hesitation in incorporating folk remedies into his writings. This fits a model of culture that was to last to the Enlightenment in which élite culture found no difficulty in borrowing from oral, popular culture – indeed, there are examples in seventeenth-century England of doctors as well as patients using folk remedies.[12] Learned medicine was always composed of different levels of complexity, and the boundaries between it and popular medicine were more permeable than they might appear at first sight. This is even more so in popularized medicine, the learned medicine available to the public at large.

To come back to Elyot's introduction. After defending himself against the College of Physicians he moved to the attack. Despite never having been 'to Montpellier, Padua nor Salern' yet, he wrote, he had found for himself 'something in Phisick, whereby I have taken no little profit concerning myne owne health'.[13] In other words, universities are not essential for a knowledge of medicine. Elyot then explained that he wrote so that 'men observing a good order in diet, and preventing the great causes of sickness they should of those maladies the sooner be cured'.[14] Empirics sold cure-all remedies, but the mark of the physicians was that they offered advice on diet and regimen as well as remedies tailored to the individual. Elyot is saying that a special part of the physicians' expertise can be written about by a layperson. Moreover, the literate public should share this knowledge. In the next sentence Elyot goes on to justify writing his book in English rather than in Latin, the language of the learned. This was the *sine qua non* of a popular medical book and was often deemed worthy of comment (or excuse if the author came from the ranks of the learned physicians):

But if Phisitions be angry, that I have written phisicke in English, let them remember that the Greeks wrote in Greeke, that Romaines in Latin, Avicenna, and the other in Arabicke, which were their owne proper and maternall tongues.[15]

And then Elyot adds bitterly:

And if they had bene as much attached with envey and covertise as some nowe seem to be, they would have devised some particular language with a strange cypher or forme of letters, wherein they would have written their science, which language or letters no man should have knowen, that had not professed and practised Phisicke: but those, although they were Paynims and Jewes, yet in this part of charity, they far surmounted us Christians, that they would not have so necessary a knowledge as phisicke is, to be hid from them, which would be studious about it.[16]

The learned physicians had invested time and money mastering Latin medical books at university, and Latin clearly helped to protect their trade. As John Securis, a Salisbury physician who had been a pupil of the staunch Galenist Sylvius in Paris, put it in 1566:

If Englyshe Bookes could make men cunnying Physitions, then pouchemakers, threshers, ploughmen and coblers mought be Physitions as well as the best yf they can reade.[17]

From English books Securis immediately went on to make a general complaint that in actual fact anyone was allowed to practise medicine. This brings out nicely the point that the assumption of a monopoly of practice through learning and Latin had no connection with the real world, despite the physicians' wishes and claims that only those with learning and Latin should be allowed to practise. Securis wrote:

Then wer it a great foly for us to bestow so much labour and study all our lyfe in the scholes and universities, to breake oure braynes in readyng so many authours . . . yea and to the greatest follye of all were to precede in any degree [i.e. take a degree] in the Universities with our great coste and charges, when a syr John Lacke latin a pedler, a weaver, and oftentymes a presumptuous woman, shall take uppon them (yea and are permytted) to mynister Medicine to all menne, in every place, and at all tymes. *O tempora, O mores* . . . and so, many tymes not only hinder and defraud us of our lawful stipende and gaynes: but (which is worst of all and to much to be lamented) shall put many in hasarde of their lyfe . . .[18]

In Elyot's introduction to his *Castell of Health* we find some of the recurrent themes of popularized English medicine in the sixteenth and seventeenth centuries: a wish to appear respectable and learned, a confidence in one's own experience and knowledge, and the desire to make medical knowledge available to a wider number of people.

How wide varied with the author. Elyot wrote for the reasonably well-to-do with servants; they could use his advice to look after their own health or as an act of Christian charity to help the poor. Nicholas Culpeper in the middle of the seventeenth century, with a much more radical approach (discussed below), reached out to a larger audience, though it had its limits for, apart from interest and price, literacy formed a natural barrier to true popularization. Another common theme hinted at by Elyot and which was used to justify popularization is the image of a medical establishment mean and monopolistic, against which the author fights the good fight. The learned physician had been associated with expense, greed and covetousness from the Middle Ages and these qualities could be countered by the Christian one of the altruistic charitable care of the sick.

But not all writers who wrote in the vernacular were against learned medicine. James Hart, John Cotta and James Primrose were staunch Galenists who wrote treatises in English in the first half of the seventeenth century that warned people away from empirics, women practitioners, 'parson-physicians' and the other rivals to the learned physicians. James Hart, a Northampton puritan physician, wrote an extremely strong condemnation of these rivals in the introduction to his *KΛINIKH, or the Diet of the Diseased* (1633), yet he went on to disseminate the secrets of his fellow physicians to the general public. He was clearly aware that Latin was the trade language of the learned physicians. He wrote that he did not set down lists of remedies (he was concerned with diet for the sick) because the public could not be instructed to relate the remedies to the constitutions and ills of individual patients (the mark of the learned physician):

> Those remedies therefore are to be sought for in the learned workes and volumes (which Empiricks and all sorts of ignorant Physitians are never able to attaine unto, and by consequent unfit to practise this profession) of the judicious and learned Physitians of all ages; and can by none but by a judicious understanding, trained up in that profession, be duly as they ought accomodated to several individuall parties; *observatis observandis*, with due observation of all the several circumstances of time, place, person etc. Hence then may easily be evinced the error and ignorance of such as divulge abroad in the vulgar tongue, their rare secrets (as they call them) against any disease whatsoever. I doe not deny, but they may sometimes be seconded by some prosperous and successful issue in some: but that is by hap and hazard (as we say) *as the blinde man throwes his staff* . . . But when I see the world use these aright, they have already, then shall I be both ready and willing to communicate further what I know. My earnest care and indeavour hath ever bin since my first setting upon this profession, is, and ever, I hope, shall be to benefit the publike: but by such a course I should rather abouse than benefit any.[19]

The force of Hart's language was designed perhaps to show that he had not broken ranks with his learned colleagues. But he did give advice on diet in English to English readers. He justified this by referring to his desire 'to doe the common-wealth most service'[20] – a typical wish of the puritan godly. He also pointed out that classical advice on diet for the sick had not been based on English experience but 'according to that countrey and climat of Greece, . . . the which how farre it differeth, even at this day, from the diet of this our Iland both in sicknesse and in health, thou who have travelled into those countries, and the learned Physitian are best able to judge'.[21] The sense of Englishness was a potent reason for going beyond foreign authority, however learned. Hart's final motive for publishing was to give the public the information that would enable them to protect themselves. He stated that he wrote 'so people may the better be enabled to detect and discover the ignorance and unsufficiency of many ignorant persons intruding upon the practice of this profession, and to prevent posture'. In general, 'My purpose is only to teach the simple ignorant sort of people, whose credulous simplicity is too often exposed as a prey to every cheating and ignorant asse'.[22] This sense of protecting and educating the public can be found in continental works such as Laurent Joubert's *Erreurs populaires au fait de la medicine et regime de santé* (1578) which Hart quoted extensively, and in the attack on uroscopists and other empirics by the Dutch physician Peter van Foreest in his *De Incerto, Fallaci Urinarum Judicio* (1589) which Hart translated as *The Arraignment of Urines* in 1623. Hart's Northampton colleague John Cotta also wrote in defence of learned medicine and attacked other practitioners.[23]

Out of this wish to protect the public medical knowledge became popularized. James Primrose originally published his book on *Popular Errors* in Latin (1638), but when in 1651 his friend Robert Wittie translated it into English, Wittie wrote that he did so because he was especially concerned that gentle-women who practised charitable medicine for the poor should learn of their errors from the book.[24] These writers were seeking to re-educate their readers away from popular practitioners and practices and turn them to learned medicine, and to do this they used the demotic instrument of the vernacular to reach their readers, and so made more permeable the barriers set around learned medicine.

However, appeals to national and demotic sentiment more often served to justify a move away from learned medicine. Timothie Bright, a Cambridge physician later turned clergy-man, extolled the virtues of native English remedies. Bright was a Cambridge physician who had put in eleven years of study for his MD and had published various works in Latin. But the College of Physicians was no friend and threatened him with prison for practising without its licence in London. He was a rebel within the ranks of learned medicine. At a time of intense national feeling Bright argued in his *Treatise Wherein is Declared the Sufficience of English Medicines* (1580) that God's providence ensured that every country produced within its borders the remedies for the diseases that were native to it. The remedies of the classical and Arabic authorities could work in Greece and Asia but only English remedies could be effective for English diseases in English bodies with English constitutions.

(Significantly, William Harrison in his nationalistic *Description of England* (1586–7) expressed the same sentiment.[25]) As Bright put it:

> The whole art of physic hath been taken partly from the Greeks and partly from the Arabians. And as precepts of the art, so likewise the means and instruments wherewith for the most part the precepts of the same art are executed: which hath bred this error in times past, now by a tradition received, that all the duty of a physician touching restoring of health, is to be performed by the same remedies, not in kind only, but even especially with those which the Grecian and Arabian masters used, who wrote not for us, but for their Greeks and Arabics, tempering their medicines to their estates.[26]

Not only should medicine be written in the local language, but its remedies were also to be local. In this way, the Anglicization of medicine was breaking the hegemony of learned medicine.

Phillip Barrough, who was licensed by Cambridge University to practise both surgery and medicine, also tried to break away to some extent from classical authority. His *Method of Physick* (1583) deals with diseases and their remedies in the traditional head-to-toe order and has additional sections on fevers, tumours, venereal disease and the making of remedies. It was a comprehensive handbook of medicine.

Barrough discussed why he wrote the book. He clearly had a religious view of the duties of a physician: 'shall not the physition looke to have a shrewd checke at Gods hand, if he either hath proudly denied his helpe to the poore, or negligently visited them?'[27] This view of uncharitable physicians who might prefer 'lying fame and vile lucre'[28] made it easier to argue that patients could treat themselves. Barrough, like other English Protestant writers,[29] stressed that the body was of God's workmanship and had to be kept in good order: 'What can be more excellent than to be able to maintaine and keepe in order that best workmanship of God, and (which is more) to correct, reforme and amend it . . . And seeing there is nothing given unto us of God more acceptable than the health of the body, how honourably must we thinke of the means by which it is continued, and restored if lost?'[30] Barrough castigated those who did not look after their own bodies so that their bodies 'have been nothing else but storehouses and mansions of disease' and they had become like 'an evil and negligent tenant' though 'God had bestowed their bodies upon them as gorgeous palaces or mansion houses, wherein the mind may dwell with pleasure and delight'.[31]

This strong religious sentiment helped Barrough to argue for self-help and treatment. He wrote that 'it behoveth every man to be cunning in his own constitution, and to know so much as may serve to forestall the coming of many ordinary diseases which commonly light upon the ignorant: yea and sometime to be able to chafe away a malady when it hath already caught hold of the body'.[32] In a sense, the physician was not needed for 'every man may judge best of his owne bodie, and preserve the declinings and alterations of the same'. More practically, Barrough pointed out that physicians were not always available when needed – an often repeated complaint used to justify such books as Stephen Bradwell's *Help for Suddain Accidents Endangering Life* (1633) and Thomas Brugis's *The Marrow of Phisicke* (1640).

The type of medicine Barrough wrote about was self-consciously aimed at the lay reader. He extolled the virtues of experience and wrote that it is not enough to read the books of Galen, for 'when they shall go into the commonwealth to practice . . . they shall meet diseases that Galen never dreamt of'. The realization of the imperfection of the art of medicine should lead the physician to accept 'that as experience was the ancient beginner of Physicke, so that now it is the true and sincere accomplisher of the perfection of the same'.[33] The emphasis on experience, especially experience not available in books or to Galen, was a liberation from authority. A stress on experience and the aim of a popular readership often went together.

A practical advantage was that experience might exclude theory and could be synonymous with remedies and treatments. In other words, the text was simpler and the reader could get more quickly to the bits that mattered – what to do about the illness. Barrough's book, in fact, was reasonably learned as well as being compendious; it had Latin marginalia and was in the tradition of the Latin *practica* or vade-mecums on therapeutics[34] which lay at the simpler end of the spectrum of difficulty in learned medicine. It gave a very brief description of the disease, its signs, and cause and then concentrated on its treatment. As Burrough put it:

> I have (good reader) for thy benefit collected out of sundry Authors, as it were a breviary or abridgement of Physick, and together with those deductions, I have enterlaced experiments of mine owne, which by long use and practise I have observed to be true. Throughout the whole book I have bin more curious in prescribing the sundrie curations and waies to helpe the disease, then in explaining the nature of them: my reason was, because if my books should come to the hands of the unlearned, a little would suffice (the former being more necessarie).[35]

Nationalism, religion, an emphasis on experience all led to the popularization of learned medicine, and to the conclusion that patients could treat themselves – which, of course, reflected what happened anyway. What we have are attempts to break down the barriers erected by learned medicine. Nationalism, religion, and experience all helped in this because of their concern with, and appeal to, the population at large.

Radical alternatives

As we have seen, the sense of anger with physicians was a motive for popularization. This was particularly so in the case of books on medicine for the poor where the Christian sense of charity was a powerful vehicle for this anger. Robert Pemel in his ΠΤΩΧΟΦΑΡΜΑΚΟΝ *or Help for the Poor* (1650) gave as his main reason for publishing 'these hard times, wherein the poor have scarse bread to eat, much less money to go to the Physition or Chirurgion'.[36] One of the celebratory poems to Pemel's work castigated physicians for their 'love of large reward' which made them deaf to the cries of the poor who 'hath no gold to grease their fists'.[37] Lancelot Coelson, 'student in Physick and Astrology', in his *The Poormans Physician and Chyrurgian Containing Above Three Hundred Rare and Choice Receipts . . . . Published for the Publique Good* (1656) referred to 'the insolency and Pride' of Greek and Roman physicians[38] and asked that 'the Physicians of our times may have contrary spirits humble, meek and lowly, visiting even the poorest of Patients when help is required, for the life of the most miserable vassal is as dear in the sight of God, as the life of the most renowned Monarch'.[39] Thomas Cocke, in his *Kitchen Physick: Or, Advice to the Poor* (1676), rather than giving low-cost medical receipts as did Pemel and Coelson, instead proferred advice on the appropriate diet for particular disorders. He deplored the fact that physicians would not visit the poor, so that neighbours and friends had to go on their behalf to get advice.[40] The poor, he reported, said 'Physick and Physicians are only made for rich men, and wait on Princes, and receive gifts of kings, but never thanks, not prayers from him who hath no other fee'.[41] There is a clear ideological and political force in these statements.

The Civil War and Protectorate was the time when the political desire to break down the barriers to medical knowledge and provision was at its most intense. Charles Webster has fully explored the calls and projects for medical reform in his magisterial *The Great Instauration*. It is clear that a Christian charitable approach that emphasized the needs of the poor came to be united with a theoretical approach at variance with Galenic medicine.[42] The latter was often based on Paracelsian, chemical, and/or astrological ideas. Galenic medicine was not only attacked because of the greed of its practitioners, but medical reformers like Noah Biggs (1651) and the Leveller William Walwyn (1669)[43] also bitterly criticized its procedures which they saw as cruel and ineffective. In other words, the arguments for medicine to be open to all were given added force by the existence of alternative medical theories. Popularization, therefore, could take place in the context of theory change. Nicholas Culpeper exemplifies the more politically pointed characteristics of the Civil War period as well as some of the earlier facets of the medical popularizer, and it is worth having a brief look at his reasons for popularizing medicine.[44]

Culpeper had fought in the Civil War on Parliament's side and had been wounded. He was clearly a political radical. In 1649 he wrote:

God gave Tyrants in his Wrath, and will take them away in his Displeasure. The Prize which We now, and They (all the Nations in Europe) within a few years shall play for is THE LIBERTY OF THE SUBJECT.[45]

This comes from the introduction to Culpeper's unauthorized translation into English of the College of Physicians' pharmacopoeia. He quickly descends to particulars. Priests, physicians, and lawyers most infringe the liberty of the Commonwealth.[46] He castigates the pride, ignorance, fearfulness, uncharitableness, and greed of the physicians:

> Would it not pity a man to see whol estates wasted in Physick, ('all a man hath spent upon Physicians') both body and soul consumed upon outlandish rubbish? . . . Is it handsom and wel beseeming a Common-wealth to see a doctor ride in State, in Plush with a footcloath, and not a grain of Wit, [knowledge] but what was in print before he was born? Send for them into a Visited House [with plague], they will answer, they dare not come. How many honest poor souls have been so cast away, will be known when the Lord shall come to make Inquisition for Blood [will try felonies, crimes deserving execution]. Send for them to a poor mans house who is not able to give them their Fee, then they will not come, and the poor Creature for whom Christ died must forfeit his life for want of money.[47]

Culpeper was perhaps a Leveller; he was certainly concerned, as his contemporary biographer assures us, to provide cheap remedies for the poor, culled from native herbs and not from expensive foreign products.[48] As Culpeper wrote, plagiarizing Timothie Bright word for word, God provided animals with remedies, so he would not forsake another part of his creation – human beings – by not providing them with remedies for their illnesses wherever they lived.[49] Culpeper's motives for publishing and making available medical knowledge to a wide public were both political and religious (the two are almost inseparable in this period) and a sense of charity was prominent. He wrote that the good of his country and the needs of the poor motivated his translation of the London pharmacopoeia of the College of Physicians:

> Pure pitty to the Commonality of England (I assure you) was the motive, the prevailing argument that set my brain and pen a work upon this subject, many of whom to my

knowledg have perished either for want of money to see a Physitian, or want of knowledg of a remedy happily growing in the garden.'[50]

Culpeper called himself 'Student in Astrology and Physick' and joined Christian charity to an astrological–chemical medical system; he saw it as his calling (bestowed by God) to provide this medical knowledge for the poor. It would, however, be ahistorical to compare Culpeper with a figure from later popular medicine, railing against medical authority and putting forward an idiosyncratic medical system underpinned by a populist and religiously based medical ethic alien to orthodox medicine. Criticism of orthodox medicine for its monopolistic, closed tendencies had already been expressed by popularizers such as Elyot and Burrough. Moreover, Culpeper was writing at a time when religious values, such as a stress on charity, were the orthodoxy and were dominating discussion of the nation's affairs. This was also a time when the Galenic consensus within learned medicine was crumbling, and it was unclear what was to be the future foundation of learned medicine. But, in any case, Culpeper himself publicized Galenic medicine in his *Treatise of the Fevers, the Method of which was Galens* (published in *Culpeper's Last Legacy* 1655) and he was involved in the commercial enterprise of translating Latin medical texts written by Galenists or by mildly radical continental medical writers.[51] Despite appearances, Culpeper was reasonably typical of his time.

In terms of this chapter, Culpeper illustrates the paradox of openness and of distinctions that informs much of popular medicine. When replying to a possible charge that by translating the pharmacopoeia, and setting out the virtues and uses of the remedies 'thereby fellows will be induced to the practise of Physick',[52] Culpeper wrote:

> All the Nation are already Physitians, If you ayl any thing, every one you meet, whether man or woman will prescribe you a medicine for it. Now whether this book thus translated will make them more ignorant or more knowing any one that hath but a grain of understanding more than a horse may easily judge.[53]

But Culpeper quickly departed from the assertion of the complete openness and universality of medical practice among the

English. He pointed out to the apothecaries that it was in their interest that he had made their work available to a larger public.

> . . . . it tends to the advancement of their trade, if they have not wit enough to know that private men cannot make up most of these compositions themselves, but knowinge the vertues of the vertues of them, will resort the more to them for physick, they deserve the name of a Company of Dunces.[54]

Not everyone could be an apothecary to their ills. Distinctions did after all exist, medicine was not open in all senses to all.

Another way of seeing the paradox is to consider Culpeper's uncertainty in his *Directory for Midwives* (1651) as to who was educating whom. He noted that he had been called by God to correct error, but he added that if a midwife thought he had got anything wrong then she should tell him and he would amend it.[55] The distinctions of knowledge both exist and do not exist in English popularized medicine of this period.

Conclusion

There is much else to English popularized medicine than the authors I have mentioned. For example, books were written publicizing the virtues of spas, often with the aim of attracting more customers. Examples of cures were advertised and medical theories set out that explained the reasons why the particular waters worked. The openness of English medical culture is here apparent, for the writings were aimed at the customers, the patients, to persuade them to come to the spas, rather than at the physicians who would then recommend the spas to their patients. William Turner in the sixteenth century hoped his work on the 'Bath of Baeth' would inform 'the manie in the North partes, which being diseased with sore diseases would gladly come to the bath of Baeth, if they knewe that there were any there, whereby they might be holped'. In a nationalistic vein, Turner added that these Northerners 'know not whether there be any [baths] in the Realme or no . . . therefore I thought good to showe the vertues of our own Bathes, for if they be able to help mennes diseases, what shall men need to goe into farre countrys to seke that remedie there which they may have here at home?[56] In the seventeenth century Michael Stanhope, Robert Wittie, Robert Pierce, and others extolled the virtues of Knaresborough, Scarborough and Bath.[57] The promotional literature on the spas (often of a high technical level) illustrates the desire to make a medical facility available to the largest number of people possible who could afford it, and shows commerce joined with medical popularization.

There were other means of popularizing medicine. Advertisements in the form of posters or bills not only advertised the services of a practitioner but also conveyed something of his or her work. But what interested people probably more than anything else were medical recipes. They were what made you better. Women were especially concerned with them. They were often the main providers of medical care and, lacking the learned theory of the physicians, they depended heavily on prescriptions. Gervase Markham, who wrote a series of how-to books (fishing, fowling, farming, the care of horses), discussed in his *English Hous-wife* (1615) the 'inward and outward Vertues which ought to be in a complete Woman'. These were: 'her skill in Physick, Surgery, Cookery, Extraction of Oyles, Banquetting stuffe, Ordering of Great Feasts, preserving of all sorts of Wines, conceited Secrets, Distillations, Perfumes, ordering of Wool, Hemp, Flax, making Cloth and Dying, the knowledge of Dayries, Office of Malting of Oates, their excellent uses in a Family, of Brewing, Baking and all other things belonging to a Household'.[58] Before the intense specialization in the provision of services and products ushered in by the consumer revolution of the early eighteenth century and then by the Industrial Revolution, the household produced many of its own goods and services – even if as with physick, surgery, or brewing they were also commercially available. In a sense, the material conditions of life in principle enabled anyone to be a distiller, brewer, textile maker, baker, etc., just as anyone could practise medicine or surgery – if the money and the apparatus were available. Markham's housewife was a well-to-do one.

Markham did make the usual nod in the direction of the physicians:

> the depth and secrets of this most excellent Art of Physick, are far beyond the capacity of the most skilful woman, as lodging onely in the breast of learned professors, yet that our House-wife may from them receive some ordinary

rules and medicines, which may avail for the benefit of her Family is (in our common experience) no derogation at all to that worthy Art. Neither do I intend here to load her mind with all the Symptomes, accidents and effects which go before or after every sickness as though I would have her assume the name of a Practitioner, but only relate unto her some approved medicines, and old doctrines, which have been gathered together, by two excellent and experienced Physitians, and in a Manuscript given to a great Countess of this land . . .[59]

Despite his patronizing tone Markham went on to give directions and recipes for the housewife to deal with the most serious illnesses such as plague, frenzy, and the different types of fever.

The large number of manuscript collections, often put together with recipes for food and cosmetics, indicates that people were not merely passive readers of medical knowledge but took an active interest in bringing it together. The collections tended to be indiscriminate and eclectic, illustrating a lack of concern with keeping to particular sources and types of medical knowledge (hence showing again that the categories 'popular' and 'popularized' were at this time ambiguous and indeterminate). The published collections of remedies often laid more stress on who had put the collection together (often a royal or noble figure) than on their medical provenance.

William Blundell and his family got their visitors to give them the details of any effective remedies which they then wrote into a book.[60] Lady Ranelagh, Robert Boyle's sister, was probably the compiler of a manuscript collection from the late seventeenth century. As well as describing how to make sugar cakes, 'Lady Essex a Cream Cheese', the collection also gave prescriptions for serious illnesses. Some are from lay people, 'Mrs Rodgers. A drink for the Rickets which never yet failed', others were from learned medicine as Dr Denham's remedy for the gout, 'commended by Galen, Avicen and Fallopius'; while yet others were from Paracelsians, the rivals of learned medicine, as 'Quercetans [Quercetanus'] Decoction for the jaundice'.[61] All types of medicine are present here without distinction.

There were some forms of medicine which did not come from lay, learned, or radical medicine. Recipe no. 617 reads:

A Receipt by way of Charm from Ague. Our Saviour Jesus
Christ seeing the Cross. He had a Agony upon him; the
Jews asked him art thou afraid and He said I am not afraid
nor have I an Ague, All those that fear the Name of Christ
and wear the Name of Christ about them shall have no
Ague, Amen, Sweet Jesus, Sweet Jesus, Sweet Jesus. Amen
Sweet Jesus, Amen. This to be sewed in a black silk and put
to the pitt of the Stomach an hour before the fitt comes
and not seen by the party but worn till all in pieces.[62]

Keith Thomas in his *Religion and the Decline of Magic* has charted
the prevalence of religious and magical healing. Not only were
wise men and women thick on the ground, offering to discover
witchcraft causing illness, and selling amulets and charms, but
the established Church also proffered means to cure illness. In
times of plague, prayer and atonement were institutionalized in
national days of prayer to God to withdraw his anger and
punishment. Godly ministers like William Perkins at the beginning of the seventeenth century not only taught (in effect,
popularizing) that God in his providence brought illness and
could take it away, but also taught what was the best type of
medicine that the ill should use (in his case, Galenic). Certainly,
magic and then religion were to decline in significance as the
Enlightenment began, but in the earlier part of our period the
existence of witchcraft, magic, and religion, all recognized by
the State and the law, meant that there were other bodies of
medical knowledge and other medical practices and practitioners that reinforced the paradox of distinction and openness. Religion, and even witchcraft and magic, the tools of
Satan, the necessary antithesis of God, in principle crossed all
social boundaries. Their effectiveness and existence were, in
terms of theological doctrine and law, universal, not popular or
élite, not high or low culture. Of course, condemnations of
witchcraft and magic did use social categories – their practitioners in England were often taken to be poor or ignorant. In
the same socially stigmatizing way, the learned physicians castigated the ignorance of empirics, 'vagabundes and ronagetes'[63]
who proffered medical care. However, the openness of English
medicine helps to drown the significance of these voices and
the existence of religious and other supernatural means of
causing and treating illness increases the eclectic and open

sense of medicine. Popular and popularized medicine are categories that, in this time, one should indeed be cautious about.

Notes

1. Roy Porter (ed.), *Patients and Practitioners. Lay Perceptions of Medicine in Pre-industrial Society* (Cambridge: Cambridge University Press, 1985); Lucinda McCray Beier, *Sufferers and Healers. The Experience of Illness in Seventeenth Century England* (London: Routledge, 1987); Roy Porter and Dorothy Porter, *In Sickness and in Health. The British Experience 1650–1850* (London: Fourth Estate, 1988); Dorothy and Roy Porter, *Patient's Progress. Doctors and Doctoring in Eighteenth Century England* (Oxford: Polity Press, 1989); Doreen G. Nagy, *Popular Medicine in Seventeenth Century England* (Bowling Green, Ohio: Bowling Green State University Popular Press, 1988). Also on medical practitioners, see Margaret Pelling and Charles Webster, 'Medical Practitioners' in Charles Webster (ed.), *Health, Medicine and Mortality in the Sixteenth Century* (Cambridge: Cambridge University Press, 1979), 164–235; on French popularized medicine, see Andrew Wear, 'Popularized Ideas of Health and Illness in Seventeenth-Century France', *Seventeenth Century French Studies*, I (1986), 229–42. On German Lutheran popular medicine, especially women's care of children, see Steven Ozment, *When Fathers Ruled: Family Life in Reformation Europe* (Cambridge Mass: Harvard University Press, 1983).

2. On literacy, see Lawrence Stone, 'The Educational Revolution in England 1560–1640', *Past and Present*, 28 (1964), 41–80; David Cressy, *Literacy and the Social Order* (Cambridge: Cambridge University Press, 1980); Margaret Spufford, *Small Books and Pleasant Histories* (London: Methuen, 1981, chap. 2); Keith Wrightson, *English Society 1580–1680* (London: Hutchinson, 1982), 183–99; Peter Laslett *The World We Have Lost – Further Explored* (London: Methuen, 1983), 228–37.

3. Laslett, *The World We have Lost – Further Explored*, pp. 232–3, states that after 1753 a little over 60% of males and 40% of females were literate. His figures are drawn from Roger Schofield's study of the consequences of the Hardwick Marriage Act of 1753 where, for the first time, both bridegroom and bride had to sign the marriage register or leave their mark.

4. Paul Slack, 'Mirrors of Health and Treasures of Poor Men: The Uses of the Vernacular Medical Literature of Tudor England' in Charles Webster (ed.), *Health, Medicine and Mortality in the Sixteenth Century* (Cambridge: Cambridge University Press, 1979), 237–73.

5. On the College of Physicians, see George N. Clark, *A History of the Royal College of Physicians* (Oxford: Clarendon Press, 1964–6), 2 vols; Harold J. Cook, *The Decline of the Old Medical Regime in Stuart London* (Ithaca and London: Cornell University Press, 1986).

6. Sir Thomas Elyot, *The Castel of Health* (London, 1580), sig. A 3r. Here and elsewhere I have often used editions of early modern works that are later than the first.

7. ibid., sig. A 3v.
8. ibid., sig. A 3v.
9. On Renaissance medical method, see N.W. Gilbert, *Renaissance Concepts of Method* (New York: Columbia University Press, 1960; W.P.D. Wightman '*Quid Sit Methodus?* Method in Sixteenth Century Teaching and Discovery', *J. Hist. Med. 19* (1964), 360–76; Andrew Wear, 'Galen in the Renaissance' in V. Nutton (ed.) *Galen: Problems and Prospects* (London: Wellcome Institute for the History of Medicine, 1981), 229–62; *idem*, 'Explorations in Renaissance Writings on the Practice of Medicine' in A. Wear, R.K. French, I.M. Lonie (eds), *The Medical Renaissance of the Sixteenth Century* (Cambridge: Cambridge University Press, 1985), 118–45; Jerome Bylebyl, 'Teaching *Methodus Medendi* in the Renaissance' in Fridolf Kudlein and Richard J. Durling (eds), *Galen's Method of Healing* (Leiden: E.J. Brill, 1991), 157–89.
10. Andrew Boorde, *The Breviary of Health* (London, 1547), sig. A 6r.
11. For an influential analysis of this culture in the later period, see N. Jewson, 'Medical Knowledge and the Patronage System in Eighteenth-Century England', *Sociology* 8 (1974), 369–85; also R. Porter, 'Laymen, Doctors and Medical Knowledge in the *Gentleman's Magazine*' in Roy Porter (ed.), *Patients and Practitioners* (1985), 282–314; Andrew Wear, 'The Meanings of Illness in Early Modern England' in Yosio Kawakita and Shizu Sakai (eds.), *Patient–Doctor Relations in History* (Tokyo: Ishiyaku Euro American, forthcoming); on Galen and patients' medical knowledge, see Galen, *De Optimo Medico Cognoscendo*, ed. Albert Iskander (Berlin: *Medicorum Graecorum Supplementum Orientale* 4, Berlin Academy of Sciences, 1988).
12. On Galen's eclectic use of sources for his knowledge of drugs, see Vivian Nutton, 'The Drug Trade in Antiquity', *Journal of the Royal Society of Medicine 78* (1985), 138–45. Reprinted in Vivian Nutton, *From Democedes to Harvey: Studies in the History of Medicine* (London: Variorum Reprints, 1981), chap. 9. The early modern reader of Galen could see how he noted lay medical practice; for instance, he set down how a 'plebeius' prepared and used fumitory either as a cathartic or as a strengthening medicine, Galen (1625), *De Simplicium Medicamentorum Facultatibus* in *Galeni Opera*, vol. 5, Venice: Junta, p. 49 v. An example from the sixteenth century comes from Thomas Cogan (1584) *The Haven of Health*: of chamomile he wrote 'And this medicine I learned of a countrey man for an Ague, which I have proved true in many though it fayled in some. Take a handful of Cammomill, washe it cleane and bruise it a little, and seeth it in a pint of Ale, till halfe be wasted, scumme it well and straine it, and drinke it an houre before the fit, and if you thinke it better put in Sugar, cover you warme and procure heate, so doing three daies together fasting' (my edition London, 1612, pp. 68–9).
13. Elyot, *Castell of Health* sig. A 3v.
14. ibid., sig. A 4r.
15. ibid., sig. A 4r.
16. ibid., sig. A 4r.

17. John Securis, *A Detection and Querimonie of the Daily Enormities and Abuses Committed in Physick* (London, 1566), sig. B 2r-v.

18. ibid., sig. B 2v.

19. James Hart, *KΛINIKH Or the Diet of the Diseased* (London, 1633), 26–7.

20. ibid., p. 24.

21. ibid., p. 25.

22. ibid., p. 26.

23. John Cotta, *A Short Discoverie of the Unobserved Dangers of Severall Sorts of Ignorant and Unconsiderable Practisers of Physicke in England* (London, 1612).

24. James Primrose, *Popular Errours or the Errours of the People in Matter of Physick* (London, 1651), trans. Robert Wittie: Wittie's Epistle Dedicatory to Lady Frances Stickland sig. A 3v.

25. William Harrison, *The Description of England,* ed. Georges Edelen (Ithaca: Folger Shakespeare Library, Cornell University Press, 1968), chap. 20, pp. 265–8.

26. Timothie Bright, (1580) *A Treatise Wherein is Declared the Sufficiencie of English Medicines. For Cure of all Diseases, Cured with Medicine* (London, 1580), 47.

27. Phillip Barrough, *Method of Physick* (London, 1634), sig. A 5r.

28. ibid., sig. A 6r.

29. See Andrew Wear, 'Puritan Perceptions of Illness in Seventeenth Century England' in Roy Porter (ed.), *Patients and Practitioners, Lay Perceptions of Medicine in Pre-industrial Society* (Cambridge: Cambridge University Press, 1985), 55–99 esp. 61–3.

30. Barrough, *Method of Physick,* sig. A 6r.

31. ibid., sig. A 7r.

32. ibid., sig. A 7v.

33. ibid., sig. A 6r.

34. On the *practica* see Andrew Wear, 'Explorations in Renaissance Writings on the Practice of Medicine' in A. Wear, R.K. French and I.M. Lonie (eds), *The Medical Renaissance of the Sixteenth Century* (Cambridge: Cambridge University Press, 1985), 118–45.

35. Barrough, *Method of Physick,* sig. A 7r.

36. Robert Pemel, *ΠΤΩΧΟΦΑΡΜΑΚΟΝ, Or Help for the Poor* (London, 1650), sig. A 2v.

37. ibid., sig. A 3r.

38. Lancelot Coelson, *The Poormans Physician and Chyrurgian* (London, 1656), sig. A 4v.

39. ibid., sig. A 5r.

40. Thomas Cocke, *Kitchen Physick: Or, Advice to the Poor* (London, 1676), 10.

41. ibid., p. 8.

42. Charles Webster, *The Great Instauration* (London: Duckworth, 1975), esp. pp. 245–323; Webster's conclusions of a puritan-Paracelsian-reform of medicine nexus must still stand for the period after 1640 or slightly before, despite Peter Elmer's revisionist thesis in his 'Medicine, Religion and the Puritan Revolution' in Roger French

and Andrew Wear (eds), *The Medical Revolution of the Seventeenth Century* (Cambridge, Cambridge University Press, 1989), 10–45. However, puritans, in the period before the Laudian reforms when they felt they constituted the real Church of England, often took a conservative Galenic line (see James Hart, John Cotta, William Perkins, William Gouge).

43. Noah Biggs, *Mataeotechnia Medicinae Praxews. The Vanity of the Craft of Physick* (London, 1651); William Walwyn, *Physick for Families: Or the New Way of Physick* (London, 1669).

44. On Culpeper, see F.N.L. Poynter, 'Nicholas Culpeper and his Books', *Journal of the History of Medicine*, 17 (1962), 152–67; *idem*, 'Nicholas Culpeper and the Paracelsians' in Allen G. Debus (ed.), *Science, Medicine and Society in the Renaissance: Essays to Honor Walter Pagel* 2 vols (New York: American Elsevier, 1972), vol. 1, 201–20; Charles Webster, *The Great Instauration*, 267–73 *et passim*.

45. Nicholas Culpeper, (1649) *A Physical Directory or a Translation of the London Dispensary Made by the College of Physicians* (London, 1649), sig. A 1r.

46. ibid., sig. A 1r.

47. ibid., sig. A 1v. The quotation 'all a man[sic] hath spent upon Physicians' is from Mark 5, 25–7: 'And a certain woman, which had an issue of blood twelve years. And had suffered many things of many physicians, and had spent all she had and was nothing bettered, but rather grew worse. When she had heard of Jesus, came in the press behind and touched his garment.'

48. Anonymous, 'The Life of the Admired Physician and Astrologer of our Times, Mr Nicholas Culpeper' in Nicholas Culpeper, *Culpepers School of Physick* (London, 1659), sig. C 4r.

49. Culpeper, *School of Physick*, 1–49.

50. Culpeper, *A Physical Directory*, 314–24.

51. Abdiah Cole in the 1660s was advertising his series of books making up 'The Physicians Library' which included texts by Sennert, Riverius, Plater, Bartholinus, Riolan, Veslingius, Fernel, etc., some of which were claimed to be translated by Culpeper. Culpeper's biographer in *The School of Physick* wrote that a member of the College of Physicians agreed 'That he [Culpeper] was not onely for Gallen and Hypocrates, but he knew how to correct and moderate the tyrannies of Paracelsus', sig. C 4v. How far this was put in to make Culpeper acceptable to a wide variety of readers and how far it represents Culpeper's own position is unclear.

52. Culpeper, *A Physical Directory*, sig. A 2r.

53. ibid., sig. A 2v.

54. ibid., sig. A 2v.

55. Nicholas Culpeper, *A Directory of Midwives Or a Guide for Women* (London, 1681), sig. A 4r-v.

56. William Turner, *The Rare Treasor of the Englishe Bathes* in Thomas Vicary, *The Englishemans Treasure* (London, 1586), 105.

57. Michael Stanhope, *Cures Without Care . . . Mineral Waters near Knaresborow . . .* (London, 1632); Robert Wittie (1660) *Scarborough Spaw*; Robert Pierce, *Memoirs of the Bath* (Bristol, 1697).

58. Gervase Markham, *The English Hous-Wife* (London, 1653), titlepage. On women and medicine, see the works by Beier, Nagy, the Porters, and Ozment in note I, and Patricia Crawford, 'The Sucking Child: Adult Attitudes to Child Care in the First Years of Life in Seventeenth Century England', *Continuity and Change*, I (1986), 23–51 and *idem* 'The Construction and Experience of Maternity in Seventeenth Century England' in Valerie Fildes (ed.), *Women as Mothers in Pre-industrial England: Essays in Memory of Dorothy Mclaren* (London: Routledge, 1990), 3–38.

59. Markham, *The English Hous-Wife*, 4.

60. T. Ellison Gibson, (1880) *A Cavalier's Note-Book* (London, 1880), 244–6.

61. 'Collection of 712 Medical Receipts with some Cooking Recipes', *Wellcome MS 1340, Boyle Family*, nos 234, 240, 85, 631, 101.

62. ibid., no. 617.

63. Boorde, *Breviary of Health*, sig. 7v.

2

Acquiring surgical know-how

Occupational and lay instruction in early eighteenth-century London

Philip K. Wilson

In a recent assessment of the accounts of 'science' and 'the public', Steven Shapin has claimed that members of the 'accredited' scientific community have historically been distinguished from the public on levels of 'cultural competence'.[1] Scientists have typically been depicted as having acquired 'cognitive and manipulative skills' which the public did not possess; a distinction demonstrable by the scientist's use of 'mathematical and technical language'. However, Shapin argued that our interpretations of a discontinuity between scientists who know something and the public who does not are superficial and exclusive. In particular, they fail to consider the sets and range of beliefs which scientists and the public share. Explaining such beliefs, he noted, is also integral to understanding which types of therapies physicians and patients have deemed appropriate throughout history.[2]

Identifying which skills and procedures the public and various types of practitioners expected particular professions or trades to possess should further our understanding of what Shapin termed 'cultural competence'.[3] Questions to be considered include: What diseases and disorders did the public believe themselves to be capable of treating? and, Whom did they rely upon to perform other medical or surgical tasks? Were certain conditions perceived, by the public or practitioners, as the exclusive domain of one particular trade or profession? And, how were the skills necessary to attain an 'occupational competence' conveyed to the public and/or to specific tradesmen or professionals?

Many physicians in early eighteenth-century England disputed over particular medical theories.[4] Some argued that such theoretical reasoning was totally unrelated to the practical treatment of patients.[5] The public, too, apparently expressed much less concern over a physician's theoretical orientation than over the immediacy and cost of the relief he provided. Still, it remains an arduous task to assess the public and professional views of physicians' competency. Rather, it appears more manageable to estimate the practical competence of a trade more oriented around the acquisition of particular skills.

More than their medical counterparts, surgeons were trained towards acquiring definite manual skills. Many English textbooks of the late seventeenth and early eighteenth centuries retained the ancient fourfold classification of surgery as an art, or craft, whose practitioners (1) joined unnaturally separated parts, (2) separated preternaturally joined parts, (3) removed superfluous parts and (4) supplied those that were wanting.[6] These texts, all written in the vernacular, also specified that surgery was a 'manual Operation' in which its practitioners 'by the Use of Instruments, or the Assistance of the Hands' would aim to 'relieve those accidental Diseases' which patients were 'externally subject to'.[7] Surgeons, so their texts would have us believe, were relied upon to incise tumours, reduce fractured bones and dislocated joints, repair ruptures and fistulae, amputate limbs, 'cut' for bladder stones, and apply topical medicines and bandages (Figure 1).

Historians have claimed, however, that the public did not overtly distinguish the disorders that surgeons treated from the treatments offered by physicians, apothecaries, barbers, wise neighbour women, and quacks.[8] Rather, they have argued that an occupational pluralism existed, both in London's medical marketplace and in the provinces, to such a degree that diverse tradesmen and professionals were relied upon to treat syphilis, the King's evil, gout, and cancer as well as to set bones, let blood and draw teeth.[9]

Following Shapin's conviction towards delineating various levels of competence, I will compare the idea of surgical competence which is unveiled in the popular literature with that claimed as exclusive to the surgical trade. First, the writings which described surgical conditions and treatments will be identified. Following this, I will discuss ways by which the skills used to treat two conditions, skull fractures and bladder stones, were communicated. Specifically, I will describe an attempt to educate surgeons in trepanning the skull, a skill in which they were

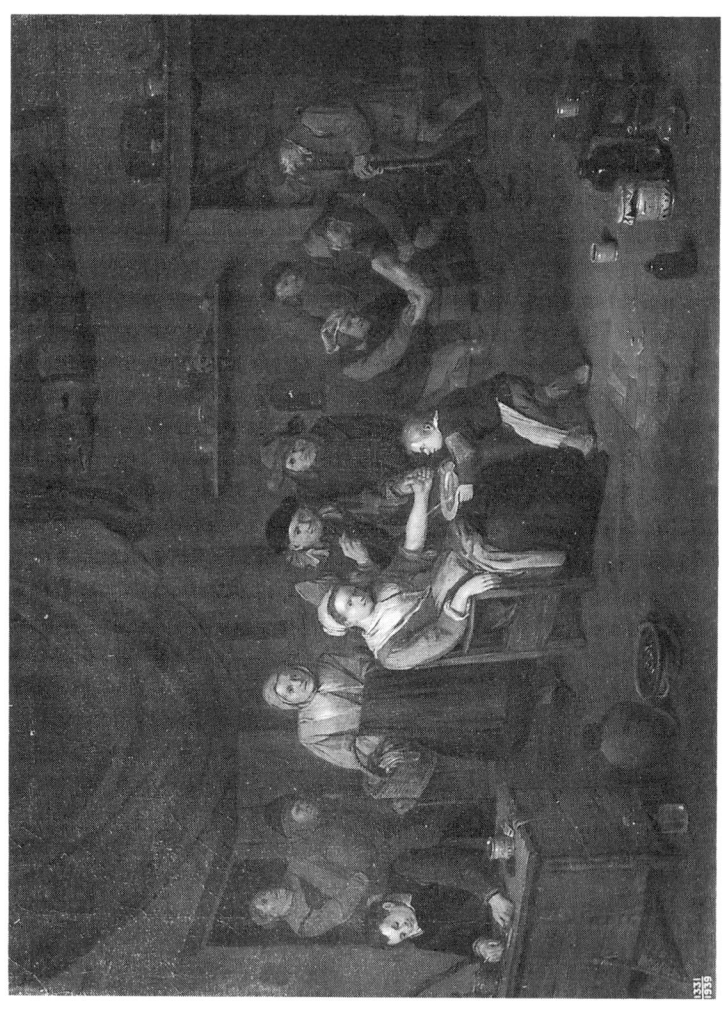

Figure 1 Egbert van Heemskerck's depiction of 'surgeons' letting blood and treating an external wound. Late seventeenth or early eighteenth century. (Reproduced by permission of the Wellcome Institute Library, London.)

apparently privileged. Additionally, ways by which diverse bladder-stone treatments were promoted will be analysed. Finally, I will describe some major difficulties in explaining any aspect of early eighteenth-century surgical practice according to twentieth-century concepts of popularization.

In whose hands? Lay practice vs. masters of an art

Between 1690 and 1740, at least ten surgical textbooks were published which recounted, in part, some aspects of surgical practice in London.[10] Although the specific content and detail varied widely, the texts typically conformed to one of two general formats. Some authors, like surgeon and later physician Daniel Turner, in his two-volume *Art of Surgery*, organized their texts under the more traditional headings of tumours, ulcers, wounds, and fractures.[11] His emphasis on external disease reflects the contemporary restrictions against surgeons treating internal disorders. Still, many surgical authors described these external conditions with reference to strategic internal body parts, stressing the importance of anatomy to their practice.

More numerous than these texts, concise, often pocket-sized, manuals of surgery were printed.[12] Sea surgeons' manuals by Hugh Ryder, John Moyle, and John Atkins exemplify this format. Brief step-by-step instructions or answers to specific questions described how to amputate limbs and treat multiple fractures or head wounds, in addition to remedying many less threatening injuries. Some, like Edward Dunn, surgeon to the Royal African Company, compiled his *Compendious and New Method of Performing Chirurgical Operations* explicitly to guide readers 'by the Hand in every Step of an Operation, in a clear, easy and succinct Manner . . . where ambiguous Circumlocutions are purposely avoided, and useless Distinctions, are dropped'.[13]

Communicating surgical know-how was not exclusive to surgical texts. During this period, at least sixteen different domestic manuals also appeared. Most of these manuals included sections of surgical remedies in addition to 'domestic concerns' such as cookery and cosmetics.[14] Although many works of this genre instructed readers in the delicate carving of game and fowl, they generally limited their instructions of operative surgery to blood-letting and bandaging (Figure 2).

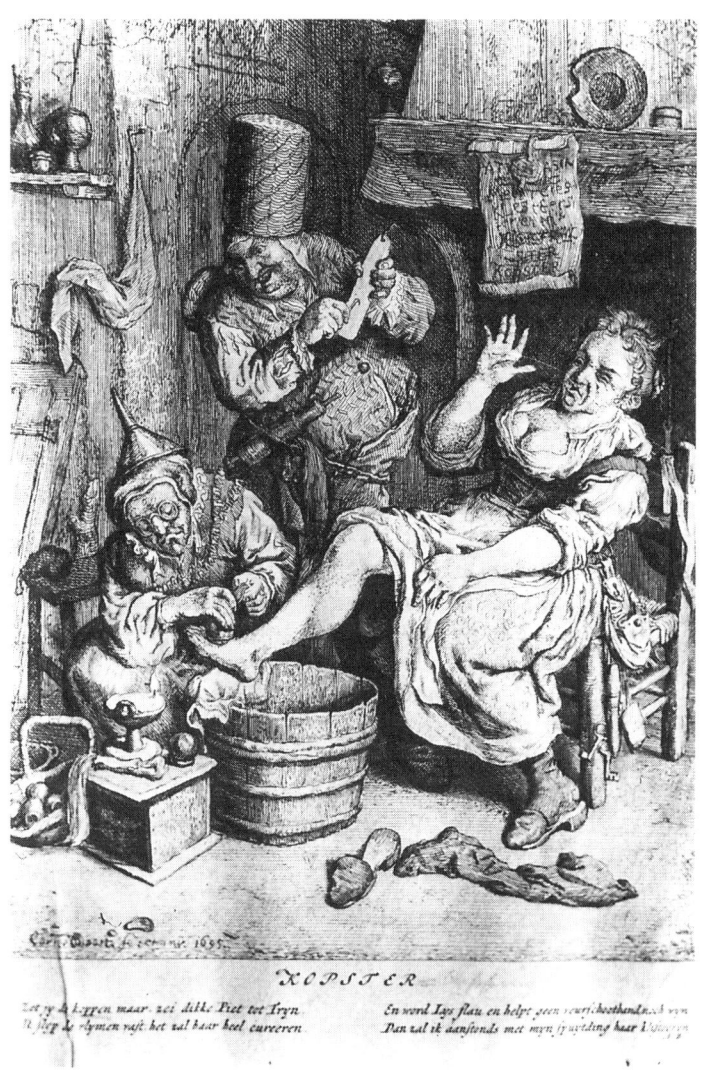

Figure 2 Cupping, a common variety of blood-letting not exclusive to the surgical trade. (Cornelius Dusart, 1695; reproduced by permission of the Wellcome Institute Library, London.)

Like surgical texts, many domestic manuals proffered remedies for treating boils, burns, corns, and piles, together with suggestions for removing moles, freckles, and the 'Pits in the Face' of smallpox.[15] Treatments, typically in the form of 'Receipts in Surgery', listed proportions for compounding and procedures for externally applying plaisters, poultices, ointments and salves. However, domestic manuals devoted only a small section of, more commonly, a few scattered pages to treating surgical conditions. Their concise 'Practical and easy Prescriptions' were often intermixed with treatments for fevers, gout, worms, and other diseases of 'physic'. Although the categorical headings of their surgical counterparts were lacking, an index or table of contents was generally provided, referring readers to specific pages.

Of the six known authors of contemporary domestic manuals, three were 'housewives', one a cook, one a lexicographer, and another a countess.[16] Although the readership of these manuals is unknown, some clues suggest the intended audiences. Eliza Smith, author of the long-running *Compleat Housewife*, composed her manual for 'those generous, charitable, and Christian Gentlewomen that have a Disposition to be serviceable to their poor hurting neighbour'. *The Complete Family Piece* offered aid to 'effectually cure' sufferers 'without the Assistance of a Surgeon (even supposing you had a good one near at hand)', while the *Family Companion for Health* instructed gentlewomen how to relieve their menials' sufferings. *The Ladies Dispensatory* distinguished itself more explicitly from textbook accounts as the anonymous author offered directions for the 'generality of women, who require plain practical Doctrine, in *English* words . . . unencumbered with numerous Definitions and Demonstrations that appear in texts written for the Learned and Contemplative'.[17] Reprintings of these manuals in up to twenty-one or more editions, far exceeding that of any contemporary surgical text, suggests that they were indeed popular. Consequently, their content was likely to have become widespread.

The potential usefulness of these manuals to literate provincial residents remote from a surgeon's care is understood. In London, however, many trade surgeons were available.[18] Yet, London's lay public had multiple opportunities to purchase domestic manuals from bookstalls on the streets.[19] After all, self-treatment provided the public with an alternative to paying surgeons' fees.[20] And as the titles of many manuals suggest, they were designed to 'Compleat' their readers' practical know-how, making them 'Accomplished' in all domestic skills including surgery.[21] In order to build readers' confidence in their abilities to treat certain surgical disorders, some authors employed rhetorical devices against surgeons in defence of their own 'tryed' and 'approved' remedies. *The Family Magazine*, for instance, boasted of a medicine which had 'cur'd an obstinate Tumour of the knee that had baffled some Chirurgeons'.[22]

Surgeons' accounts corroborate suggestions of a self-treating public. Occupational surgeons, detesting this particular practice, rebuked the proliferation of domestic manuals. Daniel Turner, among the most vocal opponents, claimed that the intent and content of such manuals fostered quackery. In particular, he despised anyone believing themselves capable, after reading any book of 'Physick', to 'set up for a Doctor or a Surgeon . . . pretending . . . to the Cure of any . . . Disease' without proper training and qualification.[23] 'More people have been Ruined', he argued, by attempting to 'set up a Physician in every Family', through 'Mistakes . . . [such as] an ill timed administration of a Good Medicine, or some other Over-sight', than would have been caused had their disease 'been left only to Nature'.[24] Another author claimed that those who pretend 'to *everything* they do not understand', let blood 'without suspecting the Nerve or Artery may ly in the way'; or, by not allowing 'putrid matter' to drain from a sinus, fistula or ulcer, they create such a condition that the very pain is 'loud enough to call the Surgeon'.[25]

Echoing many fellow practitioners, Turner leads us to believe that patients only sought a surgeon's services after their own treatments had failed. Typically, so he claimed, patients had already undergone such 'abusive' service from the hands of a series of barbers, apothecaries, and quacks before calling on a surgeon.[26] In an attempt to coax the public away from self-treatment, Turner warned them that using surgeons only as a means of last resort had already cost many patients their lives.

Some distinctions must still be drawn between the types of self-treatment which surgeons like Turner despised, and the practical guidelines laid out in domestic manuals. Indeed, it appears that the authors of domestic manuals were instructing readers towards attaining a different level of surgical competence than that found in surgical texts. One is struck by

Arabella Atkyns's elaborate recommendation for treating wounds in which large vessels had been cut. 'Pellets of lint moisten'd with oxycrate, and rolled either in white or Roman vitriol may be applied to the mouths of [such] wounds', over which 'the common Styptick' was applied; then 'covering all with a plaster of deninum'. The author concludes that 'when these gentler means will not take effect, an actual cautery may be used'.[27] Although such description is totally consistent with that in standard surgical texts, it is quite uncommon in domestic manuals. Although works like *The Accomplish'd Ladies Delight* and *The Complete Family Piece* employed standard medical and surgical terminology like 'impostumes' and 'fomentations', the treatments they recommended were strikingly simple in comparison to those found in surgical texts. Most domestic manuals merely offered a few simply compounded remedies for wounds described only as the 'Prick of a Thorn' or the 'Bite of a mad dog'.

Another distinction arises in that domestic manuals identified certain disorders as solely within the surgeon's domain. The 1739 *Ladies Dispensatory*, a work which otherwise promoted lay surgical care, warned that treatments for such conditions as gangrene of the womb must not be 'undertake[n] rashly'.[28] Rather, patients suffering from the listed symptoms suggestive of the disorder should be referred to a surgeon's care. 'Deep, winding' ulcers were also described as being so 'dangerous' that a 'surgeon's work is . . . generally necessary'.[29] Although Arabella Atkyns directed her readers to 'snip' the pustules of shingles, she warned them that attempting to cut away corns had 'often' led to 'mortifications . . . [of the] most fatal consequences'.[30] Thus, readers of domestic manuals were urged to limit the range of disorders they attempted to treat. Although they may well have read surgical texts and watched the operations of their occupational counterparts, contemporary writings suggest lay practitioners were instructed towards attaining different levels of surgical know-how from those of surgeons.

As with the serious conditions mentioned above, domestic manuals did not address the care of head wounds, particularly those wounds thought to have fractured the skull. Therefore, examining the treatments recommended for this disorder will illustrate one way by which surgical know-how was communicated among occupational surgeons.

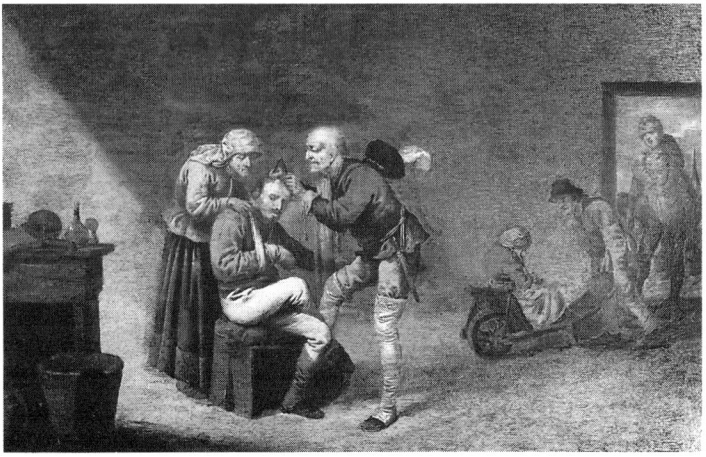

Figure 3 Surgery on a man with multiple injuries, including a head wound, while other patients are being brought forth. Seventeenth Century. (Pieter Quast; reproduced by permission of the Wellcome Institute Library, London.)

Skull fractures

It appears that surgeons were the publicly recognized caretakers of skull fractures. Extant case reports suggest that such accidents were not uncommon in the capital city[31] (Figure 3). Numerous reports state that London surgeons treated skulls fractured by the kick of a horse or a blow on the head. One described a patient whose skull was fractured by the 'Fall of a Tile from a House'; another, from an 'Iron-Pin' hitting a girl in the head as it flew from a 'machine' at the 'flying Horse' in Moorfields; and another, which a young man received by falling after being 'tripp[ed] up' by a friend.[32] Furthermore, when a 10-year-old boy fractured his skull after falling 20 feet from the 'Top of an old wall, as he was taking out a *Sparrow's* nest', London surgeon John Cagua was sought. Hugh Ryder, another local surgeon, was called in to treat the skull fracture a young carpenter received when the steeple of 'Bow-Church' toppled upon him. At another time, Ryder treated a boy's wounds from a 'Cart-Wheel' rolling over the side of his head. The exclusion of such reports from lay manuals further suggests claims that skull fractures were publicly believed to require a surgeon's care.

Methods for examining and treating patients suspected of a skull fracture are found in nearly all surgical texts of the period. Most accounts, however, only briefly identified the seemingly standard procedural sequence: clearing hair and the scalp away from the wound, determining the extent of fracture, cleansing the wound, removing loose bone fragments, and stopping any haemorrhage. Although trepanning (i.e. boring into the skull) was frequently suggested as remedial for post-fracture headache or for draining any built-up 'matter' on the brain, surgeons generally shunned this 'extremely dangerous' operation.[33]

London surgeon Daniel Turner claimed that his fellow practitioners too readily absolved themselves from handling patients with fractured skulls. He represented his colleagues 'abandon[ment]' of such 'miserable People' as failings towards their fellow man. It was, he argued, surgeons' responsibility to provide their 'utmost' for the 'Preservation' of skull-fractured patients. He pointed out that although 'Accidents of this kind' may 'seem . . . very desperate', it 'Often falls out' that many patients have 'notwithstanding been recover'd' following surgical care.[34] In particular, he sought to convince fellow surgeons of the 'Remarkable' benefit they could achieve by trepanning.

Turner regarded trepanning as the critical step in treating most skull fractures. He specified that 'three or four times' as many patients were lost by 'its not being done at all, and many others [lost] from [its] delay'. But, he discouraged a 'rash enterprise' of its performance without proper know-how. He cautioned readers that trepanning should only be performed after consultation with senior practitioners. With their aid, he claimed, a consensus could be reached as to when the patient's condition was no longer 'too hazardous' for the operation. And, in order to 'furnish Instruction' in this procedure. Turner relayed a detailed account of a 'Remarkable case in Surgery' which he had attended.[35]

Turner's case appeared as a pamphlet in 1709, and described the events following the skull fracture of Mr S.R.'s 6-year-old son.[36] This boy had been struck in the head by a misguided cat-stick thrown during a cock fight in Southwark. In recounting this case, Turner, as principal attending surgeon, provided readers with a daily diary account of his observations and actions for the '4 score and 4 days' from the time of the accident to his findings at autopsy.[37] Such an extensive and detailed account is rare among contemporary surgical case histories.

This case was also the most elaborately detailed of the more than 200 surgical case histories Turner had reported from over twenty years of practice. Furthermore, this was the only case for which Turner commissioned an engraving.[38]

Given that trepanning ranks among the oldest known surgical operations, Turner's elaboration upon this procedure at first appeared puzzling. Yet, by examining this work in the context of his later, explicitly pedagogical works, and considering the limited instructions offered in alternative texts, Turner's educative intentions become clearer.

Formerly, English surgical texts had typically described trepanning by identifying the instruments used, and offering a literal ABC procedural approach. Turner, however, elaborated upon the indications for this course of treatment and gave specific operative instructions in the context of a particular case. Turner hoped that placing his procedural instruction in a practical everyday format would prevent any misinterpretation.

The pedagogical aspect of Turner's writing is well-defined by his terminology. His use of anatomical language, particularly in identifying the anatomical points he considered most relevant to his operation, implied that his intended readers must have had some surgical experience. Indeed, he specified it as a 'Rule' that 'no Person [should] attempt to meddle' with fractured skulls 'who has not first well acquainted himself with the . . . Structure of the Cranium . . . the Meninges, and the Brain invested by them'.[39] This experience could, Turner emphasized, be gained by practising trepanning upon the skulls of the deceased, a further occupational privilege over the public.

Unlike most surgical authors who strove for brevity, Turner appears to have aimed for unambiguous clarity in instructing his readers on the anatomically precise use of a trepan. First, he described the specific anatomical regions of the skull which had been fractured. Then, he explained why any operation on certain anatomical regions was to be avoided. Although his digressive discourse was likely to have provoked much mental imagery of these anatomical regions, he also provided his readers with a fully labelled diagram to which he frequently referred (Figure 4). By reinforcing the written text with an illustration, Turner attempted to identify unmistakably which anatomical features he considered must be known in order to perform this operation.

Contemporary accounts suggest that neither physicians nor the public questioned the surgical privilege of treating skull fractures.[40] Turner's writing upheld the surgeons' responsibility to treat this common accident competently. Since many junior surgeons had disparate backgrounds,[41] Turner's instructions also served to supplement his readers' personal experiences. In this way, Turner helped to secure this particular operation as an exclusive skill of the surgical trade.

Such emphasis on instructing fellow surgeons did not apply to all the conditions surgeons treated. Instead, contemporary writings about treating other disorders centred more around competition and self-promotion. As an example, I shall examine how recommendations for treating bladder stones not only promoted surgical skills, but advertised one practitioner's competence over another.

Bladder stones

Ere Night is half spent, he wishes for Day; when Day appears, he longs for Night; Distracted with his sufferings, he lyes wakeful counting the Hours, any one of which when protracted and multiplied by raging Misery, seems a numerous Train . . . He changes his Pillow, but not his Pain, new-makes his Bed, but keeps his old Inequitudes, and though he often turns from Side to Side, he never leaves his Agonies behind.[42]

Bladder stones, like skull fractures, were not uncommon among early eighteenth-century Londoners. Thousands of bladder stones or calculi were privately displayed at Gresham College, the College of Physicians, Barber-Surgeons Hall, and in many curio cabinets. They were also publicly exhibited in coffee shops, barbershops, and on the stages of mountebanks.[43] Such displays provide evidence of the high incidence of this disorder at the time, and exemplify both the common and the extremes of size, shape, and substance of the bladder stones which 'cruelly vex[ed]' the afflicted.[44] As to the sufferers, one London physician described the 'sedentary Lawyer, the hard Student, and the inactive, indolent, and voluptuous Gentleman' as being more susceptible to this 'grievous Distemper' than the 'laborious Husbandman, and Meckanick, the daily Traveller, and [the] indefatigable Sportsman'.[45]

Although descriptive accounts abound of the various methods proffered for curing the stone, historians have not

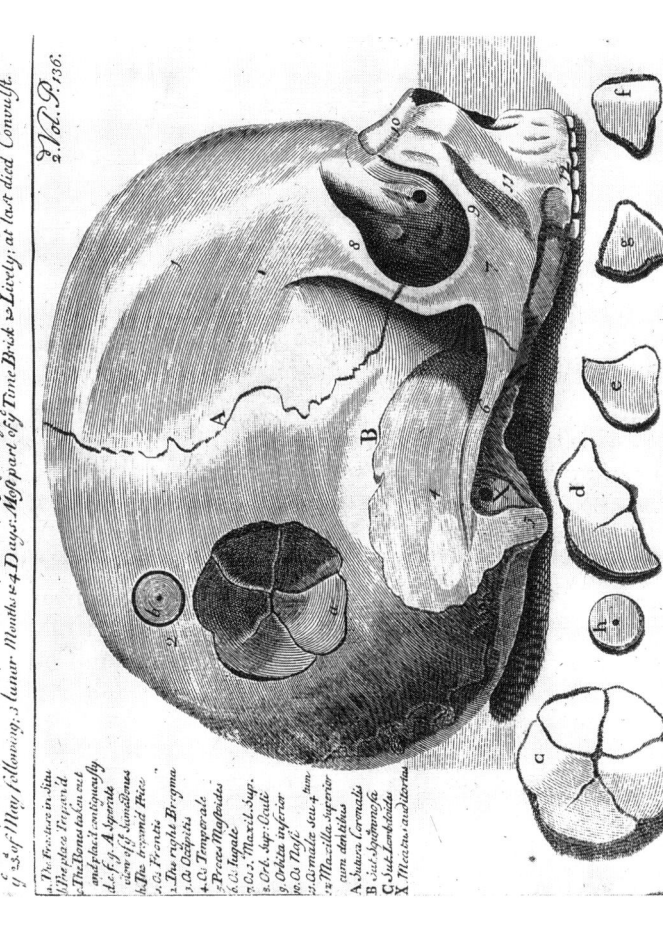

A View of a Fractur'd Skull, taken from ye Skull of Mr J. P's aged 6 years; who was wounded on ye 24th of Feb 1708, elevated to ye 23d of May following, 3 lunar Months & 4 Days: Most part of ye Time Brisk & Lively; at last died Convulsd.

2 Vol. P. 136.

T. Slater Sculp

1. The Fissure in situ
2. Plagues Triparid
3. The Bone taken out and placed continuously
   d. e. f. g. A Spicula view of ye 3 humi Bones
   h. The ye 2nd Piece
4. Os Frontis
5. Os Bregma
6. Os Occipitis
7. Os Temporale
8. Proces Mastoides
9. Os Jugale
10. Os Maxil. Sup.
11. Orb. Sup. Oculi
12. Orbita inferior
13. Os Nasi
14. Maxilla seu 4 hum.
15. Maxilla superior cum dentibus
A. Sutura Coronalis
B. Sut. Squamosa
C. Sut. Lambdoidea
X. Meatus auditorius

Figure 4 Detailed view of the fractured skull and trepanning site of the boy treated by Daniel Turner in 1709. (D. Turner, *Art of Surgery* 1732; reproduced by permission of the Wellcome Institute Library, London.)

elucidated the types of information these accounts conveyed.[46] In the early eighteenth century, bladder stones were treated by either extirpation or dissolution. In the following section of this paper, I shall first discuss how several London lithotomists (i.e. 'cutters' for the stone) advertised their surgical techniques. I will then differentiate the treatments conveyed in these accounts from the 'easements' for the stone proferred in contemporary domestic manuals and in the writings of physicians and natural philosophers. Particular attention will be drawn to how these authors tried to make special remedies known, discounting the advice of their adversaries.

John Bamber, William Cheselden, John Douglas, Joannes Groenevelt (also known as John or James Greenfield), Benjamin Marten and Josiah Paul were premier lithotomists in early eighteenth-century London. Three were surgeons, three were physicians. Of these, Groenevelt, Douglas, and Cheselden published accounts, in part, as self-advertisement of a particular procedure.

Groenevelt, a licentiate of the College of Physicians, exemplified that cutting for the stone was not 'below' the practice of a physician. Indeed, he claimed to have personally saved more than 'Two Hundred Fourscore' stone sufferers by lithotomy. He attributed his successful operation to the technique described by Francois Tolet: removing stones by cutting into the bladder wall from an incision made above the pubic bone in the lower abdominal region (the 'high operation'). Although he translated much of Tolet's writings into his own English treatise in 1710, he withheld particular aspects of the operation from the 'Eyes of the Vulgar'.[47] Such omission of detail probably contributed to his name and reputation being overshadowed by his contemporary, John Douglas.

In 1720, London surgeon John Douglas described a lithotomy method which, he claimed, would 'prevent' impotency, incontinency, and fistulae; all common 'dismal Consequences' of his competitors' lithotomy operations. Additionally, Douglas stressed that his procedure allowed lithotomists the great advantage of making their incision as large as necessary without cutting any of the 'great vessels'. Although this 'high operation' appears remarkably similar to Groenevelt's, Douglas explicitly instructed his readers in the positioning of their patients and in the use of particular instruments. Acknowledging Groenevelt only in passing reference, he proclaimed this operation as the 'Lithotomia Douglassiana'.[48]

Three years later, Douglas recounted the further successes he had achieved at the Westminster Infirmary together with those of John Bamber, surgeon at St Bartholomew's, and William Cheselden, surgeon at St Thomas's – two lithotomists who had adopted his procedure.[49] Soon, after noting a diminishing success rate from Douglas's method, Cheselden claimed that more benefit could be achieved by making his surgical incision in the lateral perineal region. Like Douglas, Cheselden fully described the method of his procedure.[50]

Cheselden's method soon became a local standard hospital practice, replacing that of Douglas.[51] He took advantage of his position at St Thomas's, advertising the success of his technique through many lectures and operations, both of which drew large crowds. A number of foreign lithotomists flocked to his operations, offering 'great Applause' and publicizing his technique in their home countries, both by word of mouth and in their writings.[52] In addition to advertising his personal success, reports of Cheselden's operation also promoted beliefs that the hospital offered both a favourable operating environment and a fruitful training centre for junior surgeons. By advertising his competence in a particular surgical technique, Cheselden also helped to secure this operation as a specialty of surgical practice.[53]

Lithotomists faced severe condemnation from those who favoured non-surgical methods of relieving stone sufferers. Daniel Turner, for example, characterized most London lithotomists as the 'vulgar' type of quacks who cut for the stone without being 'bred up in the Practice of surgery'.[54] The lithotomists' advertisements, he argued, were like the mountebanks' boasts of panaceas. In return, lithotomists like Douglas justified the necessity of his operative approach by claiming that no effective stone solvent had yet been found.[55] Groenevelt also warned readers against using the commonly peddled 'approved' solvents which were likely to 'wake [a] sleeping lion' by jarring quiescent kidney stones into the bladder where they would create much havoc.[56]

Despite Groenevelt, Douglas, and Cheselden self-promoting their competence as lithotomists, the public appears not to have shared their enthusiasm for the knife.[57] The numerous advertisements and public testimonials supporting non-surgical remedies, compared with the relatively few patients who could boast of having been successfully treated by lithotomists, suggests that the former methods had, indeed, gained much more popularity.

Nearly all domestic manuals recommended some type of medicine to 'ease' the 'racky pain' of the stone. Physician William Salmon offered a selection of twelve oral medicines to cure such patients in his *Family-Dictionary*. He claimed that these remedies could be compounded from ingredients which were few in number, cheap, common, easily compounded, effectual, safe, durable, and small in dose.[58] Bailey's *Dictionary Domesticum* offered sixteen remedies for the stone; *The Family Magazine*, twenty-six; while *The Accomplish'd Housewife* specified only three remedies. However, two of the three remedies, a beech-oil compound and Daffy's elixir, were the two most widely publicized lithontriptics (i.e. stone-breaking compounds) in London.[59]

The beech-oil compound comprised powdered and dried marshmallow leaves, the 'Herb' mercury, saxifrage, and a common pellitory. After adding beechnut oil, it was served as a tea. Eliza Smith promoted this remedy in her *Compleat Housewife*, adding the authoritative support of a local 'modern college physician'. The physician, she claimed, described a gentleman, who, drinking beer from a cup carved from a large bladder stone, had not realized the above remedy had been boiled in his refection. The cup quickly 'fell to pieces' in his hands. Such sudden 'dissolution', so the physician claimed, was attributed to the added beechnut oil. After using this story to illustrate the efficacy of her remedy, Mrs Smith informed her readers that the 'Right sort' of 'True Nut-oil' was obtainable from Mrs Goddard, at the Golden-Ball in Burleigh Street, for 1s 6d per phial. It is of little surprise that Mrs Smith's *Compleat Housewife* was also available from the same shop.[60]

Repeatedly finding the same recipes for remedies in various sources suggests they were among the more popular forms of treating the stone. Many domestic manuals, typically those with large sections on cookery, suggested that stones and gravel were preventable by diets concentrated with carrots, onions, cherry pits, and hops.[61] Numerous long-running advertisements also promoted compounds made from lime, lemon juice, sweet broom, and crushed oyster and snail shells. In combination with remedial medicine, one popular manual also claimed that stone dissolution was enhanced by 'walk[ing] up and down hastily, or rowl[ing] yourself on a Bed'.[62]

Like the lay authors of domestic manuals, most physicians and natural philosophers also promoted non-surgical cures for the stone. George Cheyne proclaimed that only 'Divine, Innocent, Indolent and Joyous Temperance' in habit and diet could prevent this malady. Although not all accounts were so morally based, many London physicians advocated particular diets to prevent and/or cure the stone.[63] For example, physician Theophilus Lobb performed 200 *in vitro* experiments to test which components of diet or 'Ailments' best dissolved, softened, or broke human calculi.[64] Based upon these experimental findings, he recommended a number of safe, natural, easily obtainable lithontriptics. Although he detailed his experiments more extensively than most of his colleagues, Lobb's expressed belief that natural substances prevented natural causes of disease was shared by many.

This experimental approach of the late 1730s represented a change in, or at least an extension of, many physicians' studies of bladder stones earlier in the century. A connection between this change and the advertisement of a particular 'cure' warrants our investigation.

Early in the 1700s, many physicians compared the formation of human stones to natural petrifaction (stone formation).[65] Indeed, their writings on human stones fill more pages of the *Philosophical Transactions* during this period than any other single surgico-medical subject.[66] Numerous separate treatises discussed the consistency of human stones and their similarity to stones or gravel of the earth or those found in animals. Nicholas Robinson provided perhaps the most extensive natural philosophical account of human stones in his *Treatise on the Gravel and Stone* (1721). Of this work, 222 pages were devoted to the nature of solids, the natural history of stone generation and the nature of urine before briefly addressing a few methods of curing bladder stones. By mid-century, however, writings on the dissolution of stones had replaced much of that on petrification.[67]

An outbreak of interest in stone dissolution occurred between 1738 and 1740. This interest was prompted by advertisements for Mrs Joanna Stephens's cure for the stone. At this time, Stephens had proposed to 'make her [secret] medicine' known to the 'publick' for the benefit of all who suffered from this 'wrath'. In exchange for this benevolence towards her compatriots, Stephens demanded £5000 from Parliament. A Parliamentary committee was set up to monitor the preparation and administration of her remedy to treat four selected sufferers of the stone over the following year. Many fragments of calculi were identified in the patients' urine throughout the treatment. At the end of the year, March 1739/ 1740, the patients claimed that their symptoms had been completely alleviated, and no stones were detected. Mrs Stephens soon received her full 'Reward' from the Office of the Exchequer, and was never heard from again. Her remedy, however, remained highly sought-after by the public.[68]

Controversy over Mrs Stephens's 'Cure for the Stone' provoked much comparative and competitive experimentation among physicians and natural philosophers. Experiments were performed in private homes, before learned societies, on patients, and, in the case of physician James Jurin, on himself.[69] Some investigators, like David Hartley, claimed their evidence supported Stephens's claims, while others, like James Parsons, claimed that their findings invalidated her claims.[70] This intensive experimentation not only produced many new remedies, but it also demonstrated the desire which experimenters shared with the public for finding effective alternatives to surgery.

Unlike attending skull fractures, treating bladder stones was not publicly perceived as strictly a surgical matter. Many physicians shared this public view, and endorsed the same compounds as those found in domestic manuals. The acceptance of Mrs Stephens's competence in providing a remedy, particularly its approval by Parliament, supports Shapin's argument that the public's perception of appropriate treatment was not necessarily 'discontinuous' with that of the professionals. Indeed, in this example, many physicians shared the public belief in the efficacy of Mrs Stephens's cure.

Self-advertisement had played a major role in making some types of treatment more popular than others. Physicians' writings, patients' testimonials, and quacks' handbills helped to endorse particular remedies for potential 'customers'. But the prolific self-advertisement still left sufferers of the stone a considerable range of choice in therapy. As one physician claimed, all the books are 'so full of Remedies . . . that it is hard for those who are not skillful to know which to chuse'.[71] As a 'consumer', the patient was likely to know of many general advertisements and may personally have known of particular products' success or failure in relieving the discomfort, but physicians did not generally believe that the public was fully capable of judging the efficacy of one medicine over another. Domestic manuals typically touted all their remedies as 'effective' or 'approved', but rarely elaborated upon measures of efficacy. Only one exception, Bailey's *Dictionary Domesticum*, suggested how patients could judge objectively whether a particular concoction was correctly prepared to dissolve the stone.[72] It was noted in an early 'History of Popular Medicine' that many physicians viewed the 'mere publication of receipts' as an 'incompetent' method of treating disease.[73] Daniel Turner had labelled this method of 'set[ting] forth advertisements' without 'knowledge of the Patient, or Enquiry into this Condition' as quackery.[74]

Medical writings of the 1730s, however, began to compare the efficacy of several claimed 'dissolvents' based on experimental results. Such comparison led physicians, more than authors of domestic manuals, to differentiate remedies according to both the constitutions of the stone and the patient. These writings soon led physicians to advertise their exclusive competence in selecting the proper cure to match a particular patient's overall constitution.[75]

The distinction between the public's and the physician's apparent views of competence suggests several related conclusions. At the basis of selecting a treatment for bladder stones, the decision was either to cut or to dissolve. Few patients attempted to cut themselves for the stone, and although lithotomists had gained competence in this skill, patients rarely opted for surgery. Instead, the public, in part through the know-how provided in domestic manuals, came to view themselves as capable of self-treatment of this disorder with various homemade compounds. Given the reaction from physicians, a large section of the public must indeed have been administering remedies to themselves. Although physicians claimed to be the ultimate guides in selecting proper therapies, a variety of widely advertised remedies persisted in the public literature. Thus, the ultimate choice between treatments appears to have remained in the hands of the populace. The extensiveness of popular medicine later in the century is evident by the legacies of Buchan and Tissot as discussed in other chapters of this book.

'Popularization' of surgery?

In an earlier draft of this paper, I attempted to explain how some surgical treatments, particularly topically applied remedies, became popularized in the early eighteenth century. Specifically, I sought to establish the extent to which Richard Whitley's model of popularization was useful for explaining the apparent demarcations between orthodox and lay forms of surgical practice. Whitley has challenged and expanded the more traditional conceptions of popularization as a diffusion or dissemination of a simplified form of knowledge from the learned (high culture) to the uneducated (low culture).[76] Although Whitley's challenge has, with some success, been used to explain the popularization of scientific knowledge in fields such as geology, relativity theory, and molecular genetics,[77] I found it quite historiographically problematic for earlier periods.

According to Whitley, knowing the reading audience is essential for explaining the 'popularization process'. Thus, our insufficient understanding of who the literate public was in periods before the nineteenth century presents a major drawback. To take an example: domestic manual authors provided instructions to a lay audience. The use of language in surgical texts suggests that they were written to an audience which was already skilled in this practice. Such depiction, however, represents only the extremes of readership. Without considering the potential breadth of the 'reading public' and identifying more precisely who read whom, an account of what knowledge actually became 'popularized' can become drastically skewed. Additionally, the proportion of lay practitioners who actively acquired their skills through an oral tradition or 'learning by doing' must not be neglected.

Popularization studies thus far have focused primarily on scientific knowledge. It remains to be determined, however, just how scientific knowledge is fundamentally distinguishable from popularized, public, common, medical, surgical, or other 'types' of knowledge. As recent criticism of popularization studies has argued, 'popularized' knowledge is only distinguishable from the whole bed of knowledge by a 'matter of degree'.[78] It could be proposed, for example, that both Douglas's and Cheselden's accounts represented attempts to popularize their knowledge of particular lithotomy techniques. The techniques did become more well-known, but whether this was popularized knowledge rather than basic, practical, or surgical knowledge is unclear. For these earlier periods, it appears to be more sound to measure the acquisition of skills than to estimate shifts from 'scientific' to 'popular' knowledge. Determining the practical know-how of a particular trade should also enhance our ability to bridge the gap between medical practice and theory as well as between technology and science.[79]

Whitley has also claimed that the form and function of popularization appear to be historically specific. The use of a popularization model should, therefore, represent specific sociohistorical contexts as well. For example, to argue that Daniel Turner popularized the use of trepanning in a 1709 treatise, when his apparent motive can be more accurately represented as instructional, would appear to be introducing an anachronism. On the other hand, Mrs Stephens's medicine appears to have become quite popular. Indeed, it represented the popular hope of avoiding surgery. Yet it became popular through a diverse number of methods more easily identifiable than popularization. The reification of popularization is, in fact, hiding a variety of processes. Newspapers advertised the product, Parliament financed the disclosure of secret ingredients, and experimentalists reported on its reputed efficacy. These factors appear to have been linked together more through contemporary advertising and self-promotion than through what we might presently identify as popularization. Labelling processes as popularization, it has been argued, more typically reflects some historians' 'flexibility' in using this term rather than conforming to specific sociohistorical contexts.[80]

Describing the spread of a technique in terms of advertising also prevents the somewhat tautological trap of determining whether popularization is more of an intention or a consequence. Although it is possible to document what know-how is being propagated to the public, the effect of its reception – even the reception of such know-how itself – remains most difficult to ascertain. Discussing popularization without being able to document the specific reception and 'feedback' of so-called 'popularized knowledge' entraps our use of the term as merely a form of dissemination; a Whiggish snare that Steven Shapin, among others, is trying to overcome.[81] At this time, the historiographic value in analysing a popularization process appears to be much more useful in specific cases than using 'popularization' as a blanket term to hide our ignorance.

Acquiring surgical know-how

Acknowledgements

I gratefully appreciate the constructive commentary and suggestions that Sandra Cavallo, Christopher Lawrence, Paola Govoni, Roy Porter, Andrew Wear, and Janice Wilson offered on an earlier version of this paper presented at the Wellcome Institute Symposium on the History of the Popularization of Medicine. Research for this work was supported by a Wellcome Trust Studentship.

Notes

1. S. Shapin, 'Science and the Public', in R.C. Olby *et al* (eds), *Companion to the History of Modern Science* (London, 1990), esp. 993–4.
2. ibid., 994. Shapin cited C.G. Helman's '"Feed a Cold, Starve a Fever" – Folk Models of Infection in an English Suburban Community, and Their Relation to Medical Treatment', *Culture, Medicine, and Psychiatry* 2(1978), 107–37.
3. In addition to N. Jewson's stimulating and provocative 'Medical Knowledge and the Patronage System in Eighteenth-century England', *Sociology* 8(1974), 169–85, much groundwork regarding patients' interaction with physicians was laid in the essays in R. Porter (ed.) *Patients and Practitioners: Lay Perceptions of Medicine in Pre-industrial Society* (Cambridge, 1985).
4. Factions divided over medical theories can be found in many of the disputes over the causes of fevers, smallpox, gout, and other maladies. Adrian Wilson has recently analysed political factions within the discourse over smallpox inoculation: A. Wilson, 'The Politics of Medical Improvement in Early Hanoverian London', in A. Cunningham and R. French (eds), *The Medical Enlightenment of the Eighteenth Century* (Cambridge, 1990), esp. 24–34.
5. Castigating mechanical-based medical theorization in favour of personal observation, eighteenth-century London surgeon and physician Daniel Turner argued it is 'One thing to talk of Cures, which may be enterpris'd by the *Ratios of Quantities, increased Momentums, by calculating the Diameters of . . . Vessels, comparing the given Force at the Heart, with the reciprocal Resistance at the Sides of those Vessels, and their Angles of Incidence; computing also the exact Degrees of Viscidity in the Fluids . . . therein circulating.* And it is a quite different thing to perform the Cure, from a constant and sedulous Observation of the same Disease'. He continued, expressing an attitude shared with many of his colleagues, that medical theorists provided no 'real Benefit or Advantage, in the Recovery of the Sick or diseased patient' in his *Syphilis* (London, 4th edn, 1732), preface.
6. This classification is found in James Cooke's *Mellificum Chirurgiae. Or, the Marrow of Chirurgery* (5th edn, 1693), Alexander Read's *Chirurgorum Comes: or the Whole Practice of Chirurgery* (1687), Richard Wiseman's *Eight Chirurgical Treatises* (4th edn, 1705), Daniel

Turner's *The Art of Surgery* (1722) and Edward Dunn's *A Compendious and New Method of Performing Chirurgical Operations* (1724).

7. Cooke and Turner (n.6) discussed the role of surgeons treating external disease, as did Richard Boulton in this quoted passage from *A System of Rational and Practical Chirurgery* (1713), 1–2. Contemporary French surgeon Pierre Dionis provided perhaps the most eloquent description of his occupation as 'a Habit of the Understanding, form'd by Study, and Reflection on Experience, by which we know the Diseases of Human Bodies; and at the same time a Dexterity acquir'd by frequent and well order'd use, in applying with the Hands, by the help of Instruments, Remedies to those Places where they are wanting' (as translated in the 1710 *Course of Chirurgical Operations*, 2).

8. Margaret Pelling's 'Medical Practice in Early Modern England: Trade or Profession?' in W. Prest (ed.), *The Professions in Early Modern England* (London, 1987), 90–128, has focused on physicians, having previously analysed the diversified practice of barber-surgeons in 'Occupational Diversity: Barber-Surgeons and the Trades of Norwich, 1550–1640', *Bulletin of the History of Medicine* 56(1982), 484–511. Harold Cook examined a significant territorial dispute between the apothecaries and physicians in 'The Rose Case Reconsidered: Physicians, Apothecaries, and the Law in Augustan England', *Journal of the History of Medicine and Allied Sciences* 45(1990), 527–55; and Roy Porter has re-evaluated the meaning and practice of quackery in *Health For Sale: Quackery in England 1660–1850* (Manchester, 1989).

9. M. Pelling, 'Appearances and Reality: Barber-surgeons, the Body and Disease' in A. Beier and R. Finlay (eds), *London 1500–1700: The Making of the Metropolis* (London, 1986), 82–112. Presently, I am investigating the demarcations between surgery and physic in early eighteenth-century London, specifically focusing upon Daniel Turner's diversified careers in both fields.

10. Surgical authors Cooke, Turner and Boulton practised medicine as well as surgery. In addition to aforementioned texts, other available surgical texts of English authors included Hugh Ryder, *New Practical Observations in Surgery* (2nd edn, 1693); John Moyle, *Chirurgus Marinus: or The Sea-Chirurgion* (1693); *idem, The Experienced Chirurgion* (1703); James Handley, *Colloquia Chyrurgica: or, The Whole Art of Surgery Epitomiz'd* (1705); John Atkins, *The Navy Surgeon* (1738); Samuel Sharp, *A Treatise on the Operations of Surgery* (1739); and William Beckett, *Practical Surgery Illustrated and Improved* (1740). Surgical writings were also offered by physicians William Salmon, *Ars Chirurgica* (1698) among others; and John Colbatch, *Four Treatises of Physic & Chirurgery* (2nd edn, 1698).

11. Turner further denominated definitions, causes, prognoses and treatments of specific diseases under each heading.

12. See, for example, Ryder's *New Practical Observations*, Moyle's *Chirurgus Marinus*, Handley's *Colloquia Chirurgica*, and Atkins's *The Navy Surgeon*.

13. E. Dunn, *Compendious Method*, 'To the Young Surgeons'.

14. Part of the popularity of domestic manuals may have been due to the cosmetic instructions they offered at a time when, it has been

claimed, beauty was becoming a commodity in London. Virginia Smith initiated studies of eighteenth-century concerns of beauty in her 'Cleanliness: the Development of Idea and Practice in Britain, 1770– 1850' (unpublished PhD thesis, University of London, 1985).

15. Such conditions were described in the numerous reprintings of Aristotle's *Family Physician*. Janet Blackman discussed the popularity of the pseudonymous Aristotle in 'Popular Theories of Generation: The Evolution of Aristotle's Works, the Study of an Anachronism', in J. Woodward and D. Richards (eds), *Health Care and Popular Medicine in Nineteenth Century England* (New York, 1977), 56–88.

16. Anonymous manuals included *Accomplish'd Female Instructor* (1704); *Family Companion for Health* (1729); *Young Lady's Companion* (1734); *Complete Family Piece* (1736); *Ladies Dispensatory: or Every Woman Her Own Physician* (1739); and *Accomplish'd Housewife; or the Gentlewoman's Companion* (1745). Three 'housewives' completed works: *Accomplish'd Ladies Delight* by Hannah Wooley (1696), Mary Kettilby, *A Collection of Above Three Hundred Receipts in Cookery, Physick and Surgery* (1714), and *Compleat Housewife: or Accomplish'd Gentlewoman's Companion* by Eliza Smith (9th edn, 1739). The Countess of Kent, Elizabeth Grey, collected *A Choice Manual of Rare and Select Secrets in Physick and Surgery* (21st edn, 1708). Charles Carter, a cook, wrote *Compleat City and Country Cook* (1732). Nathaniel Bailey, the compiler of *Dictionary Domesticum* (1736), was a lexicographer. See also John Shirley, *The Accomplished Ladies Rich Closet of Rarities* (3rd edn, 1691). Pseudonymous authors included Aristotle's *Family Physician* (1723), and Arabella Atkyns, *Family Magazine* (1741). R. Bradley's *Country Housewife and Lady's Direction* (6th edn, 1732) contained no medico-surgical content, and *Adam's Luxury and Eve's Cookery* (1744) devoted only five pages to the 'Physical Virtues of all Sorts of Garden-Roots and Herbs'. Despite similarity in the title of Thomas Fuller's *Pharmacopoeia Domestica; or, The Family Dispensatory* (1739) with the above works, the content was not of similar domestic basis, and this work was intended 'for the Use of Physicians in the Country'. Doreen Nagy discussed the contents of some of these works in *Popular Medicine in Seventeenth-century England* (Bowling Green, 1988), esp. 55, 63, 68–71.

17. *Compleat Housewife*, preface; *Complete Family Piece*, v; *Family Companion*, 'To the Reader'; and *Ladies Dispensatory*, v.

18. I have recently re-examined Sidney Young's estimation, not challenged or confirmed for over a century, that between 1670 and 1745 there were, on average, 75 freemen in London's Barber-Surgeons' Company. See S. Young, *Annals of the Barber-Surgeons* (London, 1890), 259.

19. Given the large number of popular riotous uprisings, numerous accidents derived from both daytime trade and night-time preoccupations, the many injured men returning from war, and the squalor of the increasingly crowded living conditions in London's growing conurbation, surgical disorders and diseases probably abounded in great variety. See, for example, J. Stevenson, *Popular Disturbances in England 1700–1870* (London, 1979), esp. 53–90. Summaries of London's social conditions by Geoffrey Holmes, Roy Porter,

and Lawrence Stone are known to many. A social history of sea surgeons, however, is awaiting an author.

20. London's expanding wealth among the middling set is brilliantly discussed in Peter Earle's *The Making of the English Middle Class: Business, Society, and Family Life in London 1660–1731* (London, 1989).

21. Although William Buchan's motto, allowing everyone to 'be their own physician and surgeon', is directly taken from later in the century, its implications were present in domestic manuals long before.

22. Atkyns, *Family Magazine*, 238. Eliza Smith vouched that her *Compleat Housewife* contained many 'family-receipts' which 'cured when all other means have failed'. See preface.

23. Turner, *The Modern Quack; or, the Physical Imposter, Detected* (London, 1718), 157; and Turner, *Discourse Concerning Fevers* (London, 1727), 14.

24. Turner, *Fevers*, 14.

25. *Present State of Physick & Surgery in London* (London, 1701), 14.

26. Daniel Turner claimed that it was 'very rare' for surgeons to treat anyone who had not been 'spoyl'd' by the workmanship of others, particularly the meddlesome neighbourhood women practitioners. See his *Apologia Chyurgica. A Vindication of the Noble Art of Surgery* (London, 1695), 107–8.

27. Atkyns, *Family Magazine*, 267.

28. *Ladies Dispensatory*, 157.

29. ibid., 301.

30. A. Atkyns, *Family Magazine*, 70, 65. Of all the domestic manuals, the surgical prescriptions and restrictions discussed in this pseudonymous work have been the most difficult to characterize. At times, the author, after claiming a condition as 'belonging properly to the surgeons', offers no instructions whereas, at other times, the surgeon's duties are explicitly revealed, as seen in the treatment of a wounded artery, discussed above. My speculation is that disorders which were perceived as needing more emergency care were described in domestic manuals, whereas less life-threatening conditions were not detailed.

31. It is most difficult to determine the incidence and prevalence of many surgical disorders, including skull fractures. Few case studies, if they were recorded, have survived, and such disorders are rarely distinguishable from mortality lists. J. Cagua, *Phil. Trans.* v.42 (1739), 495, and H. Ryder, *New Observations*, 19, 76.

32. Cases taken from W. Wood, 'Practical Chirurgery', Royal College of Surgeons (England), MS Tract A297 (3), case 29; W. Beckett, *Practical Surgery*, 124; Turner, *Art of Surgery*, v.2, 204, 218. Surgeon Richard Wiseman reported, in a slightly earlier period, eighteen head wounds, many of which were derived from war. His contemporary, London surgeon Joseph Binns, claimed that most of the thirteen skull fractures he treated resulted from civil violence, often 'crimes of passion'. As cited by L. Beier, *Sufferers and Healers: The Experiences of Illness in Seventeenth-century England* (London, 1987), 65, 73. Perhaps Prince Rupert, the nephew of Charles I, was the most

renowned skull fracture patient of the period. The most recent, though not completely accurate, account of his treatment is by G. Martin, 'Prince Rupert and the Surgeons', *History Today* 40 (1990), 38–43.

33. Although numerous works address particular palaeo-pathological evidence of trepanning, the persistence of this treatment and its modification in trepanation have not received recent socio-historical analysis.

34. Turner, *Art of Surgery*, v.2, 205–6.

35. ibid., 209.

36. D. Turner, 'A remarkable case in Surgery. Wherein an account is given of an uncommon Fracture and Depression of the *Skull*, in a child about Six years old; accompanied with a large *Abscess* or *Aposteme* upon the *Brain*' (London, 1709). Turner later added an abridged form of this work to his *Art of Surgery*. As the original pamphlet is quite scarce, I have cited pages from its later printings.

37. Turner's patient was wounded on Shrove Tuesday, 24 February 1708/09.

38. The only other illustrations Turner included in any of his works, other than his engraved portrait, were a copy of anatomist William Cowper's diagram of his ligation of a Gastrocnemius muscle tendon (*Art of Surgery*, v.1, 505) and an engraving of an 'eighteen-tailed bandage' used in treating compound fractures (*Art of Surgery*, v.2, 151).

39. Turner, *Art of Surgery*, v.2, 219.

40. Turner's 'Remarkable case' prompted St Thomas Hospital surgeon William Beckett's critical reply with 'Chirurgical Remarks, Occasioned by the Death of a CHILD, whose Case was printed in that Year by Daniel Turner, surgeon', (London, 1709). Beckett's argument, however, was not over Turner's method of trepanning. Rather, he disagreed with Turner's account of the 'true cause' of death, and identified the particular course of therapy which, he claimed, had 'obstructed' Turner's 'methodical . . . Procedure' from achieving 'a Cure'. Beckett's mechanist theorization, however pertinent to his argument, and Turner's probable reception of it are beyond the scope of this paper.

41. Some were trained by various lengths of apprenticeship, whereas others gained their surgical experience as ship's surgeons or hospital 'cubbs'.

42. R. Blackmore, *Dissertation on a Dropsy, a Tympany, the Jaundice, the Stone, and a Diabetes* (London, 1727), 155.

43. Hans Sloane, in a letter to Marquis de Caumont, stated that he had 'some Hundreds' in his 'Collection of such kind of Curiosities'. See *Phil. Trans.* 40(1734–38), 374, 376. Fishmonger Samuel Leek of Swinthin Alley had his stone cut, and a 1710 treatise remarked that the stone 'may now be seen at Mr. Kelton's, a Barber, against the Salutation-Tavern, in Exchange-Alley'. J. Groenevelt, *A Complete Treatise of the Stone and Gravel* (London, 1710), 55–6. This was much expanded from his *Treatise on the Stone and Gravel* (London, 1677). Similarly, Mrs Wheatley, a glassier's wife, Smithfield Bar, without, 'carefully preserve[d]' a large stone she had passed for those who, like

HRH Mary II, expressed a desire to see it. J. Colbatch, *Physico-Medical Essay Concerning Alkaly and Acids* (London, 1698), 99–100. Hans Sloane and other natural curiosity collectors reportedly received a number of rarities of bladder stones as well. Perhaps the most noted English collection, containing many examples from the eighteenth century and earlier, ended up much later in the Museum of the Royal College of Surgeons (England). Unfortunately, much of this collection was destroyed in the 1940s.

44. N. Robinson, *Treatise on the Gravel and Stone* (London, 1721), 132. Unfortunately, no 'ostensible records' of the lithotomies performed in London hospitals during the eighteenth century were preserved. Alexander Marcet first noted this lack of records in 1817, but he uncovered the records of 506 lithotomies performed in Norwich between 1772 and 1816. See O.H. Wangensteen and S.D. Wangensteen, *The Rise of Surgery* (Folkestone, Kent, 1978), 600, n.2.

45. Robinson, *Treatise on Gravel*, 173.

46. Among the most thorough accounts are H. Shelley's 'Cutting for the Stone', *Journal of the History of Medicine* 13 (1958) 50–67; *idem*, 'Intravesical Destruction of Bladder Stone', *Journal of the History of Medicine* 19(1964) 46–60; A. Viseltear, 'Attempts to Dissolve Bladder Stones by Direct Injection', *Bulletin of the History of Medicine* 43(1969) 477–81; O.H. Wangensteen, S.D. Wangensteen, and J. Witta, 'Lithotomy and Lithotomists: Progress in Wound Management from Franco to Lister', *Surgery* 66 (1969), 929–52.

47. J. Groenevelt, *Treatise on Stone*, x–xi, 278–9. Tolet's work had already been introduced to English readers by A. Lovell in his translation of Tolet's *Treatise of Lithotomy* (London, 1683). Groenevelt claims to have worked closely with Benjamin Marten, with whom he also 'shared all the fruits of his own years'. Harold J. Cook has recently discussed Groenevelt's controversial reputation in 'Medical Innovation or Medical Malpractice? or, A Dutch Physician in London: Joannes Groenevelt, 1694–1700', *Tractrix* 2(1990) 63–91.

48. J. Douglas, 'Lithotomia Douglassiana; or, An Account of a New Method of Making the High Operation . . . to Extract the Stone', (London, 1720), 21–2, title page.

49. In a revised version of 'Lithotomia Douglassiana' (London, 1723), 62, Douglas claims that his three successful patients were 'shewed before the Royal Society, soon after their Recovery'. (60) Paul had cut two patients, and Cheselden, eight, before August 1722.

50. W. Cheselden, *A Treatise on the High Operation for the Stone* (London, 1723). He further discussed his change of methods in 'A Short Historical Account of Cutting for the Stone', appended to his *The Anatomy of the Humane Body* (London, 4th edn, 1730).

51. Standard in England, for Cheselden acknowledged that his method was adopted from the standard method of Leiden anatomist, Johann Rau.

52. James Douglas, John's brother, discussed Cheselden's popularity as a lecturer and lithotomist in his *Appendix to the History of the Lateral Operation for the Stone* (London, 1731), 2. By the aid of

attendants at Cheselden's performance, his procedures became disseminated in French, Dutch, and German.

53. By expressing his operative success in numerical rates of patients saved per patients cut, an uncommon format for describing positive results in contemporary writings, Cheselden emphasized the extent to which he had mastered the skill of performing a special operation. Cheselden listed 46 patients by name, age, date of operation, and the outcome in his 'Short historical account', 344–6. J. Douglas, *Appendix to History of Lateral Operation*, 2, claimed Cheselden had 'saved 50 Patients out of 52, whom he had cut'. And Cheselden later tallied only 20 deaths of 213 patients he had cut in his *Anatomy of the Human Body* (5th edn, 1740), 333. Wangensteen *et al.* compared Cheselden's 'statistics' with those of earlier and later lithotomists in 'Lithotomy and Lithotomists', 936–7, 947.

54. D. Turner, *De Morbis Cutaneis*, 351.

55. Douglas, *Lithotomia Douglassiana*, 1723, 9–10.

56. Groenevelt, *Treatise on Stone*, 277.

57. Although there were isolated reports of the lay public surgically removing their own stones, such 'advice' is not found in any of the literature. See J.J. Murphy, 'Self-performed Operations', *British Journal of Urology* 41 (1969), 515–29.

58. W. Salmon, *Family-Dictionary* (London, 1696), preface.

59. *Accomplish'd Housewife*, 316–17. One or both of these compounds was also promoted in Smith, *Complete Housewife*, 251–2, 264–5; *Complete Family-Piece*, 12; Atkyns, *Family Magazine*, 221; Bailey, *Dictionarium Domesticum*, under 'STONE'; and the *Compleat City Cook*, 261–2. Groenevelt also claimed these remedies were 'much talk'd of in Town', *Treatise on Stone* (1710), 231–2.

60. Smith, *Compleat Housewife*, 265–6.

61. According to several accounts, like the one in *Family Companion for Health*, 150, much controversy arose over whether hops caused or cured the stone.

62. *Accomplish'd Female Instructor*, 146.

63. G. Cheyne, *An Essay on the Gout* (London 1720), 97, as cited by Robinson, *Treatise on Gravel*, 140.

64. T. Lobb, *Treatise on Dissolvents of the Stone, and Curing the Stone and Gout by Ailment* (London, 1739).

65. Apart from the bladder, stones were reportedly found, usually during post-mortems, in the muscles, lungs, stomach, liver, gall bladder, bowels, tongue, brain, heart, and in the blood itself. See Blackmore, *Dissertation on Dropsy*, 157.

66. My tallies indicate that 27 cases of bladder stones totalling 338 stones and much gravel were reported.

67. Among the experimental accounts were H. Bracken, *Lithiasis Anglicana, or a Philosophical Enquiry into the Nature and Origin of the Stone* (London, 1739); S. Hales, 'An account of some experiments and observations on Mrs. Stephens's medicines for dissolving the stone', (London, 1740). Among Hartley's 'Ten cases of persons who have taken Mrs. Stephens's medicines for the stone', (London, 1738).

James Jurin, who later gained renown for his 'Lixivium Lithnotripticum', first wrote on the stone in an 'Account of the effects of soap-lye taken internally, for the stone', (London 1742). Brown Langrish described the effects of lime water as a 'method for dissolving the stone' in his *Physical Experiments Upon Brutes* (London 1746) as did R. Whytt in his 1752 *Essay on the Virtues of Lime-water in the Cure of the Stone*. J. Parsons contributed a *Description of the Human Urinary Bladder, with Animadversions on Lithotriptic Medicines* in 1742 with anatomical significance similar to W. Rutty's *Treatise on Urinary Passages* (London, 1726). John Greene Crosse listed publications on the stone as Appendix III of his *Treatise of the Formation, Constituents, and Extraction of the Urinary Calculus* (London, 1833), 166–211. I have encountered but few earlier publications which were not included in this remarkable compilation.

68. A. Viseltear recounted much of this case in 'Joanna Stephens and the Eighteenth Century Lithontriptics; A Misplaced Chapter in the History of Therapeutics', *Bulletin of the History of Medicine* 42(1968), 199–220. Mrs Stephens's medicine was frequently discussed in the newspapers, in separate medical pamphlets, and domestic manuals such as Atkyns, *Family Magazine*, 218–19.

69. Jurin, 'Abstract of the case of James Jurin . . . as far as it relates to the taking of his lixivium for stone and gravel', (London, 1752), and Lobb, *Dissolvents of the Stone*, 255.

70. One physician, S. Morand, advertised Stephens's claims internationally when he took his experiments before France's Académie Royale des Sciences. David Harley is currently re-examining the disputes over this controversial therapy.

71. Groenevelt, *Treatise on Stone*, 235–6.

72. 'You may know whether this water [distillate] be well prepar'd or not, by putting a piece of mutton and a small stone into it; for if the water be right, the stone will dissolve . . . but the flesh will remain of a vermilion hue, without receiving any injury', Bailey, *Dictionarium Domesticum*, under 'STONE'.

73. R. Reece, 'History of Popular Medicine' in *A Practical Dictionary of Domestic Medicine* (London, 1808), 15.

74. Turner, *Modern Quack*, 152. Typical of such treatments was Kettilby's recipe for a particular 'Oyl' to treat 'any Bruise or Wound' and an ointment that was claimed as 'good for any Ach [*sic*]or Swelling in Man or Beast', *Collection of Three Hundred Receipts*, 98, 116–17.

75. Dr William Rutty claimed that the cure of the stone regarded 'the *Physician*, . . . only whilst the *Calculus* is small enough to be forc'd through the *Urethra* by [a] medicinal Process, . . . and if it is grown to any considerable size, it is the *Surgeon's* Province, and requires the *Operation*', *Treatise on Urinary Passage*, 54. R. Blackmore reserved the 'manual Operation' as a 'last Refuge', *Dissertation on a Dropsy*, 205. The only mention of the operation in domestic manuals was in Bailey. *Dictionarium Domesticum*, under 'BLADDER', which stated that 'if none of these [recommended] medicines succeed, then recourse must be had to cutting'.

76. Whitley claimed, for example, that by analysing the forms and apparent functions of scientific exposition, one finds a variety of ways in which scientific knowledge has been popularized between different groups (e.g. teachers–students, specialists–generalists). Additionally, he claimed that the 'popularization process' is inseparable from the generation and development of scientific knowledge. As evidence, he has shown, in limited case studies, that 'feedback' generated from popularization has functioned both to challenge and to validate existing scientific knowledge, together with promoting the production of new knowledge. The fullest explanations of this model are presented in R. Whitley, 'Knowledge Producers and Knowledge Acquirers: Popularization as a Relation Between Scientific Fields and Their Publics', in T. Shinn and R. Whitley (eds), *Expository Science: Forms and Functions of Popularization* (Dordrecht, 1985), 3–28; and J. Bunders and R. Whitley, 'Popularization within the Sciences: The Purposes and Consequences of Inter-Specialist Communication', in Shinn and Whitley, *Expository Science*, 61–77.

77. Also in Shinn and Whitley, *Expository Science*, see S. Yearley, 'Representing Geology: Textual Structures in the Pedagogical Presentation of Science', 79–101; M. Biezunski, 'Popularization and Scientific Controversy: The Case of the Theory of Relativity in France', 195–207; and E. Yoxen, 'Speaking Out about Competition: An Essay in *The Double Helix* as Popularization', 163–81.

78. S. Hilgartner, 'The Dominant View of Popularization: Conceptual Problems, Political Uses', *Social Studies of Science* 20 (1990), 528.

79. Barry Smith is among the few who have begun to specify meanings of 'practical' knowledge. See his 'Knowing How vs. Knowing That', in J. Nyiri and B. Smith (eds), *Practical Knowledge: Outlines of a Theory of Traditions and Skills* (London, 1989), 1–16.

80. ibid.

81. Shapin, 'Science and the Public', 990–1007.

3

Readers, texts, and contexts
Vernacular medical works in early modern England
Mary E. Fissell

When we look at the large body of works considered 'popular' medicine, one of the few things that we know about them is that they were printed and reprinted. We assume from this that these little books were read fairly widely. Until recently, historical analysis has ceased here, focusing on book ownership and stopping short of questions about how reading happened. This paper explores how popular health books were read, and how those contexts of use influenced the kinds of knowledge that these books purveyed.

In particular, I focus on a text called the *Erra Pater*, sometimes mistranslated in the eighteenth century as 'The Errors of the Father'.[1] It is also often referred to as *The Book of Knowledge.* This is a work of popular health and divination; it most closely resembles a sort of perpetual almanac. Next to the Bible, almanacs may have been the most common form of the printed word found in English households.[2] It is estimated that in the 1660s through the 1680s, there were over 400,000 almanacs sold in some years, which was more than one for every four households.[3] Almanacs thus represent one of the most widely distributed sources of health information in the seventeenth and eighteenth centuries.[4] They provided agricultural advice, political comment, a calendar, and advice on health and climate and the weather. Both Bernard Capp and Keith Wrightson have noted that almanacs, often written by physicians or members of the gentry, have to be understood as a bridge between popular and élite cultures, however defined.[5]

At the cheap end of the market, almanacs were challenged by works such as the *Erra Pater*, which provided a permanent equivalent. The *Erra Pater* went through forty-two different editions in the eighteenth century; almost half of these were North American. It was published in the British Isles in London, Glasgow, Edinburgh, Belfast, Paisley and Gosport. In North America, it was published in Boston and Philadelphia, as well as smaller towns such as Exeter and Portsmouth in New Hampshire and Hartford, New Haven, New London and Suffield in Connecticut.

North American and British versions of the *Erra Pater* are similar but patterns of publishing differ. In Britain, the book was published and republished steadily throughout the century. In the New World, however, publishing was almost exclusively in the 1790s. The Britain publishers who produced the *Erra Pater* included it in a list of chapbooks and didactic works. For example, during the 1720s, Thomas Norris published forty works of fiction or amusement such as *Valentine and Orson*; seventeen didactic works such as *Arithmetic Made Easie;* eight books on popular medicine including two editions of *Erra Pater*; and fourteen religious or devotional books such as *A Token for Children*.[6] In other words, publishers who printed *Erra Pater* often specialized in works typical of the lower end of the book market.[7]

However, the *Erra Pater* had a long history by the time it appeared in the eighteenth century. There is an edition of 1535, containing similar advice. For example, it lists the dangerous days of the year, and makes predictions based upon what day of the week starts the year.[8] Compared with later versions, this is rudimentary, but it has the same basic function, to keep men and women healthy by providing guidance about the body and the weather. The eighteenth-century texts, however, claim to be translated by the seventeenth-century astrologer William Lilly, although there is no evidence to suggest that Lilly actually had a hand in its composition.

Like many others of its type, the *Erra Pater* is broken into sections, enabling the reader to consult the text on particular issues even though it lacks an index. Part 1 deals with astrology and predicting the future; Part 2 is a series of prognostications for health and recipes for remedies. These are followed in Part 3 by discussions of physiognomy, palmistry, and dream interpretation. Part 4 consists of a farmer's calendar and the Compleat Gardener, a compendium of remedies for animals and directions for planting and harvesting. Finally, almost all editions include the Dealer's Directory, a sort of tradesman's ready reckoner, which includes tables of troy and avoirdupois weights, charts for bakers who live in various corporations as to the weights of loaves, lists of principal towns, roads, fairs, and markets. Various legal documents are given as forms to follow, such as bonds, bills of sale, wills, and indentures. The book usually closes with a calendar of fixed feasts, and a list of historical events up to the present, including such memorable moments as the first use of guns, the first printing in England, the plague, etc.

Obviously, a text such as this was not primarily about medicine.[9] Nevertheless, the medical component is included in every edition I've seen (most are virtually identical to each other) and, like the almanac, such a work represents a kind of lowest common denominator of medical advice book. More generally, such works are about man's – and sometimes woman's – relation to the natural world, and are revealing of attitudes towards healing and health care.

Before examining the text's relationships with its reader, two contexts may be of use. The first is consumption – how was this book bought, sold, used, re-used, thrown away? Implicit in this query is the exploration of the relationship between this book and other books. Second, what can we know of the experience of reading in the early modern period? What are the preconditions structuring potential interactions between reader and text?

Historians of medicine look at a book like the *Erra Pater* and assume that it is in some way 'popular' – it is small, the print quality is poor, and it has rather grubby woodcuts – it is similar to a lengthy chapbook. However, as Margaret Spufford has shown, and Roger Chartier further developed, we cannot know the social location of the book's readers from such evidence.[10] For example, Spufford has shown that chapbooks – long assumed to be 'popular' and thus the province of non-élites – were often read by upper-class schoolboys. So, too, one of the best-known collections of chapbooks is that assembled by Samuel Pepys. Thus, just because a text looks 'popular' does not mean that we can infer its readership. Indeed, we cannot even assume that such a book was not used by medical practitioners. Perhaps practitioners did not consult the *Erra Pater* in order to acquaint themselves with the rudiments of astrological medicine – but in an era in which many health-care workers pursued multiple occupations, medical personnel could have used the book for agricultural advice, or for its tables of weights and measures, or its lists of fairs.

Unfortunately, evidence about the actual cost of various editions of the *Erra Pater* is scarce. I have not yet found any prices for the *Erra Pater* itself. Similar works appear to have cost one or two shillings.[11] Estimating secondhand cost is even more difficult, but secondhand cost is a much better indicator of the limits to ownership – although, of course, not to readership. From fragmentary evidence, I would estimate that the secondhand price might have been at least as low as sixpence. Sixpence represents, very roughly, about half of a day's wages for a labourer, so we can guess that this book was fairly widely available to most of the literate.

Attempts to investigate actual book-ownership have been equally problematic, especially for small and presumably inexpensive books such as the *Erra Pater*. For instance, probate inventories, one of the main sources for book-ownership, may not have listed such books individually. Very few items worth less than a shilling or two seem to have been recorded in inventories, which eliminates most of the lower end of the book market.[12] Nor was will-making so extensive as to provide a good indication of book ownership in lower social strata.

Thus, we can suggest that this book was probably within the means of artisans and above. In addition, the text itself proclaims that it is available to those 'of the meanest capacities'. However, this rhetorical strategy should not be taken at face value to imply that this book was therefore read by cowherds and clodpates. The phrase 'of the meanest capacities' is very often used and probably speaks as much to a certain epistemology as to any specific implied readership. In other words, the context of consumption requires further detailed work on plebeian book-ownership and patterns of publishing before it can illuminate the role of texts such as the *Erra Pater*.

The other context which we must pursue is that of reading itself. How did people engage with texts such as the *Erra Pater*? This question seems of particular significance for books such as medical works, where our imaginations can dream up a plethora of potential encounters between reader and book. Perhaps the *Erra Pater* served as a do-it-yourself guide, with an individual reading the text and looking at an ill person simultaneously. Or maybe the book was read as entertainment, or used as a sort of seed catalogue by gardening enthusiasts – the potential range is very wide.

In general terms, reading in early modern England varies from our current experiences in certain crucial ways. First, reading took place within a culture still partially oral in nature. Certainly newspapers, novels, shop signs in words rather than pictures, lending libraries, and a host of other features of print culture began to flourish in the first half of the eighteenth century. But paper and ink were not cheap, and people listened to sermons, memorized lists, heard town criers declaim the news, participated in religious disputations – in sum, engaged in all sorts of practices at the interface of print and oral culture.[13]

So too, the meaning of the printed word as cultural artifact had different resonances in the early modern period than in our own. Specifically, words could have magic potential, could function as charms. Within the *Erra Pater* words sometimes assumed quasi-magical qualities. For example, a range of methods of divination was recommended which relied upon manipulation of the letters of a person's name. Some of these methods required the individual's name in Latin rather than English. This practice probably owes more to the magical qualities associated with foreign words than it does to any learned qualities of the implied reader. In a work related to the *Erra Pater*, the reader's attention is drawn to the different functions of words and writing because the book opens with 'Several Secrets of Art and Nature', namely, how to make coloured and invisible inks.[14] Texts might thus have thaumaturgic or totemic value somewhat independent of their content.[15]

Nor was the printed or written word consumed in the cloistered quiet of individual privacy. Rather, the gap between the fully and the functionally literate, and the literate and illiterate, was constantly bridged by the association of words with images and by the practice of reading aloud. Thus broadsheets, ballads and fly sheets, as well as chapbooks and medical works, were illustrated by means of woodcuts, which aided the reader's interpretation of the text and provided an alternative means of participation for the unlettered.[16] The actual repertoire of woodcuts was somewhat limited, which meant that texts referred to each other by means of images, perhaps unintentionally, providing the non-literate with curious connections among a variety of works.

So, too, reading was often reading aloud. Natalie Davis and others have shown how early modern reading was often a group activity, households gathered round the fire of an evening, listening to tellers of tales and readers of texts, or artisans hiring one of their number to read aloud in the workplace.[17] Indeed, it has recently been argued that the word 'reading' in the eighteenth century usually implied reading aloud, even in literate circles; only when modified did it suggest a solitary activity.[18]

Historians refer to such early modern habits as 'intensive reading'.[19] Intensive reading implies access to very few books, which are read and re-read, meditated upon, consumed in ways unfamiliar to us, often as a group activity of the kind described by Davis. What little we know about reading habits in late seventeenth- and early eighteenth-century England suggests that intensive reading was not the dominant style. Eager readers might well have access to quite a number of books through networks of borrowing and exchange. Indeed, J. Paul Hunter has recently described the typical reader of late seventeenth-century proto-fiction as a young, lonely, urban, ambitious person who read in private, seeking guidance about how to live in exemplary tales and fictions.[20] Nothing could be more removed from the convivial peasant gatherings predicated by intensive reading. However, aspects of intensive reading lingered on, and the contexts in which the *Erra Pater* was bought, borrowed, read and re-read owe something to this older style of reading as well as that described by Hunter.

These brief sketches of the contexts of consumption and of reading itself remind us of what literary theorists already knew: that reading books is not always the scholarly, sequential activity which is rumoured to occur in our studies or in the reading room of the British Library – if, indeed, such structured activities take place at all. Hence, as Roger Chartier has argued, our models of reading books from the beginning to the end, with strong attention to the development and unfolding of the plot, may not apply to early-modern experiences at all. With reference to texts simplified for cheap editions, Chartier has posited a distinct style of reading for early moderns who were not scholars – readers, but with different expectations of texts from those who read expensive humanist editions or full-length novels. He suggests that this group employed a form of reading characterized by self-contained sequences, often discontinuous, aimed at the inexperienced or infrequent reader.[21] For instance, he draws upon Carlo Ginzburg's analysis of the Friulian miller Mennochio's idiosyncratic reading of various religious and philosophical works, illustrating how this form of reading depended upon short items which were not read as part of a narrative sequence, but were made sense of individually. These items could then be combined in various satisfying ways.

Chartier develops his analysis from the bibliothèque bleue, the collection of French chapbooks which were simplified and modified in order to appeal to a wide audience. However, Lisa Jardine and Anthony Grafton have recently shown that dis-junctive styles of reading were not the sole prerogative of the partially literate or the infrequent reader. They analyse the reading practices of the sixteenth-century humanist scholar Gabriel Harvey, showing how he read many books simul-taneously, reading small bits of a number of books in con-junction, cross-referencing and comparing. Although Harvey should not be compared directly with a reader of the *Erra Pater*, the more general point – that styles of reading differ greatly over time – is of use. Moreover, Jardine and Grafton suggest that modes of reading which do not stress continuity and narrative flow were widespread in early modern England among a range of social groupings.[22]

If we look at the *Erra Pater* and contemporaneous English chapbooks, such theories about reading styles can help to explain some of these texts' seeming peculiarities. Typical chap-books are usually twenty-four small pages long and yet are broken into chapters. Often those chapters are free-floating incidents in the main character's life rather than a progressive unfolding of narrative.

Take, for instance, the story of Tom Hickathrift. The edition I have used was printed in Whitehaven by one Ann Dunn, sometime in the mid to late eighteenth century, but the story had been published since the mid-seventeenth century.[23] It is a series of short chapters, each headed by an italicized sentence which tells what is going to happen in that chapter. In each one, Tom vanquishes the latest in a long series of enemies. It is not clear why and how these men came to be Tom's enemies; it is the fighting scenes which matter. In addition to the very common feature of one event per chapter, this text shares with many others a tendency to repetition on a theme. In this case, repetition concerns symbolic and dramatic elements to the demise of Tom's enemies. For instance, in one chapter, Tom

strikes a man on his neck, whereupon the fellow's head flies off
into the air and strikes down one of the leaders of an insur-
rection. A few pages later, after Tom has been insulted by a rude
suitor, he kicks the suitor, who flies into the air, bounces off a
ridgepole, and into a fishpond. Such parallel and repetitive
actions are typical of this type of book. Another element of
repetition occurs at the end of this text. As is so often the case,
a verse summarizes the tale for the reader:

He conquered armed men and giants too
And did run Bears and Lions thro' and thro'
Affording to his Native Land Relief
Yet after all he died with very Grief.

But what seems to us repetitive was obviously an important
element to this kind of text.

Repetition and re-working are significant structures in the
Erra Pater. The actual techniques of repetition sometimes vary
from those of chapbooks, but their underlying function is much
the same. As in fiction, verses often remind the reader of crucial
details. For example, the *Erra Pater* describes the parts of the
body ruled by different signs of the Zodiac. This information is
presented in three ways: by means of a woodcut, a prose discussion and a verse which sums up the basic points. The verse is
as follows:

Man's Head and face Heaven's ram obey,
His Neck the neck-strong Bull doth sway;
The Arm twining Twins guide hands and Arms,
Breast, Sides, and stomach Cancer charms:

And so on, and so on. Obviously, the function of this verse is to
fix the basic points into the reader's memory, by means not only
of rhymes but also visual and punning images and emblems.
Thus the neck is ruled by a neck-strong bull, and we can
remember that the arms are governed by the twins if we think of
them twined arm in arm.

These kinds of memory devices were common and important
in an era in which writing things down was not a matter of
frequent recourse. Many items in early modern life involved just
this kind of symbolic representation. Rather than proceeding by
narrative unfolding, or by progressive exposition of a theme, a

range of devices such as shop signs, broadsides, and religious images used emblems which summed up the logical relationship between various elements at a glance. The intricacies could be explored or not as the viewer wished. In either case, the means by which the viewer understood the emblem were different from the progressive solitary reading of a text.[24]

Verses such as those in the *Erra Pater* must have been familiar to readers who had undertaken any formal education. Whatever rudimentary schooling basic readers received was very likely to have stressed rote memorization. David Cressy has emphasized that even learning to read was an oral process; children in schools chanted letters and combinations of letters out loud. Since writing was taught after reading, children did not use writing as an aid to reading; instead they were trained to rely upon memory.[25] Thus verses such as the one about the signs of the Zodiac should not be understood as purely repetitive; instead, they served as summations of the text, as elegant emblems containing verbal and visual elements in a form easily understood and appreciated by early-modern readers or listeners.

Even aside from the frequent verses, the *Erra Pater* is a very repetitive book by our standards. It opens with a range of possible forecasting methods, based upon when certain days fall in the calendar. If New Year's Day falls on a Monday, for example,

> expect a hard and cold Winter, and a wet Summer, and as a Consequent of that, many Diseases; the Fruits of the Earth very indifferent, which will produce great Scarcity in some Places. It also denotes the Downfal of the Gentry, and many Marriages among the common People.[26]

This analysis is followed by predictions by means of the day of the week Christmas falls upon, and a range of other similar devices. So, too, quite a variety of methods to divine various questions are offered, based upon manipulating the letters in the individual's name.

But such repetition seems to have been a big seller. In part, people read books differently from the way they do now and repetition was not construed as a problem. If we understand reading, not as a process of exploration, an individual voyage of discovery, but rather as a form of memory, then repetition becomes a positive advantage. It is that moment of satisfied recognition which an audience displays when it applauds after the first few bars of a piece of music that provides a key to understanding the functions of repetition in these books. Often, repetition is across texts, from one work to another – and on multiple levels, from thematic to narrative to factual – but it also functions within one text. Hence, for example, the repetition of Tom beating up his enemies, or the repetition within the *Erra Pater* of ways of knowing what the year will bring, serves to validate knowledge through familiarity and to fix it in readers' minds.

Repetition was also an important element to religious works, although it functioned somewhat differently. David Hall has argued that writers of religious works intended their books to be read and re-read, combed for meaning and partially committed to memory, like scripture. Therefore the repetitive quality of vernacular religious works was made by the intended reader's style of interaction with the text; re-reading and memorizing texts created repetition. In some ways, despite startlingly high literacy rates, Hall's New Englanders continued to employ features of intensive reading in their interactions with religious works.[27]

Thus, the contexts of reading in the early modern period suggest ways of understanding the structures of popular medical works. Indeed, an understanding of such contexts might provide clues to the author's or publisher's perceptions of his or her audiences, and the intended uses of medical texts. For example, the rhetorical structures of repetition and versification are absent from S.A. Tissot's and William Buchan's texts but are familiar indeed to readers of certain editions of Aristotle's *Masterpiece*. While we cannot know who actually read these works, we can infer intended readership from the author's use of conventions associated with certain forms of reading, and then ask how knowledge contained within those texts was mediated by forms of reading.

Close readings of two sections of the *Erra Pater* suggest the ways in which the author attempted to create certain relationships between the text and its reader, which imply how such a book was intended to function. For one section, I employ a form of literary endeavour called reader-response theory; in particular I rely upon the work of Stanley Fish. In part, this is an exploration of method: can popular health texts, often resistant to traditional forms of medical-historical analysis, be interpreted as works of literature?

Reader-response theory, as its name implies, focuses attention upon the reader and the process of reading.[28] In particular, Stanley Fish argues that the temporal flow of reading must be crucial to an understanding of the interpretive process. He shows how the minute structure of texts can serve to reinforce the reader's certainty of him/herself, of the text's (and the world's) order and rationality – or can do quite the opposite. In particular, he advocates a method which serves to, as he puts it, 'slow down the reading experience' so that the micro-events of reading which escape our normal attention can be understood.[29]

There are undoubted problems with this method for historians. First, to what extent does a text structure responses to itself? Is textual determinacy absolute? Here the experiences of Ginzburg's Friulian miller suggest that historians would be well advised to take a relaxed attitude towards textual determinacy, and accept, along with Fish, that we cannot know the answer to this problem. However, there is another more pressing problem for historians. Fish's position implies a certain common set of reading experiences, a shared grammar of perceiving and absorbing texts. While a literary critic is presumed to be making analytical statements about texts within an interpretive community often temporally distinct from that of the text's original author, historians are seeking a closer link to the context of a book's production. In other words, can a late twentieth-century reader use a late twentieth-century method of textual analysis to any purposeful end on a late seventeenth-century text?

The utility in Fish's method lies in the difficulties we have in reconstructing early-modern reading practices. Roger Chartier relies, at times, on texts which are self-referential; they explicitly discuss how they are themselves to be read. Lisa Jardine and Anthony Grafton use marginalia and a reader's own comments on what he has read in order to reconstruct his patterns of reading. Robert Darnton is able to utilize the letters of a Rousseau reader as well as Rousseau's own comments on how he wished to be read. But for the historian of the *Erra Pater* or the *Compost of Ptolmaeus* or the *Arcandum*, such strategies are less useful. Hence my interest in the methods of reader-response theory, which focus on the actual process by which a text is read, actualized, brought into being, by the reader. If Chartier is right, and early-modern reading is very different from our own experiences, perhaps a close reading of texts will begin to suggest to us how their authors attempted to structure their readers, tried to constrain their readers' attempts to inscribe themselves in the text. Those very attempts, of course, also reflect the author's assessment of his or her reader's desires.

A close reading of the prologue to the *Erra Pater* reveals many of the qualities Chartier enumerates, but on the micro-linguistic level, rather than that of structure or narrative flow. In addition, it suggests that the reader is inevitably confronted with the curious epistemological status of the reader and the book he or she is reading. Finally, attention to the fine structure of the text highlights the difficulties which secular writers encountered in persuading their readers in an era in which sacred publishing laid claim to truth.

Fish advocates slowing down the reading process so that the inevitable ambiguities and confusions engendered by sequences of words, which may be subsequently resolved and forgotten, can be recovered and understood as a part of the interpretive process. Application of this technique to the prologue of the *Erra Pater* suggests that nothing is certain in this passage; meaning is always multiple and potentially alterable. Such fluidity derives from the structure of the sentences themselves: they are very long, containing many clauses delimited by commas or semi-colons seemingly chosen at random. Hence the text is a morass of indirect or multi-direct reference, especially for the novice reader. Indeed, one is tempted to suggest that these clauses function almost as individual statements by themselves. In literary terms, the axis of meaning has been shifted from syntagmatic to paradigmatic. In non-jargon, these phrases have meaning, not as a sequential chain, but rather as a series of signs with equivalent and interchangeable meanings. The function of this shift is, in part, a certain degree of repetition and a sense of the text functioning as variations on a theme. However, it also serves to create ambiguity; the reader expects the various clauses to have an equivalent function, but this is not always the case.

For example, the first sentence repeatedly moves the reader between the status of the divine and the sinful by means of a long series of equally weighted clauses. The clause 'infus'd by its Almighty Maker' never resolves the ambiguity present from its start. It modifies 'Spark of Immortality' which is equivalent to 'The Soul of Man'. But does it suggest that it is God himself who does the infusing, or is it the divine which is the substance infused into the soul? Confusion continues with 'does still retain a relish of its Original'. Here again, Fish's attention to temporal sequence suggests that the initial meaning of 'Original' refers back to the Almighty Maker himself. But then the next clause implies quite the reverse: 'that it covets Knowl- edge'. The word 'covets' shakes the reader off course by enter- ing the domain of sin, indeed, of Original Sin.

While claiming some form of textual authority, the text undermines itself by referring to Christian ambiguity about profane knowledge. David Hall has shown how New England religious texts of this period used the authority of the Word, the Scripture, to convince the reader of their legitimacy, even if such works were sermons or other non-scriptural texts. He argues that such religious works denied any mediation between text and reader; they presented themselves as direct access to the Divine.[30] But such a technique was less successful for writers of secular works. The author of the *Erra Pater* used scriptural images and references, perhaps, as Hall discusses, to augment his or her authority, but the technique keeps breaking down in the face of the secular text.

The same kind of radical disjuncture happens a line or two later: 'it searches out the Stars and all their various Influences; nay, rifles all the heavenly Constellations'. The word 'nay' is first read as a negative, preparing the reader for the opposite of searching out all the stars. What follows is both opposite and same. Where the actions described (rifling the constellations) are roughly equi- valent to the earlier clause, their connotations are dramatically different. Indeed, from the word 'rifling' the reader's expectation of a negative is enhanced – 'rifling' implies a form of theft or, at least, some kind of illicit activity. It is only as the rest of the clause is reached that it becomes apparent that 'nay' serves here as an intensifier as much as a negative. The positive connotations of the quest for knowledge in the first clause are undercut by its negative and sinful aspects in the second.

Such ambiguity is heightened by the author's repeated use of sexual metaphors for knowledge. For example, in the verse, the author compares knowledge to the 'hidden Birth of Things' and refers to 'Dame Nature's secret Workings'. Again, such references remind the reader of original sin and underline the curious status of the knowledge which this text promises to purvey. Where does this leave the reader? As in the rest of the prologue, he or she is floating between error and salvation, never certain if knowledge is sinful or sacred.

However, the reader is not powerless. He or she is free to make meaning of these long chains of equivalent clauses, to embark on the process of interpretation which is the focus of the entire book. This text appears to be less deterministic, less directive of the reader's experience than later classics of popular medicine which take control of the reader more directly. For example, both William Buchan and S.A. Tissot use the beginning of their books to display a variety of styles which make their own textual authority apparent. *Domestic Medicine* and *Advice to the People* confront the reader with an array of prefaces, dedications, introductions, and the like.[31]

Buchan, for example, has two Latin quotations – one from Cicero, one from Celsus – on the obverse of his title page. This is no 'Dear Reader'; instead, these quotations emphasize Buchan's claim to learning, to gentility, to scholarship. This is followed by an advertisement for another of Buchan's works, and then a dedication to Sir John Pringle. Like the opening lines of the *Erra Pater*, Buchan's dedication utilizes a long string of clauses:

> The character which you justly sustain in the literary world, your laudable and successful endeavours to extend and improve the art of medicine, the confidence reposed in your skill by the Public, and the important station you hold in the care of the Royal Family, all conspire to point you out as a most proper Patron of a Performance which has for its object the HEALTH of the inhabitants of Great Britain.[32]

However, unlike the *Erra Pater*, all these clauses are the same; each one enumerates another virtue belonging to John Pringle. Each clause starts with a positive attribute: character, laudable and successful endeavours, confidence, important station. At no point is there any ambiguity, any space where readers must make meaning themselves. Instead, the text's authority is sustained by the payoff of the end of the sentence, which serves to emphasize the writer's control over his material.

Tissot was also given to lengthy sentences, but his prose style, as translated by J. Kirkpatrick, creates and maintains control in a different way. Take this sentence from his preface:

> To consider such Success with Indifference, were to have been unworthy of it, which Demerit, at least on this

Account, I cannot be justly charged with; since indifference has not been my case, who have felt, as I ought to, this Gratification of Self-Love; and which, under just and prudent Restrictions, may perhaps be even politically cherished; as the Delight naturally arising from having been approved, is a Source of that laudable Emulation, which has sometimes produced the most essential good Consequences to Society itself.[33]

In this sentence, the clauses are subordinated to each other, with the result that ambiguity is minimized. Semi-colons serve to divide the major parts of the sentence from each other, so that even if the reader is temporarily puzzled by one of the subordinate clauses, the semi-colon restores order. So, too, the sentence moves from Tissot's individual feelings to the good of society as a whole; the meaning reinforces the sense of order created by its structure.

Tissot and Buchan use very different styles from these literary ones when they come to the beginning of the substance of their books, namely the introduction. Both use a similar technique – indeed, Buchan may have copied Tissot. Both open their introductions with the statement of a fact, whose truth is underlined by the structure of the sentence itself. Tissot, still fond of long sentences, confines himself to:

The Decrease of the Number of Inhabitants, in most of the States of Europe, is a fact, which impresses every reflecting Person, and is become such a General Complaint, as is but too well established on plain Calculations.[34]

The simple declarative structure of the first half of the sentence denies the reader any hermeneutic freedom and gives the author control. Buchan uses the same strategy:

The improvements in Medicine, since the revival of learning, have by no means kept pace with those of the other arts.[35]

Again, the reader's consent is assumed; no persuasion is deemed necessary. The straightforward prose style, especially after Buchan's flowery dedication and prolix preface, emphasizes the simple truth, the factual nature, of what is to follow.

In other words, close attention to the ways in which these texts are written can suggest how readers were expected to respond to them. Where the *Erra Pater* created ambiguity for its readers, it also permitted a certain interpretive latitude. Buchan and Tissot, however, employed a variety of prose styles to the same end: the creation and maintenance of authority and control. In part, these differences are due to the contexts of publication. When the *Erra Pater* was first published, it addressed an audience familiar with the authority of writings on religion. Some of its hesitations and lack of authority result from uncertainties about secular texts. Tissot and Buchan are early examples of a very different type of textual authority based on scientific knowledge.

The prologue to the *Erra Pater* also needs to be understood in specific contexts of reading. Fish's theory predicates a unitary reader, of no specific class or gender or race or history. Certainly, from what we know of the patterns of literacy in the early-modern period, access to this text was strongly shaped by gender and social status. More men than women could sign their names, and the ability to sign one's name varied directly with social standing.[36] While imperfect, the ability to sign one's name appears to be the most useful proxy for estimating comparative levels of literacy although some people who could read could not sign their names. Recently scholars have noted that women may be particularly under-represented as readers when signing ability is used as an indicator of literacy.[37] As it happens, the copy of the *Erra Pater* which I've used most often appears to have been sold by one woman to another. This copy, in the John Rylands Library, has a printed bookplate on which is written 'Mary Curry', and has an advertisement pasted in it for a bookseller in Exeter, one Jane Pring, who also sold ink, paper, maps, prints, medicines, and wallpaper. Although we cannot currently move beyond such individuals to good quantitative evidence about men's and women's patterns of literacy, we can make inferences about differential reading habits.

For example, the curious structure of the prologue to the *Erra Pater* might have been read differently by men and women. Girls were almost never taught Latin; nor were most boys. But those boys who started at a grammar school, even if they did not progress very far, would have read the prologue distinctively. First, studying Latin meant an attention to grammar, as the name of the school suggests. This attention to the structure of language – especially as developed for Latin, where the order of the words does not determine their meaning in the way in which it does in English – meant that the prologue's multiplicity of clauses might be read in specific ways by grammar school boys. Perhaps the interpretive freedom which the text's structure predicated was more limited if the reader were paying close attention to the structure of the entire sentences; perhaps the shift from the syntagmatic to the paradigmatic was more difficult to achieve.

Second, the long strings of clauses of the prologue would not have been unfamiliar to a grammar school boy. Latin scholars were familiar with a vast range of equivalent phrases which meant the same thing. As Walter Ong has pointed out, this tendency derived in part from Renaissance humanists' desire to teach their pupils oral fluency in Latin; elegance in spoken Latin demanded a ready supply of eloquent phrases. Thus collections of commonplaces flourished, providing a novice with literally hundreds of ways of saying the same thing.[38] Perhaps a reader used to these elegant ways of saying the same thing might have paid less attention to the inconsistencies and contradictions of the clauses in the *Erra Pater*, might have expected and found consistency where others found ambiguity.

Obviously, these differences in reading styles can only be suggested; we lack direct knowledge of men's and women's encounters with this small book. However, we can imagine a spectrum of readers' responses structured by educational experience. Women and those men who did not go to grammar school would be at one end of the spectrum while highly educated university men are at the other. David Cressy's work implies that, even at the less-educated end of the spectrum, men and women may have been differentiated. He analyses the records of an early eighteenth-century orphanage whose records included details of the standards of literacy attained by the children on entry and while educated in the institution. Girls as a group were less fluent readers than boys.[39] If such patterns were widespread, literate women may have read less fluently, and tended towards styles of reading which emphasized discontinuity. Such reading afforded them greater interpretive freedom, especially with a text such as the *Erra Pater*.

While the *Erra Pater* is nowhere explicit about how it should be read, it does provide the reader with clues about how knowledge functions. For example, as the prologue suggests, knowledge is multivalent, neither fully good nor bad, but full of the potential for good and evil. Since the text itself is knowledge, such insights cannot help but be in some way self-referential, directing the reader towards certain relationships with the text. In part, the prologue is a come-on, titillating the reader with promises of secret knowledge unveiled. But the ambiguities go further. The text functions simultaneously to promise the reader knowledge and to undercut its own authority to convey that knowledge.

Perhaps the clearest indication of this paradoxical attitude to knowledge is the section on dream interpretation. Dream interpretation was a significant element in many early modern chapbooks and, indeed, in individuals' lives.[40] However, in the *Erra Pater*, dream interpretation is not an easy or unambiguous process. In terms of health, the text had already advised the reader to stick to 'the Rule of Contraries', in other words, to interpret a bodily sign as requiring its opposite.[41] Disorders involving an excess of cold humours were to be treated with warm remedies. However, the rule of contraries operated only partially in the world of dreams. To dream of black coffins and mourners meant that the death of a loved one would follow. But to dream of the death of a close friend was not a cause for alarm; it meant that the friend was in good health.[42] Most dreams worked by likes or contraries, but there were no clear guidelines as to which to follow. Other dreams worked synecdochically: dreaming that your teeth fell out or were taken out implied the loss of children or relations.[43]

Advice on dream interpretation functioned also as wider comment on interpretation; indeed, this section can be understood as a more general hermeneutics, advice on reading the book of nature and the book itself. Much of the text deals with means and methods of interpretation – physiognomy, palmistry, astrology, etc. This type of interpretation was common to a range of vernacular literature, especially in the later seventeenth century. 'Fiction' in the form of chapbook stories and 'fact' in the form of almanacs, news stories about prodigies, and political pamphlets which discuss dreams all provided the reader with large numbers of hermeneutic models.[44] Nor should we presume that such interpretive strategies were those of the plebeian. Barbara Shapiro has noted how the creation and dissemination of natural theology from the middle of the seventeenth century made the metaphor of reading the book of nature a commonplace. Such worthies as John Tillotson or John Wilkins sought proof of God's existence in his providences, revealed in the quirky incidents so beloved of cheap literature.[45]

The complex and mixed messages about the potential for interpreting nature which the text conveyed lent it a certain self-referential quality, a quality enhanced by the curious status of knowledge itself in this period. The kinds of knowledge these texts convey, the hermeneutic strategies they implicitly recommend to the reader, and responses which they attempt to construct in the reader are all related to beliefs about knowledge itself.

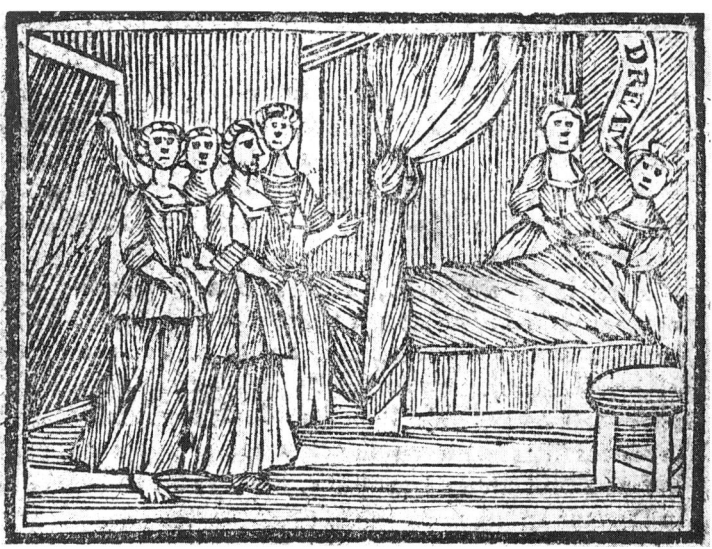

Figure 5 A dreamer and her dream (*Erra Pater, The Book of Knowledge* 1753; reproduced by permission of the Wellcome Institute Library, London.)

For example, Nancy Armstrong and Leonard Tennenhouse have recently analysed the seventeenth-century Essex clergyman Ralph Josselin's dreams in terms of a pre-modern understanding of selfhood. Josselin, they claim, dreamed about himself in ways which did not admit of separation between self and God, between self and body politic.[46] Everything in Josselin's diary is recorded in relation to Josselin himself; the subject/object division with which we are familiar did not operate. In a much less subtle form, the dream and the dreamer were sometimes connected in works of dream interpretation. As the *Newest, Book . . . Book of Knowledge* put it, a dream was 'a Fiction of the Soul . . . signifying either Good or Evil to come'.[47] But the significance depended upon the dreamer:

> To Dream of having a Great Head to a Rich Man signifies Dignity; to a Poor Man, Riches; to a Champion, Victory; to a Usurer, Hopes of Money; to a Servant, long servitude; to him that hath chosen Quiet, Pain and Anger.[48]

Thus the same dream meant different things to different dreamers; the subject permeated the object of inquiry.

Much historical attention has been paid to the creation of the subject/object divide, in terms of the creation of scientific objectivity, the death of nature, or the decline of magic.[49] However, little thought has been given to the status of knowledge in an era in which knowledge and knower, book and reader, were more intimately connected than they are now. Clearly, knowledge contained in such works did not attain the kind of facticity which we associate with modern medical works. Instead, knowledge had a much more personal dimension.

For example, in sections on astrology, the *Erra Pater* reverses the usual relationship between astrological chart and reader. The text describes the physical and emotional characteristics of individuals born under each sign of the Zodiac. Thus, for example, Virgos are melancholic, very courteous, but very self-serving, with spare bodies, brown complexions, black hair and large eyes.[50] From this information, the reader is invited, 'By these Things Persons may come to know under what Signs they were born, if they will compare themselves with what is written'.[51] Similar injunctions accompany discussions of what house the Sun was in and what planet ruled the hour of the reader's birth.[52] In part, the usual relationship of knowing sign and thus learning qualities is reversed because not everyone knew their birth date in early-modern England. But the reversal goes deeper than that. It indicates the way in which subject and object were utterly mixed up. The sign under which you were born might indicate your character, but then it seemed that your character might determine what sign was yours.

In a similar manner, dreams could not therefore be read according to some sort of differential diagnosis; like astrological signs, the meanings of dreams were shaped by their dreamers. In the same way, I am suggesting, books like the *Erra*

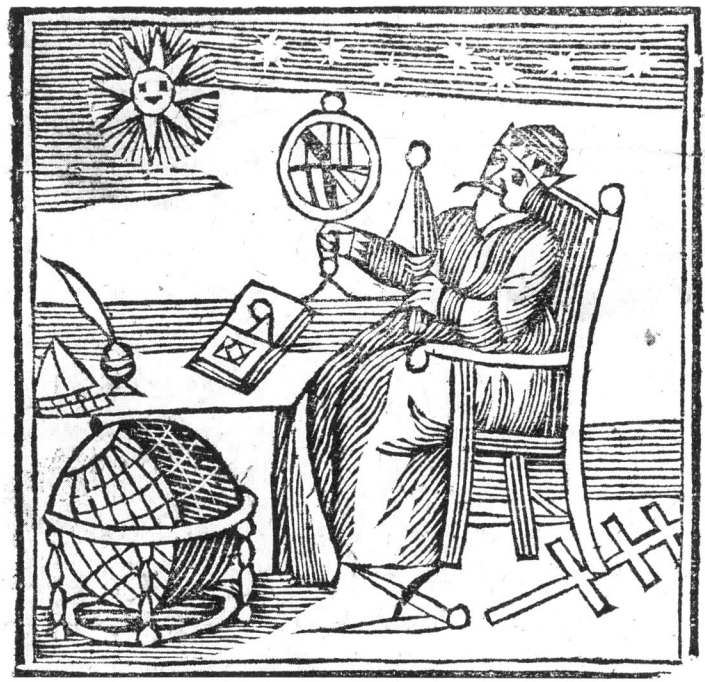

Figure 6 The astrologer (*Erra Pater, The Book of Knowledge* 1753; reproduced by permission of the Wellcome Institute Library, London.)

Pater were shaped by their readers. The forms of interpretation which the book itself advocated were riddled with the paradoxes engendered by non-sacred knowledge which could not be read directly and unproblematically.

By way of conclusion, I have argued that we cannot read eighteenth-century popular medical books without understanding something of the nature of reading in that period. These little books did not always claim the authority of factual knowledge which we associate with medical works. Instead, they functioned in a variety of ways: as entertainment, as memory devices, as statements about man's (and sometimes woman's) relationship to the natural world, and as instructions on how to manipulate that world. As one reader wrote in the front cover of a book similar to the *Erra Pater*, 'Apply thy mind such things to learn as virtue may advance so shalt thou live in sure estate not subject to chance'.[53] While readers sought power over their lives through knowledge, such knowledge did not function unambiguously or objectively. In both the fine structure of sentences and the larger structure of content, the *Erra Pater* denies itself absolute authority, denies that scientific knowledge can be unmediated. Such an analysis must prompt us to ask how subsequent popular medicine invented scientific and objective knowledge claims for itself.

Acknowledgements

It is a pleasure to acknowledge my thanks to Marie Barbieri for introducing me to reader-response theory and to David Cantor, Roger Cooter, Ann Hughes, and Roy Porter for their comments on earlier drafts of this paper.

Notes

1. The pseudonymous author – the Wandering Father – seems to be a reference to the widespread tale of the Wandering Jew. The book claims to be written by 'a Jew out of Jewry, a doctor in Astronomy and Physick' or, as the earliest edition has it, 'A Jew born in Jewrye'. Keith Thomas links this claim to the proverb 'If one affirm he learned it of a Jew, The silly people think it must be true'. Thomas traces the origins of the work to the perpetual prognostication of Esdras, widely circulated in the Middle Ages. Keith Thomas, *Religion and the Decline of Magic* (New York, 1971), 350.

2. John Sommerville, 'The Distribution of Religious and Occult Literature in Seventeenth-century England', *The Library* (1974), 221–5.

3. Bernard Capp, *English Almanacs 1500–1800: Astrology and the Popular Press* (Ithaca, 1979), 44; Cyprian Blagden, 'The Distribution of Almanacks in the Second Half of the Seventeenth Century', *Studies in Bibliography* (1958), 109–16.

4. Capp, *English Almanacs*; Patrick Curry, *Prophecy and Power* (London, 1990); Thomas, *Religion and the Decline of Magic*, esp. chapters 10–12.

5. Keith Wrightson, *English Society, 1580–1680* (London, 1982), 197; Capp, *English Almanacs*, 283 and Appendix.

6. These figures are derived from a survey of the ESTC of all works published by Norris in the 1720s. Norris also published numerous addresses to the House of Lords, speeches of the King, and abstracts of acts of Parliament under licence.

7. For example, the types of books published by Norris fit well into the typologies discussed by J. Paul Hunter, *Before Novels: The Cultural Contexts of Eighteenth Century Fiction* (New York, 1990). See also, Margaret Spufford, *Small Books and Pleasant Histories. Popular Fiction and Its Readership in Seventeenth-century England* (Cambridge, 1981).

8. Erra Pater, *A Pronostycation for ever of Erra Pater. A Jew borne in Jewrye, a doctoure in Astronomye and Physicke. Profytable to kepe the bodye in helthe. a Ptholomeaus sayeth the same.* (n.p., n.d.) This version consists of some of sections 1 and 2 of the eighteenth-century editions, including brief discussions of the four humours, the zodiac, and advice on health and agriculture month by month, all of which is virtually identical with later versions, although many sections and details appear only in the later versions. But this early version lacks discussions of physiognomy, dreams, and much of the agricultural and trade information. The earliest text that closely resembles the eighteenth-century versions of the *Erra Pater* is *The Compleat Book of Knowledge Treating the Wisdom of the Ages* (London, 1698). This followed a 1694 edition published by Thomas Basset *et al.* which combined features of the 1535 edition with aspects of the trader's directory which future editions often included.

9. The most obviously 'medical' contents are in section 2, 'Prognostications for ever, necessary for keeping the body in Health':

- Of the Disposition of Humours in the Body of Man
- Of the Spring Quarter
- Of the Disposition of Humours in the third Quarter
- Of the Disposition of Humours in the fourth Quarter
  (these four sections are advice on health and regimen according to the four seasons)
- Of the Body of Man from the four Parts of the World
  (more on regimen, some remedies)
- Directions for letting Blood (with diagrams)
- Choice Receipts in Physick and Surgery
  (this includes recipes for remedies and directions for treating fractures)

Obviously, the discussions of astrology and the prognostications for the weather include a great deal of information on health and medicine.

10. Spufford, *Small Books*, 71–5.

11. See, for example, prices included in advertisements in *The Compleat Book of Knowledge* (London, 1698). Aristotle's *Book of Problems* (London, 1725) says that it costs 1s on the title page, and lists others from 4d to 7s, mostly in the 1s–2s range.

12. Spufford, *Small Books*, chap. 3.

13. For disputations, see Ann Hughes, 'The Pulpit Guarded: Confrontations between Orthodox and Radicals in Revolutionary England', in Anne Laurence, W.R. Owens, and Stuart Sim (eds.), *John Bunyan and His England, 1628–88* (London, 1990), 31–50.

14. *The Newest, Best . . . Book of Knowledge* (London, 1764).

15. David Cressy, 'Books as Totems in Seventeenth-century England and New England', *Journal of Library History* (1986) 92–106.

16. On this point, see especially Roger Chartier (ed.), *The Culture of Print* (Cambridge, 1989).

17. Natalie Zemon Davis, 'Strikes and Salvation at Lyon' and 'Printing and the People' in *Society and Culture in Early Modern France* (Stanford, 1979).

18. Patricia Howell Michaelson, 'Women in the Reading Circle', *Eighteenth-century Life* (1990), 59–69. Michaelson's argument focuses on the patriarchal control of women's reading, but for the more general point see esp. pp. 62–3. However, see Hunter, *Before Novels*, for the argument that plebeian reading was almost always a private activity.

19. The term originates with Engelsing: Rolf Engelsing, *Der Burger als Leser: Lesergeschichte in Deutschland 1500–1800* (Stuttgart, 1974). For a recent exploration of intensive reading, see Marie-Elisabeth Ducreux, 'Reading unto Death: Books and Readers in Eighteenth-century Bohemia', in Chartier, *Culture of Print*, 191–229.

20. Hunter, *Before Novels*.

21. Roger Chartier, 'Texts, Printings, Readings' in Lynn Hunt (ed.), *The New Cultural History* (Berkeley, 1989), 154–75, see esp. 164.

22. Lisa Jardine and Anthony Grafton, ' "Studied for Action": How Gabriel Harvey Read his Livy', *Past and Present* (1990), 30–78.

23. On chapbook literature, see Spufford, *Small Books*; Susan Pederson, 'Hannah More Meets Simple Simon: Tracts, Chapbooks, and Popular Culture in Late Eighteenth-century England', *Journal of British Studies* (1986), 84–113; Victor E. Neuberg, *Popular Literature, A History and Guide* (London, 1977); Bernard Capp, 'Popular Literature' in Barry Reay (ed.), *Popular Culture in Seventeenth Century England* (London, 1985), 198–243.

24. On an earlier use of emblems, see Alain Boureau, 'Books of emblems on the public stage: coté jardin and coté cour' in Chartier, *Culture of Print*, 261–89.

25. David Cressy, *Literacy and the Social Order* (Cambridge, 1980), 20–2.

26. Erra Pater, *The Book of Knowledge Treating the Wisdom of the Ancients* . . . (London, [1726]), 2. (hereafter EP, 1726).

27. David D. Hall, *Worlds of Wonder, Days of Judgment. Popular Religious Belief in Early New England* (New York, 1989), 29.

28. For an introduction to reader-response, see Jane Tompkins (ed.), *Reader Response Criticism From Formalism to Post Structuralism* (Baltimore, 1980); Susan Suleiman and Inge Crosman (eds), *The Reader in the Text: Essays on Audience and Interpretation* (Princeton, 1980). See also Robert Darnton, 'Readers Respond to Rousseau: the Fabrication of Romantic Sensitivity' in his *The Great Cat Massacre and Other Episodes in French Cultural History* (London, 1984), 215–56.

29. Stanley Fish, 'Literature in the Reader: Affective Stylistics' in Tompkins, *Reader Response Criticism*, 74.

30. Hall, *Worlds of Wonder*, 24–8. Robert Darnton sees Rousseau as re-creating a form of direct and unmediated access to the word – but it is Rousseau, not God, who is the author. Darnton, 'Readers Respond to Rousseau', 232.

31. On Buchan, see Charles E. Rosenberg, 'Medical Text and Social Context', *Bulletin of the History of Medicine* (1983), 22–42; C.J. Lawrence, 'William Buchan: Medicine Laid Open', *Medical History* (1975), 20–35. On Tissot, see especially Ludmilla Jordanova, 'The Popularization of Medicine: Tissot on Onanism', *Textual Practice* (1987), 68–79.

32. William Buchan, *Domestic Medicine, or a Treatise on the Prevention and Cure of Diseases by Regimen and Simple Medicines* 7th edn (London, 1781), vii.

33. S.A. Tissot, *Advice to the People in General with Regard to Their Health* trans. by J. Kirkpatrick (London, 1765), xix.

34. Tissot, *Advice*, 1.

35. Buchan, *Domestic Medicine*, xix.

36. Cressy, *Literacy and the Social Order*; Spufford, *Small Books*, 19–44.

37. Both Spufford and Hobby note that girls were likely to be taught reading and needlework, spinning, knitting and the like whereas boys were taught reading and writing and possibly arithmetic. Spufford, *Small Books*, 34–5; Elaine Hobby, *Virtue of Necessity. English Women's Writing 1649–88* (London, 1988), 190–2. J. Paul Hunter has pointed out that women would have had much less need to learn to sign their names, since far fewer occasions arose in which a woman needed to sign legal documents, at least prior to Lord Hardwicke's Marriage Act of 1753. Hunter, *Before Novels*, see esp. 69–75.

38. Walter J. Ong, *Rhetoric, Romance, and Technology* (Ithaca, 1971).

39. Cressy, *Literacy and the Social Order*, 30–4.

40. Peter Burke, 'L'Histoire sociale des rêves', *Annales E.S.C.* (1973), 329–42.

41. EP 1726, 40.

42. EP 1726, 65.

43. EP 1726, 66.

44. See Capp, 'Popular Literature', particularly 228–9.

45. Barbara Shapiro, *Probability and Certainty in Seventeenth Century England* (Princeton, 1983), 94.

46. Nancy Armstrong and Leonard Tennenhouse, 'The Interior Difference: a Brief Genealogy of Dreams, 1650–1717', *Eighteenth-Century Studies* (1990), 458–78.

47. *Newest, Best . . . Book of Knowledge*, 43.

48. ibid. 43.

49. Carolyn Merchant, *The Death of Nature: Women, Ecology, and the Scientific Revolution* (New York, 1980); Brian Easlea, *Witch-hunting, Magic and the New Philosophy* (Sussex, 1980); Thomas, *Decline of Magic*; on the process by which scientific knowledge and certainty were made, see, for example, Steven Shapin and Simon Schaffer, *Leviathan and the Air Pump* (Princeton, 1986); Shapiro, *Probability and Certainty*; Lorraine Daston, *Classical Probability in the Enlightenment* (Princeton, 1988).

50. EP 1726, 15.

51. EP 1726, 17.

52. EP 1726, 23–30; 31–4.

53. Godfridus, *The Knowledge of Things Unknown* (London, n.d.) This inscription is in the copy in the John Rylands Library, and is signed Jonathan Bowden, and dated 1701.

4

The popularization of medicine in France, 1650–1900

Matthew Ramsey

The popularization of medical knowledge is, in one sense, timeless; physicians have never completely monopolized the secrets of their craft. In another sense, however, it may be argued that the popularization of medicine is a specific historical phenomenon. If, following Jacques Poirier, we define medical popularization as making the concepts and techniques of scientific medicine, the cognitive field of medical professionals, accessible to non-professionals so as to allow them to promote their own health,[1] then we are dealing with a much more restricted, though still very large, domain. Poirier stresses two criteria: the existence of 'an identifiable scientific corpus' to which the popular work refers, and the transformation of this corpus to appeal to a broad audience, through what he calls the dual process of 'reduction/seduction'. (Recent work in the sociology of science, as Philip Wilson notes elsewhere in this volume, has questioned the model of popularization as the one-way diffusion from scientists to laymen of simplified and therefore distorted versions of esoteric knowledge;[2] much the same argument could be made for physicians and the lay public, since the expectations of non-physician patients and readers arguably have some influence on medical practice and writing at all levels. But the distinction made within modern medical discourse between its 'technical' and 'popularized' forms, and the differences between the rules that govern them, are clear enough to justify retaining the model here.) A third crucial element is that medical popularization in the strongest sense – unlike the popularization of science – implies not merely the satisfaction of intellectual curiosity but the practical application of that knowledge in diagnosis and therapeutics. By these criteria, many vernacular works dealing with medical subjects do not qualify as popularizations. An example would be the writings of Raspail, one of the best-selling medical authors of nineteenth-century France, who promoted not an attenuated version of official medicine but a rival system; for this reason, Poirier argues, he can be considered only a 'pseudo-popularizer'.[3]

Medical popularization in this narrow sense is the characteristic product of a particular period in Western history, extending very roughly from the late seventeenth century through to the end of the nineteenth. The print revolution of the fifteenth century resulted in a growing body of vernacular books on medicine, surgery, and pharmacy, which disseminated a much older corpus derived from the interaction of manuscript and oral traditions; works drawing on this corpus remained in print, and new variants appeared, for four centuries. For much of the early modern period, though, the boundary between professional and lay (or even popular and élite) medical cultures was so blurred that it would be misleading to present a text as an instrument of transmission from one discrete realm to another; most educated people knew a little and sometimes more than a little medicine, while physicians and surgeons, for all their protestations of special competence, drew on a widely shared empirical tradition. Many of the domestic handbooks, moreover, were essentially recipe books, not far removed from the manuscript compendia kept by literate households; they shared secrets rather than taught medicine. We would do well to follow Roger Chartier in rejecting rigid distinctions between popular and learned, written and oral, or (it could be added) lay and professional, together with the attempt 'to establish exclusive relationships between specific cultural forms and particular social groups'; better to recognize, with Chartier, 'differentiated uses and plural appropriation of the same goods, the same ideas, and the same actions'.[4]

At least from the mid-seventeenth century, however, one can trace the development of a self-consciously scientific medicine, represented in the teaching of the faculties, that sought to break free of the Aristotelian heritage, create a rationally founded pathology and therapeutics, and critically re-examine the empirical tradition.[5] There developed in parallel a medical profession that strove to establish clearer boundaries between itself and non-professionals (including members of competing health-care occupations) and to base its claim not only on experience but also on the mastery of a scientific medicine not accessible even to educated laymen. Although the subject has not yet received the systematic study it deserves, a similar cleavage gradually appeared within medical literature. Chartier, for all his cautions against distinctions between popular and élite and against the commonplace notion of a seventeenth-century watershed separating an age of free, flourishing, and widely shared popular culture from an age of repression that followed, points to the increasing disjuncture in France, after about 1660, between texts for the élites and texts for the common people.[6] Within the medical domain, texts for the élites were themselves increasingly differentiated into 'technical' texts for professionals and 'popular' texts for laymen – which is not to say, of course, that no laymen read the former and no physicians read the latter. Where once the use of Latin (and abundant citations to authorities reaching back to classical Antiquity) had set *learned* works apart from *vernacular* works intended for a broader audience, by the end of the eighteenth century technical works in France were written predominantly in French and distinguished by their use of the vocabulary and methods of modern science.

The texts that most centrally concern us here are those that physicians wrote expressly for the use of laymen. Recognizing that only a privileged few would have direct access to their services, professionals sought to improve the health care available to the larger population, particularly in the countryside where medical personnel were scarce, by using popularization to raise the level of self-help and charitable assistance by educated laymen; a radical minority (as Roy Porter observes for Britain) contended that the dissemination of medical knowledge might make it possible to dispense with the services of professionals altogether, while the great majority insisted that difficult cases should remain the exclusive province of the expert. By the end of the nineteenth century, though, with the growth of the profession, the beginnings of third-party systems of payment, and the tightening nexus of medicine, laboratory, and hospital, this programme had lost much of its *raison d'être*, even if physicians continued to recognize that a well-informed laity would be better equipped to maintain health, prevent disease, and know when to summon the doctor. The late eighteenth and nineteenth centuries, on which most of the essays in this volume focus, were the heyday of medical popularization – though also of resistance to medical popularization, since the same forces that shaped a self-confident profession with strong claims to special expertise made it increasingly unsympathetic to the idea of the layman as a sort of permanent locum tenens for the absent professional.

This paper seeks to trace the working out of this paradox in France over the *longue durée;* a very similar story could be told about other Western countries (as several other contributions to this volume confirm), even if the experience of the Revolution gave a peculiar intensity to French debates over the wisdom of popularization. The present discussion will focus on texts and producers of texts rather than readers and reception, though Mary Fissell's interesting suggestions on the reading of medical texts in early modern England would be well worth pursuing in the French context; suffice it to say that, before the nineteenth century, ownership of the books considered here would have been largely restricted to an educated and fairly affluent élite. The narrative that follows divides the period it surveys into three broad phases. The first, which had its origins in the sixteenth-century Catholic Reformation, produced a spate of manuals for charitable persons, some by laymen, others by physicians, increasingly distinguished from less specialized works that might also contain medical advice; a few might arguably qualify as popularizations in the narrow sense of the term. The Enlightenment generated a far more explicit attempt to establish a new popular or domestic medicine on a scientific basis; its characteristic texts sought to correct the errors contained in previous generations of handbooks. With the early nineteenth century came a clear turn against diffusionism, associated in part with the reaction against the 'medical anarchy' of the French Revolution. At the same time, medical books and journals proliferated as never before, helped along by the general expansion of the publishing industry and by growing numbers of young practitioners struggling to make a living and hoping to eke out their meagre income from fees with the proceeds of their literary efforts. The Enlightenment tradition of medical popularization continued, but its leading exponents were widely condemned by name for, at best, overstimulating the imagination of the hypochondriac and, at worst, encouraging the inept amateur to practise medicine.

I

The vernacular literature of medical advice already constituted a substantial corpus by the end of the sixteenth century; it was, indeed, one factor that prompted the physician Laurent Joubert to write his celebrated treatise on popular medical errors, the founding text of a rich genre whose career closely paralleled that of the vernacular literature itself.[7] This Renaissance corpus, whose key texts were frequently reprinted into the seventeenth and even the eighteenth century, may be sorted into four loose and partly overlapping categories. They include the old literature of secrets, which derived from the medieval manuscript tradition and mingled medical remedies with a host of occult formulas and miscellaneous information about the properties of animals, vegetables, and minerals, and three other genres increasingly differentiated from it: magic books, which emphasized conjuring but continued to include some medical remedies; household manuals, which mixed a little medicine with a good deal of advice on cooking, housekeeping, agriculture, and animal husbandry; and the genre that most directly concerns us, handbooks devoted entirely to medicine, surgery, and pharmacy, which began to proliferate in the second half of the seventeenth century. The books of secrets were great hotchpotches of empirical lore, most of it ultimately derived from the natural philosophy of the Middle Ages and Antiquity.[8] The extensive compilations of materia medica found in most of these writings drew heavily on animal products and the old pharmacy of excrements; certain other remedies involved the use of amulets, talismans, and magical rituals and incantations.

Among the collections devoted exclusively to medicine and health, two subgenres stand out, derived, like the secrets literature, from an unbroken tradition reaching back to the late Middle Ages. The classic texts were those generally attributed to Peter of Spain (Pope John XXI, d. 1277) and Arnald of Villanova (d. 1311). On the one hand, the reader might study a regimen or art of living a long life, represented in the Arnaldian corpus by the *Rule of Health* and a commentary on the *Regimen of the School of Salerno*, which went through several French-language editions in the sixteenth century.[9] Such works emphasized living well to preserve health, though they typically included a good deal of medical and pharmaceutical information as well. On the other hand, the reader might consult Peter's

101

Treasury of the Poor, a standard medical compendium of the later Middle Ages, which listed the various parts of the body from head to foot, described the ailments to which they were subject, and recommended remedies.[10] Physicians of the French Renaissance took up and continued the health maintenance genre (though they sometimes stressed intervention rather than prevention)[11] and collections of remedies appeared among the works of the major contributors to the secrets literature, such as the physician Jean Liébault.[12]

The seventeenth century saw an even greater profusion of self-help manuals emphasizing hygiene, as well as compendia of remedies.[13] The royal midwife Louise Bourgeois (*c.* 1563–1636), for example, published her medical and cosmetic secrets, as did the surgeon – later royal physician – Nicolas de Blégny (*c.* 1646–1722). The Bourgeois is a representative guide to the old armamentarium: powdered skull as a remedy against epilepsy; an ointment prepared with herbs and dog dung and inserted on the tip of a candle into the male urethra as a treatment for gonorrhoea; burning old shoes under a *chaise percée*, against haemorrhoids; a human afterbirth applied, while still warm, to remove spots on the face.[14] (Bourgeois also published on obstetrics; but this work, like that of the eighteenth-century midwife Le Boursier du Coudray, arguably constitutes less a popularization than a textbook designed to raise the standard of practice in an occupation not yet fully professionalized.)[15]

The bulk of this literature was conceived in the spirit of the great revival of charity that flowered in the Catholic Reformation, which we associate with the familiar figure of Saint Vincent de Paul.[16] Some publications were the work of ecclesiastics, others of pious laymen without medical training, still others of philanthropic physicians. The authors nearly all felt impelled to present their efforts as gifts to the poor or, increasingly, as guides to medicine, surgery, and pharmacy for charitable persons. The French contribution to this genre provided a model for all Europe. It would be possible, but misleading, to arrange these texts along an imaginary continuum: at one extreme, works by medical laymen for laymen, in which charitable care for the poor essentially expressed Christian piety; at the other, works by physicians and surgeons whose sole object was to improve public health, especially in the countryside, by vulgarizing the principles of medicine and surgery. Even the manuals by medical men, however, sometimes mingled religious and medical concerns, notably the *Physician* and *Surgeon of the Poor* attributed to the physician Paul Dubé. The *Surgeon of the Poor*, for example, invited 'rich and charitable ladies' to care for the poor as a form of *imitatio Christi*.[17] The most prominent of the charitable handbooks, and perhaps the most successful of its kind in early modern Europe, was the *Charitable Remedies* of Madame Fouquet or Foucquet (1590–1681), mother of the celebrated superintendent of finance, Nicolas Fouquet.[18] Widely reprinted, this work was to remain in use in the countryside into the nineteenth century. In her dedication, the devout author enjoined priests to follow the example of Jesus Christ in caring for the sick; equally significant, the compendium carried the enthusiastic endorsement of a physician. The armamentarium of Mme Fouquet was an undifferentiated hotchpotch of traditional pharmacy (excrement, animal oils, echoes of the old astrological medicine), with some more recently fashionable remedies, such as mercury and antimony, thrown in for good measure. One formula, a cataplasm for burns, called for taking seven or eight droppings from a black horse that had been allowed to graze for two weeks in the month of May and fricaseeing them in lard. Another, against rabies, called for gathering a dozen different herbs in June or July during a full moon.[19]

Among physicians, Mme Fouquet's most active rival was Philibert Guibert or Guybert (1579?–1633), doctor regent of the Paris medical faculty and author of a frequently reprinted collection of little 'charitable' works.[20] Despite the titles, these texts do not have much to do with charity; they concern medicine, surgery, and pharmacy, especially the last. Guibert hoped to induce patients to prepare their own remedies under a physician's direction, thus reducing their expenditures and increasing the authority of doctors, while undermining that of the rival apothecaries. Other works, like the *Physician of the Poor* by Lazare Meysonnier (1602–72), a royal physician under Louis XIV, best remembered for his almanacs and magic books, the *Operator of the Poor* by the surgeon Vaussard, or the *Medicine of the Poor* by Praevotius (1585–1631), were more clearly intended to facilitate self-help, at least when no medical man was available.[21] Dubé, who saw himself as a successor to Guibert and Praevotius, thought that his handbook, unlike theirs, was specifically adapted to the needs of the isolated rural poor and relied on materia medica that would be available to them in the French countryside.[22] Though these works may have reflected divergent views of therapeutics, they shared a common purpose: to make medicine accessible, easy, and cheap. Some represent early examples of physicians expressly attempting to popularize what they took to be the best official medicine of their day, though the inertia of the old empirical tradition is even more apparent.

The popular medical literature of the first half of the eighteenth century continued the by now well-established genres, including works on health maintenance and handbooks for charitable persons. Mme Fouquet had her counterpart in dom Nicolas Alexandre (1654–1728), a Maurist father with Jansenist sympathies, and Guibert in the slightly younger Philippe Hecquet (1661–1737), doctor-regent of the Paris faculty (which he served as dean), physician of the Charité Hospital, and also a devout Jansenist (he once held an appointment as physician to the abbey of Port-Royal-des-Champs). Alexandre's highly successful *Medicine and Surgery of the Poor*, whose editions spanned a century and a half, was a practical handbook for charitable persons, listing diseases by parts of the body and describing time-honoured remedies and simple surgical treatments.[23] Thus for the bite of a mad dog, as an alternative to bathing in the sea (which he evidently accepted when it was convenient), he proposed the customary omelette with calcified oyster shell, for both internal and external use. Here, too, are recommended fricaseed cow dung for swollen testicles and an infusion in white wine of the droppings of a grass-fed gosling, against jaundice. Or the patient suffering from jaundice might 'piss on nettles, or on horse dung [that is] new and still warm . . . .' Some prescriptions had an astrological basis: remedies against worms, for example, should be given when the moon is waning. Others took the form of amulets: the root of the male peony, for example, suspended from the neck to prevent epilepsy.[24] The emphasis throughout was on inexpensive plant and animal products that might readily be found in the countryside – simple remedies that were frequently effective, the author argued, but which the rich rejected out of vanity; often patients who had received no benefit from the medical art were 'promptly cured by a remedy indicated by a peasant or mere woman [*femmelette*]'.[25]

Hecquet's pious intentions matched those of the Benedictine. Knowing that death was near, he offered his work as a gift to the poor, hoping in return to receive their prayers, which would stand him in good stead on the day of judgement.[26] But Hecquet aimed higher than Alexandre. Even a quick glance confirms that these volumes are more than a crude compendium of remedies. Hecquet dwelt on the underlying principles of medicine, surgery, and pharmacy, producing in effect a set of little primers; he did not hesitate, when necessary, to use a technical vocabulary, promising the reader a glossary of medical terms for assistance (ultimately added by the editor of the 1749 edition). The armamentarium remained traditional, however, if less baroque than Alexandre's. The ingredients for domestic medicine included crayfish, frogs, and snails, and the formula for a swallow's nest cataplasm to be applied to sore throats called for *album graecum* – dried and pulverized dog dung – in addition to the ingredient that gave the remedy its name.[27]

Forty years younger than Hecquet, the Orléanais physician Louis-Daniel Arnault de Nobleville (1704–78) brought out a rival *Manual of the Ladies of Charity* in 1747, less than a decade after the posthumous first publication of the Hecquet.[28] Where the latter had simply treated charitable persons as self-sufficient (warning them only to call in surgeons for all surgical procedures except blood-letting), Arnault added a strong injunction to consult physicians. 'It would be tempting God and violating the order [of things] not to consult them, because it is ordinarily through them that diseases are cured.'[29] But this is not yet a work of medical Enlightenment. Arnault included a selection of traditional therapies from the *Ephémérides d'Allemagne* of 1742: 'among these remedies, there are a few that may seem peculiar; but their efficacy is so well attested that we did not believe we should omit them'. They included fried sow's genitals as a remedy against incontinence; amulets against haemorrhoids, or, alternatively, the roots of a certain plant – as many as the number of haemorrhoids – suspended between the shoulders and allowed to dry; the shirt of a menstruating woman worn as an emmenagogue; oil of earthworms for contusions; burnt mole as a remedy against urinary incontinence; goose droppings against jaundice; horse dung against pleurisy; ivy gathered during a waning moon, against atrophy; and pounded cockchafers, against rabies. Elsewhere he recommended for the treatment of pleurisy a live pigeon split in half and applied to the patient for eighteen to twenty hours 'until the bad smell makes it necessary to remove it'.[30]

II

The older medical advice literature continued to be reprinted into the later eighteenth century and beyond, taking its place alongside new titles that mined the same traditions or proposed novel medical systems to a wide public. The era of the Encyclopedists and their epigones was also a great age of medical empiricism and the occult, inhabited by Cagliostro, Mesmer, and such lesser-known figures as François-Amédée Doppet (1753–99), medical doctor, future revolutionary general, and author of a book on magical medicine, as well as a treatise on the erotic uses of the whip and works on animal magnetism.[31] Other publications promoted self-help as a way of defeating the pretensions of the medical élite; John Wesley's *Primitive Physick*, essentially a compendium of empirical remedies with a few rules for hygiene, appeared in French translation in 1772.[32] A more abundant literature promoting parallel medicine con- sisted of the handbooks and pamphlets published by owners of proprietary remedies, some of whom were authorized medical practitioners. The surgeon Louis-Étienne Gachet's book on self-treatment of gout and rheumatism owed its existence to the author's interest in puffing an anti-gout elixir.[33] One extreme case from the end of the century was a remedy-seller's catalogue masquerading as a 'medicinal manual, which is accessible to everyone'. According to the author,

> Each person . . . will become his own physician, [and] that of his relatives and friends, since each article indicates (1) the name of the remedy; (2) the conditions for which it is suited; (3) the method of using it; (4) the regimen to follow during the use of the remedy and the course of the disease.[34]

The Enlightenment did not create a radically new popular medical literature; instead it took up and refashioned each of the old genres. The campaign against vulgar errors called forth expurgated and philosophical versions of the old compendia, sometimes corrected beyond recognition. The reformed popular books were purged of magic, archaic natural science, and references to aphrodisiacs, abortifacients, and other 'indecent' topics. A 'modern' version of the old *grimoire* or magic book attributed to Albertus Magnus and known in French as the

Grand Albert appeared in 1768, the work of Pons-Augustin Alletz (1705?–85), a prolific author of potboilers, many of which, like his *Handbook of the Man of the World*,[35] he designed to appeal to the upwardly mobile middle class. The new *Albertus* contained a great deal of information on medicine (though not sexual matters, well covered in its predecessors) and other practical subjects, all more or less in accord with contemporary natural science.[36] So, too, a version of the sixteenth-century domestic handbook known as the *Rustic House* appeared at the end of the eighteenth century 'purged of its errors'.[37]

The campaign to cleanse popular medical books of superstition and the old polypharmacy went hand in hand with a renewed emphasis on hygiene and health maintenance; the conjunction of these two programs marked the medical Enlightenment throughout Europe, as Maria Szlatky's essay in this volume on the Hungarian case would suggest. An ancient tradition identified regimen and the six non-naturals with philosophy, whereas remedies of the sort collected by Pliny the Elder belonged to the vulgar domain. The idea that we should first of all live correctly to avoid ill-health accorded with the neo-Hippocratic outlook of the physician–*philosophes*, and as professionals they naturally argued that hygiene was the area in which self-help was most clearly appropriate. It is not surprising that Diderot's *Encyclopédie* gave a prominent place to the articles by Arnulphe d'Aumont (1720–82) on health, regimen, and the non-naturals,[38] or that in the second half of the eighteenth century the presses spewed forth new works on health maintenance and re-editions of the old ones. Luigi Cornaro's *Advice for Living a Long Time*, for example, was reprinted in French translation.[39] Other works included a *Guardian of Health* by Le Bègue de Presle (1735–1807), who was Rousseau's physician, a translation of George Cheyne's Latin treatise on conserving the health of the infirm (his *Essay of Health and Long Life* had been translated earlier in the century), and even an *Almanac of Health* that emphasized the non-naturals.[40]

The manuals on health maintenance did not, however, supplant medical advice literature, much of it by physicians; indeed, it proliferated even more rapidly than before. Young and ambitious doctors, it was said, joined hands with enterprising small publishers to make a reputation for the one, and profits for the other.[41] (Roy Porter's observations on the commercialization of medicine in Georgian England could apply to

Old Regime – though better still to nineteenth-century – France.) Recipe collections continued to appear as well, and formulas were published in the provincial and local journals that started life in the second half of the century.[42] Many of these works, like their predecessors, spoke to the needs of priests and other charitable persons in rural areas, though others aimed at a middle-class audience. One explicitly addressed 'the ladies of charity in the countryside'.[43] More typically, the word 'charity' did not appear in the title, which in this age of enlightened *bienfaisance* might refer instead to self-treatment, domestic medicine, or medicine or pharmacy for the people.[44] Some books claimed to be useful as well to country surgeons, implicitly demoted to subprofessional status.[45]

How much medical instruction did such works offer? Some titles suggested that readers would learn how to be their own physician, though closer inspection often reveals that the author had more modest intentions. A 1759 portable dictionary of health, which has been attributed to Charles-Augustin Vandermonde (1727–62), a doctor-regent of the Paris medical faculty, made such a promise but at the same time served, according to the author, to establish the 'importance and necessity of [the physician's] art'.[46] When Jean-Nicolas Jadelot (1738–93), the most distinguished professor of the medical faculty of Nancy, published his *Pharmacopoeia of the Poor*, he wrote that he had bowed reluctantly to the public taste for 'familiar and domestic medicine', which had reached the point where it was necessary to have books that 'teach how to treat diseases without being a physician'. He hoped simply to reduce abuses and facilitate charitable medicine by making available a few simple and reliable formulas.[47]

Perhaps the farthest-reaching proposal for a popular medical publication surfaced at the end of the revolutionary decade, in the spring of 1799, when the father–son team of Jean Verdier (1735–1820), physician and specialist on medical jurisprudence, and Jean-François Verdier-Heurtin (1767–1823), surgeon and contributor of articles on medical jurisprudence to the *Encyclopédie méthodique*, issued a prospectus for a journal of popular medicine, education, and economics. They took as their motto, 'Esto tibi medicus', 'thou shalt be thy own physician', although in translating the phrase they weakened it to 'Let each man be his first physician'. Like all the enlightened reformers, they made it their primary goal to purge popular medicine of error and superstition, but they added a more grandiose programme, directed, as they put it, towards the health and perfection of man.[48] The most typical popular works by physicians still sought to supplement rather than replace the services of trained practitioners. The *Mountain Physician*, published at Grenoble in 1762 with the approbation of two local medical men, no doubt won their consent because the author proposed only inexpensive remedies suitable for the poor; he expected that the rich would always consult physicians when they were sick and that the poor would do so in serious cases – when they had been bitten by a mad dog, for example.[49] Some texts offered only a limited discussion of therapeutics. The *New Advice to the People*, for example, published in 1789 by Petit-Radel (1749–1815), was essentially a first-aid handbook; the *Manual for the Service of the Sick* by the royal physician Carrère (1740–1802), which secured the imprimatur of the Société Royale de Médecine, dealt mainly with nursing care.[50] Books that did more were meant to fill the regrettable gaps in the network of licensed practitioners. Pierre Roussel (1742–1802) warned his readers at the outset of his *Domestic Medicine*:

We do not pretend here to teach medicine to people who have never made a particular study of it – that would be to deceive them . . . It would put in their hands a dangerous weapon, all the more deadly in that it would inspire them with a false sense of security.[51]

The profession generally accepted modest works of this kind, if they were well made.

Of all the enlightened popular medical handbooks, two quickly emerged as classics of the genre: the *Advice to the People* by the Swiss physician Samuel-Auguste Tissot (1728–97), first published in 1761,[52] and the *Domestic Medicine* (1769) of William Buchan (1729–1805), which first appeared in French translation in 1775.[53] Tissot's work, as Antoinette Emch-Dériaz notes, was translated into at least thirteen European languages; although Buchan's work largely supplanted it in the English-speaking world, it held its own on the Continent. In France, Spain (as Enrique Perdiguero indicates), and probably elsewhere in western Europe, the two shared pride of place as models of their kind; in eastern Europe, Maria Szlatky's essay would suggest, the prestige of francophone culture allowed Tissot to predominate. It is hard to speak of one without mentioning the other. Almost exact contemporaries and fellow Calvinists, the Scotsman and the Swiss greatly admired each other. Indeed, Buchan presented his book as an extension of Tissot's, while Tissot, in a treatise on perfecting medical education, warmly recommended both his own work and Buchan's as a vade-mecum for country surgeons.[54]

Tissot clearly stated his intentions at the outset of his handbook. He had not written a medical text for physicians, but rather a practical work for the benefit of the rural poor, or, more precisely, for the educated persons who might assist them, as well as rural surgeons and midwives who needed a manual to reinforce their rudimentary training. This handbook was very different from a compilation of remedies to take down from the shelf when someone fell ill. Tissot provided simple but precise clinical descriptions and explanations of diseases and criticized earlier writers on charitable medicine, such as Mme Fouquet, for failing to do so. Although he omitted chronic disorders, believing that their causes were too complex to allow non-physicians to deal with them, his work provided a comprehensive little course on medicine and pharmacy.

Tissot's object in explaining medicine was not to turn every layman into a physician. Although he did not provide the detailed consideration of regimen that could be found in the works on living a long life, he did stress the value of hygiene and prevention, and he enjoined his readers to summon a trained professional in serious cases. Rather than multiply the number of practitioners, he hoped that an acquaintance with the field would promote respect for the medical art and discourage incompetent meddling by the unqualified. Indeed, like all his enlightened colleagues, Tissot saw a negative or critical side to his enterprise: to disabuse the people of their superstitious errors and discourage them from employing dangerous domestic remedies and consulting empirics. Better no medicine at all than a destructive medicine.

Tissot's contribution won wide, if not universal, acclaim from enlightened physicians in France and elsewhere; indeed, the chief reason that Buchan gave for bringing out a new manual only a few years after Tissot's had appeared in English translation[55] was simply that his Swiss colleague, by choosing to omit a discussion of chronic disorders, and by neglecting the details of hygiene, had robbed his important work of much of its value. The parallels between the two works are striking. Both combined practical advice on remedies and health care with an introduction to the principles of medicine. Buchan, like Tissot, laid a Rousseauian emphasis on temperance and exercise, calling regimen the most important part of medicine. Like Tissot, moreover, Buchan did not mean

that all men are to be made physicians. This, according to the present acceptation of the word, would be an attempt as ridiculous as it is impossible. We only mean that they should be taught the importance of due *care* for the preservation of health, and of a proper *regimen* in diseases.

In serious cases, patients should consult qualified practitioners whenever possible. Yet both authors recognized that it was not always possible to do so:

Nothing is farther from the design of the following pages, than to induce ignorant persons to tamper with dangerous medicines, or trust to their own skill, where better assistance can be obtained. But where something must be done, and no medical assistance can be had, it is certainly better to direct people what they ought to do than to leave them to blunder on in the dark.

The alternative would be to allow quacks and popular superstitions to retain their hold over the masses.[56]

Although he shared Tissot's conception of the limits of popular medicine, Buchan brought a stronger sense of mission to his campaign for the diffusion of medical knowledge. Inspired by the Scottish Enlightenment's enthusiasm for popular education and the political radical's distrust of established monopolies (as Roy Porter stresses in his essay for this volume), he sharply attacked the notion that medical learning should be confined to the profession. Secrecy aroused suspicion among the public, hindered scientific progress, and encouraged abuses, including quackery. Starting with the second edition (1772), Buchan spoke of 'laying medicine open', a phrase borrowed from a 1770 work by his friend, colleague, and fellow diffusionist, John Gregory.[57]

The French version of Buchan, by J.-B. Duplanil (1740–

1802), a medical graduate of Montpellier and physician to the comte d'Artois, appeared in 1775 and by 1789 had attained a fourth edition.[58] An enthusiastic popularizer, Duplanil added extensively to Buchan's discussions of diseases and therapies and even appended a supplement, a sort of dictionary and abbreviated textbook of medicine; later, after the Revolution, he published his own medical handbook for travellers.[59] In his preface, Duplanil praised Buchan as superior to Tissot, because he covered hygiene and chronic diseases. Defending the book against critics of popularization, he reiterated Buchan's argument that education would counteract popular errors and the influence of quacks and confidently maintained that the work would prove invaluable in the countryside. Certainly the text enjoyed rapid success and, although in France its popularity never rivalled that of Tissot, French-speaking physicians ranked it with the *Advice to the People* as an exemplar of the genre of enlightened medical popularization.

The reasons for the prestige of Tissot and Buchan are not far to seek. Their works were more than a guide to hygiene, on the one hand, or a recipe book on the other; they had written, in Charles Rosenberg's phrase, 'both a book to read and a book to use'.[60] They aimed, moreover, at the highest level of *haute vulgarisation*, describing and explaining diseases and basing their recommendations on the best recent work in medicine.

Not all of the new wave of authors who purported to initiate laymen into the secrets of medicine were so careful, or so well-informed; even Buchan and Tissot, moreover, had their detractors. There is no space here to consider in any detail the controversies over enlightened medical handbooks,[61] but the central paradox should be underscored: the same developments in medical thinking and practice that led some physicians to produce increasingly sophisticated texts for laymen impelled many of their colleagues to question the popularization of medicine and, indeed, the very conception of self-help. Justifications of domestic medicine had rested on three related assumptions that the sceptics could no longer accept without reservation: the value of self-knowledge and instinct; the predominance of hygiene and regimen over therapeutics; and the autonomy and relative simplicity of practice (such as a surgeon might learn) as opposed to theory (such as a physician might learn). On the first point, it was said that a seriously ill patient might be unaware of his own state.[62] Hygiene, too, had its limits;

Pinel, for one, saw 'presumptuous incompetence' behind the notion that through natural regimen every man could be his own physician.[63] The new clinical medicine, finally, demanded a mastery of pathology and physiology as the foundation for therapeutics.[64] By the beginning of the nineteenth century, a consensus seems to have emerged among the French medical élite that the use of popular medical books needed to be more sharply circumscribed. The physician Laurent Bodin (1762–1839), himself an active publicist and promoter of a proprietary 'tonic-stomachic pill', offered this disclaimer in a work of the Year VIII (1799–1800) that provided a digest of other medical publications:

> Those who are not masters of the anatomy and physics of the human body, of chemistry and all the sciences that make up [medical] theory, cannot suppose, without danger, that by using a work such as the *Advice to the People* by Tissot, the *Domestic Medicine* of Buchan, etc., you can decide the character of a disease and try to apply remedies.

The laity should learn only hygiene, preventive measures, and first aid, together with information on the dangers of quacks and popular errors. Only in this way could one make medicine 'domestic and popular' and successfully teach it in the schools, or through books for the cultivated reader.[65] Indeed, one has to search hard among the nineteenth-century French medical élite to find wholehearted and unapologetic defenders of Tissot and Buchan. It is no doubt significant that the last French editions of Buchan appeared at the beginning of the nineteenth century, whereas the work lived on in its native tongue for nearly seven more decades.[66] Similarly, Tissot's *Advice to the People* petered out in the nineteenth century, while publishers still eagerly reissued his *Onanisme*.[67]

III

That the medical élite of the nineteenth century mostly condemned popular medical books, even enlightened ones, did not, of course, stem the flow of new ones from the presses; the output, indeed, swelled considerably, thanks to rising literacy, new technologies that lowered the cost of the printed page, and the continued development of the consumer society.[68] Some popularizers took up the Verdiers' idea of a medical journal for laymen and, although the early attempts ended in failure,[69] at least eighteen such periodicals, by one count, were published in the three decades from 1825 to 1858.[70] In addition, some more serious journals, such as the *Gazette de santé,* were aimed in part at a lay audience, and few 'professional' journals could claim a readership composed exclusively of medical men.[71] The *Gazette*'s editor at the beginning of the nineteenth century, P.-J. Marie de Saint-Ursin (1763–1818), was himself the author of an enlightened handbook for laymen and an eloquent defender of popularization and of Tissot, a great man who had been persecuted for doing the right thing; but he had to acknowledge, somewhat testily, that no one 'had not had the danger of popularizing medicine dinned into his ears'.[72] At a more demotic level, new almanacs and even broadsides gave basic advice on routine ills and some less routine ones, such as cholera.[73] For all the doctors' aspersions, popularization flourished in the nineteenth century as never before.

In this vast corpus, it is not hard to recognize descendants of the various early modern genres. Here, for example, are works on health maintenance and the art of living a long life, including translations of the major foreign contributions: Hufeland's treatise on 'macrobiotics', for example, in which he insisted (*pace* Rousseau) that culture could help men live longer in society than in a state of nature,[74] or Anthony Willich's work on diet and regimen, abridged, adapted, and put into French by Dr Itard (1775–1838) of the National Institute for Deaf–Mutes, better remembered as the tutor of the wild child of Aveyron.[75] So, too, one finds some traditional books of secrets and charitable medicine, with many of the old recipes intact: dried and pulverized magpie brain, against epilepsy, or an infusion of chicken droppings in white wine as a *vin de chute,* for accident victims.[76] The latter recipe also appears as a remedy against pleurisy in an 1839 version of dom Alexandre's *Medicine of the Poor,* a work presented as a compromise between old and new.[77]

The more modern texts, often called *Medicine Without a Physician*[78] or *Domestic Medicine,*[79] typically offered systematic advice for dealing with the most common diseases and injuries; some, including an imposing *Catechism of Health* (far removed from Bernhard Christoph Faust's earlier work of the same title, which emphasized hygiene), proposed to give the layman a more general grasp of the principles of medicine.[80] Without necessarily claiming that their readers could dispense with the physician's services entirely, the more outspoken authors insisted that medicine could be vulgarized – it was accessible to anyone with good sense, argued the author of *Medicine within Everyone's Reach*[81] – and that where physicians were unavailable, enlightened self-help and charitable medicine were preferable to no treatment at all. The *Popular Almanac of Health* of Jean-Louis-Auguste Clavel (1808–*c.*1876), ecclesiastic and medical graduate of the Paris faculty, managed to combine injunctions against usurping the profession's prerogatives with detailed descriptions of the use of vesicants, cupping glasses, leeches, cataplasms, sinapisms, and the like.[82] (Despite the plethora of over-the-counter remedies available in the late twentieth century, the nineteenth-century home medicine chest would have boasted a much larger proportion of the standard armamentarium.) Descriptions of diseases were often remarkably complete. Many such works were still aimed at the literate élites of isolated rural areas, including, in some cases, inexperienced practitioners, although industrialization inspired a few proposals for teaching hygiene and a fear of charlatans to the working class,[83] and one author counted manufacturers among his potential readers.[84] But it should be stressed that these publications were often cheap, typically priced between one and three francs; lower costs and the rising literacy rates made possible by the spread of primary education, starting with the Guizot reforms of the July Monarchy, resulted in a more genuinely 'popular' readership than in the past. In short, the eighteenth-century project of diffusing medical enlightenment was still very much alive; indeed, several of these works were presented as perfected or updated versions of Tissot and Buchan.[85] The title of one work, *New Advice to the People on Its Health*, recalled Tissot, while another, *The French Buchan*, candidly proclaimed the source of its author's inspiration.[86]

When the writers justified their enterprise, however, they expressed themselves in self-consciously defensive tones. 'The truly educated professional [*homme de l'art*] is not afraid to popularize his language and procedures', declared Joseph-Marie Audin-Rouvière (1764–1832), physician, critic of Broussais's excessive use of leeches, and author of a highly successful *Medicine without a Physician (Médecine sans médecin)*, who lived well from the proceeds of his book and of his purgative 'grains of health' until a greater purgative, the cholera, carried him off.[87] For the current of professional opinion that condemned popular medical books could not be ignored; the publications that won the approval of the profession's intellectual leaders were those that sharply circumscribed the medical information they made available to laymen.

Something of this characteristic *pudeur* can be seen in several works published under the Consulate and First Empire, such as the *Almanac of Health* of 1811. The frontispiece depicted volumes of Tissot, Buchan, and the *Gazette de santé*, together with Rousseau's *Émile*, but, in keeping with Tissot's own intentions, the text stopped well short of teaching medicine to the people:

> Entrusting the practice of medicine to the people would be, as everyone keeps repeating, like putting a blade in the hands of a blind man, with the risk that he might strike the patient instead of the disease . . . We wish to teach each person, not how to cure his diseases, but how to prevent them through a wise regimen, and how to act when he is indisposed.[88]

Similarly, Auguste Caron, in his *Manual of Health* of 1805, while he still hoped to enlighten the people, proposed to give them, not Tissot – a work suitable only for doctors – but merely the elements of hygiene and the means of avoiding illness.[89]

This was to be the model for the next several decades and beyond. The modern domestic medical handbook taught hygiene, routine first aid and limited self-help, disdain for quacks and superstitions, and respect for the profession. 'A patient', intoned one *Popular Almanac of Health*, 'should be visited by his physician early and often'.[90] The influence of Tissot's *Advice to the People* was perhaps less in evidence than that of his *Onanisme:* avoidance of masturbation was one of the salutary precepts of hygiene and preventive medicine that could be, nay had to be, taught to the people.[91] Treatment would be limited to minor remedies in routine cases,[92] even if the book's title sometimes suggested otherwise (as was true of the work misleadingly called *Surgery without a Surgeon*).[93] One author prudently decided to limit himself to 'generalities' to prevent misuse of his book.[94] And readers were reminded, *ad nauseam*, that in all but the most trivial cases they should summon a trained physician; one manual was even intended, among other things, to aid patients in discussing their case with their physician.[95] Some of the presumably underemployed physician–authors thoughtfully provided their addresses and office hours in their books.[96] Why, then, write such a volume? To attract clients, cynics suggested. Above all because bad ones existed, the authors maintained; their fond hope was that in this domain Gresham's law would be inverted, and the good coin would drive the bad out of circulation. Some people would always continue to meddle in the medical domain, and in the homely metaphor of the *Weekly Gazette of Health*, an ill-starred project of 1823, 'it is, after all, wiser to guide a blind man who insists on walking at the edge of a precipice, than to abandon him to the terrible fate that awaits him'.[97]

The popular medical journals in general followed a similar approach, with the notable difference that their periodical format allowed them to keep readers abreast of the most recent developments in the world of medicine by reviewing technical books and reporting on the proceedings of the Academy of Medicine: no updated version of Buchan or Tissot could hope to perform this function.[98] *Health: Journal of Medical and Scientific Popularization*, founded under the Second Empire, argued that 'science until now has lacked a truly popularizing journal' and went so far as to list courses offered at the faculty of medicine.[99] It had much to say, in addition, about hygiene and first aid, but the scientific information was meant to divert and instruct rather than to turn laymen into medical practitioners. A predecessor entitled *Health: Journal of Public and Private Hygiene*, edited by the physician G. Richelot, carefully distinguished between a health journal and a medical journal destined for physicians; it described prevalent diseases without recommending therapies and reported on Morton and Jackson's experiments with ether while insisting on the risks of this procedure and the need to leave anaesthesia to the professionals. Self-treatment was limited to such innocuous therapies as the application of acetic acid to warts.[100] This broadly humanistic thrust is most apparent in the journals that mingled medical with non-medical news and book reviews, such as the polemical journal *Hygie*, which in 1826 published an admiring account of the abolition of the death penalty in Brazil, a notice on John Lingard's history of England, and a review of a play entitled *A*

Recipe for Marrying One's Daughter – though there was also room, the next year, for an account of a report presented to the Academy of Medicine on a new uterine speculum.[101]

The authors of popular medical books that deviated sharply from the accepted wisdom came, on the one hand, from the ranks of promoters of secret remedies and heterodox medical systems, and, on the other, from a much smaller number of writers, both physicians and laymen, who, like the eighteenth-century English trio described by Roy Porter, objected on more general principles to the profession's secrecy and exclusiveness.

The success of proprietary remedies obviously depended on widespread self-medication and required advertising directed to a lay public. As in the eighteenth century, certain entrepreneurs brought out popular books of medical advice as vehicles for their publicity; some contemporaries, indeed, asserted that the scribblings of the 'pill merchants' accounted for the bulk of popular medical publications.[102] This estimate may be exaggerated, but the works of successful remedy vendors such as Audin-Rouvière, Giraudeau, and Leroy were undoubtedly among the most prominent handbooks of the early nineteenth century.

In his *Medicine without a Physician*, Dr Audin-Rouvière, despite his strictures upon popular medical errors, did not hesitate to tout the virtues of his toni-purgative and grains of health.[103] Giraudeau 'de Saint-Gervais' (1802–61), who exploited the supposed vegetable remedy against syphilis known in the Old Regime as the rob Laffecteur, together with another, 'regenerative' rob, promoted his specialities in books with titles like *The Manual of Health* and *The Art of Curing Oneself.*[104] In its heyday, his organization produced a *Medical Gazette* in French, Spanish, Greek, Russian, Italian, Dutch and English editions, whose real purpose seems to have been to provide lists of his agents in France and various foreign countries.[105] Similarly, the health officer Jean Pelgas and his son-in-law Louis Leroy, whose aptly named purgative and vomi-purgative were the most notorious and among the most dangerous proprietary medicines in early-nineteenth-century France, turned out a variety of popular medical publications, including a periodical;[106] the principal work, a book entitled *Curative Medicine*, sold very cheaply by mail order, defended regular purging as the panacea for human ills. The Pelgas/Leroy system rested on a view of the human body and disease not far removed from popular humoralism; the body contained within itself a germ of innate corruption that developed at certain periods of life, vitiating the blood and humours. This corruption was responsible for all diseases; the patient was like a cask with foul dregs that needed to be rinsed several times before the wine that was kept in it would stay good.[107] Pelgas's appealingly simple system also inspired popular medical books by other hands, though not everyone shared his exclusive devotion to his cure-all.[108] Similar principles informed the system of James Morison (1770–1840), self-appointed president of a British College of Health and promoter of Morison's Pills and other purifiers of the blood, whose works in French translation, like those of his French disciples, gained wide currency in the middle decades of the century.[109] The undeniable popularity of these publications, and of the powerful purgatives and emetics that they promoted, despite the condemnation of the Royal Academy of Medicine, drove one Paris physician, D.J. Goblin, to counterattack with a *Physician without Medicine (Médecin sans médecine)*; in this inversion of the usual title, 'medicine' referred, as it often did in popular speech, to a laxative.[110]

Other radical diffusionists drew on the standard liberal arguments against censorship to justify the dissemination of medical knowledge, though not necessarily medical practice by laymen. The author of a *Little Household Physician*, a medical doctor (or so the title page claimed) identified only by his initials, suggested that at a time when serious study was widespread, and the mass of the people had acquired an 'almost prodigious' fund of general knowledge (he was writing in 1828), one should not be too fearful of mishaps caused by reading popular books; in difficult cases the amateur could turn to a professional for advice (though the author did not hesitate, for example, to recommend ergot to speed childbirth).[111] A similar line of argument appeared in *True Medicine without a Physician* by J. Morel de Rubempré, physician, active supporter of the Revolution of 1830, and prolific author. (His other publications included an adaptation of Hufeland's macrobiotics, various works on venereal disease, treatises on such subjects as impotence and masturbation, Lavater's system of physiognomy, and prostitution, and a handbook of eugenics called *The Secrets of Generation* – a title recalling a section of the *Grand Albert* – which revealed techniques that supposedly enabled readers to predict the sex of their unborn offspring and endow them with intelligence and beauty; he also wrote extensively on politics and medicine.)[112] Morel's object was not to make readers completely independent of the physician; his models (and, in his view, the only authors of truly useful works) were Tissot and Buchan. But patients could not always find a physician when they required one, and, quite apart from the occasional need for self-treatment, Morel insisted on extending medical learning beyond the official medical corps. 'Why concentrate in one body alone', he asked, 'knowledge that is precious and necessary for the happiness of all?'[113]

The greatest contribution to the diffusionist cause came later in the July Monarchy and from outside the professional camp: Raspail's *Natural History of Health* of 1843,[114] which defended freedom of medical instruction (but not practice); his *Family Physician* of the same year, which publicized his camphor cigarettes and related panaceas;[115] and above all his *Annual Handbook of Health*, which first appeared in 1845 and was then reissued every year, or nearly so, for decades thereafter (a seventy-seventh edition, by then greatly altered, came out in 1935).[116] To these works must be added the popularizations by his admiring disciples.[117] Like Morel de Rubempré, Raspail (1794–1878) was a veteran of the Revolution of 1830.[118] Morel edited a *Friend of the Peoples* in 1830; Raspail, a more specifically political *Friend of the People* in 1848 (both titles echo the title of Jean-Paul Marat's newspaper of 1789).[119] Raspail was the more radical proponent of self-help: 'The author's goal in writing this book has been to teach the patient to dispense with the pharmacist's services and the physician's attendance, at least in the most ordinary cases'. The only sort of medicine that could not be popularized was not real medicine, but scholastic fakery: 'any practice that is not based on an idea that is accessible to the vulgar is an irrational practice . . . People have been getting well more surely and more quickly ever since medicine has become less learned and has sought to popularize itself'.[120] But Raspail, unlike Morel, was not a physician. Not content to write medical books, he ran a dispensary where he gave consultations, under the cover of a licensed practitioner named Cottereau. The profession and the authorities intervened, and in 1846 Raspail was tried for illegal medical practice and convicted, though the only penalty was a minor fine.[121] For Raspail, science and democracy, theory and practice, were inseparable, and the popularization of medicine became an act of defiance. A similar role was played later in the century by the celebrated healer known as the zouave Jacob, who called Mesmer a martyr, damned the medical profession, and promoted his own brands of natural hygiene, humoralist medicine, and herbal remedies.[122]

Popular medical literature continued to flourish into the Third Republic and beyond, stimulated rather than stifled by the Pasteurian revolution and the growing prestige of medical science. The new medicine called forth new and more scientific works of vulgarization, such as the *Popular Dictionary of Current Medicine and Public and Private Hygiene*, by the positivist and anticlerical physician Paul Labarthe (1844–94), hailed by Jules Guérin of the Academy of Medicine for 'popularizing without lowering [standards]'.[123] Other, more modest, publications continued to emphasize routine hygiene and first aid. One text from 1905, quaintly entitled *Popular Medicine for the Use of Man and Animals*, evenly divided between human and veterinary medicine, chiefly offered advice on the measures to take 'while waiting for the man of science', who might be several kilometres away (though like many other medical publications, it also carried advertisements at the end for proprietary remedies).[124] From more recent periods, together with family medical handbooks fully endorsed by the profession, we find works that appeal to an interest in homeopathy, natural forms of healing and *la médecine douce*.[125] But such texts are offered either as modest adjuncts to professional medical treatment or as alternatives to regular or 'allopathic' medicine; they do not purport to teach laymen the essentials of medical theory and practice. Even the celebrated *Larousse médical*, first published on the eve of World War I by Dr Émile Galtier-Boissière (1857–1919), professedly technical enough 'to be useful even to physicians', celebrated popularization only as a means to promote hygiene and to remind the reader of the necessity of consulting a physician in the early stages of an illness. The *Larousse* was not intended to replace the doctor but rather 'to make the reader a physician's assistant'; the medications that it mentioned were to be prepared only by pharmacists, and only in accordance with a doctor's prescription.[126] The profession's position was neatly summarized in a banquet address on 'la vulgarisation médicale' delivered in 1893 by Dr Ernest Monin to a society of scientific journalists. Medical popularization, which should emphasize prevention over treatment, could reassure the patient, inspire confidence in the medical art, and discourage the use of quacks and patent remedies. It might even serve the profession by reaffirming basic principles and rescuing physicians from a narrow specialization. But it would not turn laymen into their own physician.[127]

As the long view taken in this paper suggests, the corpus of popular medical literature is remarkable for its continuity; it is possible, however, to discern three broad and overlapping developments stimulated in part by programmes of reform. The first of these movements, in the sixteenth but even more the seventeenth century, attempted to extract the most useful medical advice from an empirical tradition reaching back to Antiquity to create a specifically medical guide to self-help and charitable treatment. The second, in the Enlightenment, sought to improve and rationalize the established genres of popular books and produced a substantially modified version of one of them, an enlightened medical handbook that would base amateur practice firmly on the principles of medical science. The third, visible in the Enlightenment and then emerging with increasing force after the Revolution, sharply challenged the idea of popularizing anything more than hygiene, preventive medicine, and first aid, even for educated readers. Thanks especially to the rapid growth of the periodical press, innovations in medical science were more widely reported than ever before, but the reader was meant to admire rather than emulate.

All these developments had their parallels outside France, even if the charitable impulse of the Catholic Reformation and the nineteenth-century reaction against self-help achieved a peculiar intensity there: one of the overarching themes of this volume might be the international character of medical popularization, as the large number of translations readily attests.[128] None of these developments was wholly favourable to medical popularization narrowly defined. The last condemned it; the first subordinated medical science to the empirical tradition, on the one hand, and religious faith on the other; and the second attacked popular error with greater vigour than it promoted self-help. Nor should this surprise us. Professionalization and popularization are not, in the end, fully compatible enterprises. Yet they coexisted, and that story forms a crucial chapter in the history of modern medicine.

Notes

Unless otherwise indicated, the place of publication of books is Paris.

1. 'Raspail, pseudo-vulgarisateur', in Poirier and Claude Langois (eds), *Raspail et la vulgarisation médicale* (1988), 103–27. See also J. and J.-L. Poirier, 'La Vulgarisation médicale: Considérations philosophico-historiques', *Revue d'éducation médicale* 6 (1983), 184–90.
2. See, for example, Richard Whitley, 'Knowledge Producers and Knowledge Acquirers: Popularisation as a Relation Between Scientific Fields and Their Publics', in Terry Shinn and Whitley (eds), *Expository Science: Forms and Functions of Popularisation*, Sociology of the Sciences, 9 (1985), 3–28.
3. 'Raspail, pseudo-vulgarisateur', 115–18.
4. Chartier, *The Cultural Uses of Print in Early Modern France*, trans. Lydia G. Cochrane (Princeton, 1987), 3, 6.
5. See L.W.B. Brockliss, *French Higher Education in the Seventeenth and Eighteenth Centuries: A Cultural History* (Oxford, 1987), chap. 8, 'Medicine'.
6. Chartier, *Cultural Uses of Print*, 8, 181, and *passim*.
7. Laurent Joubert, *Erreurs populaires et propos vulgaires touchant la médecine et le régime de santé . . .* (Bordeaux, 1579). See Natalie Zemon Davis, 'Proverbial Wisdom and Popular Errors', in her *Society and Culture in Early Modern France* (Stanford, 1975), 260.
8. For a guide to this literature, see John Ferguson, *Bibliographical Notes on Histories of Inventions and Books of Secrets*, 2 vols (London, 1959).
9. *Le Régime très-utile et très-proufitable pour conserver et garder la santé du corps humain (exposé par maistre Arnoul de Villeneuve et corrigé par les docteurs régens à Montpellier* (Loudun, n.d.); *Regimen sanitatis en françoys . . .* (Lyons, 1501).
10. Peter of Spain, *Thesaurus pauperum . . .* (Antwerp, 1497, and later edns); cf. the treasury of the poor attributed in part to Arnald, *S'ensuit le trésor des povres qui parle des maladies qui peuvent venir au corps humain et des remèdes ordonnez contre icelles . . .* (1512).
11. See, for example, Jean Goeurot, *Le Sommaire et entretènement de vie très singulier de toute médecine et cirurgie . . .*, trans. from the Latin by Claude Grivel (n.d.); the earliest dated edn is from 1530.
12. Jean Liébault, *Thrésor universel des pauvres et des riches, ou Recueil de remèdes faciles, pour toute sorte de maladies . . .* (1651).
13. On the underlying medical ideas, see Andrew Wear, 'Popularized Ideas of Health and Illness in Seventeenth-century France', *Seventeenth-century French Studies*, 8 (1986), 229–42.
14. Louise Bourgeois (Boursier), *Recueil des secrets de Louyse Bourgeois, dite Boursier . . . auquel sont contenues ses plus rares expériences pour diverses maladies, principalement des femmes, avec leurs embellissemens* (1635), 2, 77, 89, 163, and *passim*. Nicolas de Blégny, *Secrets concernant la beauté et la santé, recueillis et publiez par ordre de M. Daquin . . . , premier médecin de Sa Majesté . . .* , 2 vols (1688–9). Blégny, an ambitious surgeon of uncertain reputation, began as a bandagist/hernia specialist and wound up as a royal physician; he was stripped of his title in 1693 and imprisoned at Angers for fraud.
15. Louise Bourgeois, *Observations diverses sur la stérilité, perte de fruict, foecondité, accouchement et maladies des femmes et enfants nouveaux*

naiz . . . (1609 and later edns); Angélique-Marguerite Le Boursier du Coudray, *Abrégé de l'art des accouchemens* . . . (1759 and later edns). Alison Kairmont Lingo is now working on the Bourgeois and related texts, and Nina Gelbart is preparing a book-length study of Le Boursier du Coudray.

16. On the 'medicine of the poor', see Mireille Laget, 'Les Livrets de santé pour les pauvres aux XVIIe et XVIIIe siècles', *Histoire, économie, et société*, 3 (1984), 567–84. On charitable care and the Catholic Reformation, see the essays in Colin Jones, *The Charitable Imperative: Hospitals and Nursing in Ancien Régime and Revolutionary France* (London, 1989).

17. Dubé, *Le Chirurgien des pauvres, qui enseigne le moyen de guérir les maladies externes par des remèdes faciles à trouver* . . . (with *Le Médecin des pauvres* in 1 vol., 1669), 'L'Autheur aux dames riches et charitables'. See Jean Emelina, 'Le Médecin des pauvres et le chirurgien des pauvres: un témoignage sur les aspects et l'esprit de l'éducation médicale populaire au temps de Louis XIV', *Le XVIIe siècle et l'éducation*, supplement to *Revue Marseille*, no. 88 (1972), 85–95.

18. Marie de Maupeou, Mme François Fouquet, *Recueil de receptes choisis, expérimentées & approuvées* . . . (Villefranche, 1675, and many subsequent edns at Paris, Lyons, and Dijon; title varies).

19. *Les Remèdes charitables de Madame Fouquet* . . . (Lyons, 1681), 97–8, 136–8, 198–200.

20. Guibert, *Le Médecin charitable* . . . (1624), *L'Apothiquairie du médecin charitable* . . . (1625), reprinted separately and together with other works in collections with varying titles.

21. Lazare Meysonnier, *Le Médecin charitable* . . . , 2nd edn (Lyons, 1668); G. Vaussard, *L'Opérateur des pauvres* . . . (1636); Jean Prévost (Praevotius), *Medicina pauperum* . . . (Frankfurt, 1641) and *La Médecine des pauvres* . . . (1646).

22. Dubé, *Le Médecin des pauvres* (1671), 'Avis au lecteur'.

23. Alexandre, *La Médecine et la chirurgie des pauvres, qui contiennent des remèdes choisis, faciles à préparer et sans dépense* . . . (1714). See Mireille Laget and Claudine Luu, eds, *D'après le livret de Dom Alexandre: Médecine et chirurgie des pauvres au XVIIIe siècle* (1984), which gives excerpts and a biographical sketch.

24. Alexandre, *Médecine des pauvres* (1758), 463, 157, 159 (quotation), 229, 217, 17.

25. ibid., preface, a iiR.

26. Hecquet, *La Médecine, la chirurgie, et la pharmacie des pauvres*, new edn, 4 vols (1749), 1: 2. On Hecquet's medicine, see L.W.B. Brockliss, 'The Medico-Religious Universe of an Early Eighteenth-Century Parisian Doctor: The Case of Philippe Hecquet', in Roger French and Andrew Wear, eds, *The Medical Revolution of the Seventeenth Century* (Cambridge, 1989), 191–221.

27. *Médecine* . . . *des pauvres* (1749), 4: 42, 193. For the glossary, see 3: 164–242.

28. Louis-Daniel Arnault de Nobleville, *Le Manuel des dames de charité, ou Formules de médicamens, faciles à préparer, dressées en faveur des personnes charitables, qui distribuent des remèdes aux pauvres dans les villes et*

dans les campagnes . . . (Orléans, 1747). The Bibliothèque Nationale assigns joint authorship to the Orléans physician François Salerne, one of the signers of the dedication in subsequent edns. At least five new edns appeared in the next two decades.

29. *Manuel,* preface, p. xii.

30. ibid., 5 and 334–63.

31. Doppet, *Médecine occulte, ou Traité de magie naturelle et médicinale* (1791); *Aphrodisiaque externe, ou traité du fouet et de ses effets sur le physique de l'amour* (Geneva, 1788); *Traité théorique et pratique du magnétisme animal*. . . (Turin, 1784).

32. Wesley, *Médecine primitive, ou Recueil de remèdes choisis & éprouvés par des expériences constantes, à l'usage des gens de la campagne, des riches & des pauvres* . . . (Lyons, 1772); *Primitive Physick: or, An Easy and Natural Method of Curing Most Diseases* (London, 1747).

33. Gachet, *Manuel des goutteux et des rhumatistes, ou l'Art de se traiter soi-même de la goutte, du rhumatisme, et de leur complication*. . . (1786).

34. Catalogue of Belle, calling himself a physician of Paris and Montpellier, quoted in Louis Faligot, *La Question des remèdes secrets sous la Révolution et l'Empire* (1924), p. 139.

35. Alletz, *Manuel de l'homme du monde, ou Connaissance générale des principaux états de la société et de toutes les matières qui sont le sujet des conversations ordinaires* (1761).

36. Alletz, *L'Albert moderne, ou Nouveaux secrets éprouvés et licites, recueillis d'après les découvertes les plus récentes* . . . 2 vols (1768; subsequent edns in 1769, 1773, 1780, 1782). Medicine constitutes one of three classes of secrets; the others are the useful (household and gardening hints, for example) and the agreeable (painting, flowers, and so on).

37. Louis Liger, *La Nouvelle Maison rustique,* La Bretonnerie (ed.), 11th edn, 2 vols (chez Samson, 1790); earlier edns date from 1700. Cf. *L'Agriculture et maison rustique de M. Charles Estienne*. . . (1564). Estienne died in 1564; Jean Liébault completed and extended the work, and later edns carry his name.

38. See William Coleman, 'Health and Hygiene in the *Encyclopédie:* A Medical Doctrine for the Bourgeoisie', *Journal of the History of Medicine and Allied Sciences* 29 (1974), 399–421.

39. Luigi Cornaro, *Conseils pour vivre long-temps, traduits de l'italien de Louis Cornaro*. . . (1783), reprint of 1701 translation by de Prémont.

40. Achille-Guillaume Le Bègue de Presle, *Le Conservateur de la santé, ou Avis sur les dangers qu'il importe à chacun d'éviter, pour se conserver en bonne santé et prolonger sa vie* (1763). George Cheyne, *L'Art de conserver la santé des personnes valétudinaires, et de leur prolonger la vie*. . . (1755), trans. of *Tractatus de infirmorum sanitate tuenda* (London, 1626, and Paris, 1742); *Essai sur la santé et sur les moyens de prolonger la vie* (1725), trans. of *An Essay of Health and Long Life* (London, 1724, and later edns). *Almanach de santé* (1774).

41. *Gazette de santé,* 1785, no. 1, and 1787, no. 15, cited in Harvey Mitchell, 'Rationality and Control in French Eighteenth-Century Views of the Peasantry', *Comparative Studies in Society and History* 21 (1979), p. 100, n. 48.

42. See, for example, Pierre Rambaud, *La Pharmacie en Poitou jusqu'à l'an XI* (Poitiers, 1907), 41, on the *Affiches du Poitou*; and A. Baudot, *Études historiques sur la pharmacie en Bourgogne avant 1803 . . .* (1905), 527, on the *Affiches de Dijon.*

43. *Lettres adressées aux dames de charité de la campagne, par M. Martin, ancien apothicaire de l'hôtel de l'École royale militaire & des hôpitaux de l'Armée*, 2nd edn (Auxerre, 1786).

44. See, for example, Daniel Langhans, *L'Art de se traiter et de se guérir soi-même dans les maladies les plus ordinaires et les plus dangereuses . . .* , trans. from the German by Marc-Antoine Eidous, 2 vols (1768); *La Médecine domestique: Ouvrage très-utile & très-nécessaire à toutes sortes de personnes, & particulièrement aux gens de la campagne . . .* (Nantes, 1780); Jean-Nicolas Jadelot, *Pharmacopée des pauvres, ou Formules des médicamens les plus usuels dans le traitment des maladies du peuple . . .* (Nancy, 1784).

45. See, for example, Vignon, sieur de Vignoles, *Essai de médecine-pratique, pour l'usage des pauvres gens de la campagne, afin qu'ils puissent se secourir eux-mêmes, et pour l'instruction des jeunes chirurgiens qui s'y établissent*, 2 vols (1745).

46. Vandermonde, *Dictionnaire portatif de santé dans lequel tout le monde peut prendre une connoissance suffisante de toutes les maladies, des différens signes qui les caractérisent chacune en particulier, des moyens les plus sûrs pour s'en préserver, ou des remèdes les plus efficaces pour se guérir, et enfin de toutes les instructions nécessaires pour être soi-même son propre médecin . . .* , 2 vols (1759), 1: iii.

47. Jadelot, *Pharmacopée des pauvres*, 'But de l'auteur en publiant ces formules'.

48. Prospectus for *Journal de médecine populaire, d'éducation, et d'économie . . .* (1799).

49. *Le Médecin des montagnes* (Grenoble, 1762), cited in Madeleine Rivière-Sestier, *Remèdes populaires en Dauphiné*, 2nd edn (Lyons, 1943), 3, 25–8.

50. Philippe Petit-Radel, *Nouvel avis au peuple, ou instructions sur certaines maladies qui demandent les plus prompts secours . . .* (1789); Joseph-Barthélemy-François Carrère, *Manuel pour le service des malades, ou Précis des connaissances nécessaires aux personnes chargées du soin des malades, femmes en couches, enfans nouveaux-nés, &c.* (1786).

51. Roussel, *Médecine domestique*, 3 vols (1790–92), 1: 1.

52. Samuel-Auguste-André-David Tissot, *Avis au peuple sur sa santé . . .* (Lausanne, 1761, and at least 25 subsequent edns and printings); the expanded 3rd edn in 2 vols (Lausanne, 1767) was the basis for later edns. See Lazare Benaroyo, '*L'Avis au peuple sur sa santé*' *de Samuel-Auguste Tissot (1728–1797): la voie vers une médecine éclairée*, Zürcher medizingeschichtliche Abhandlungen, 195 (Zürich, 1988), and Antoinette Emch-Dériaz, 'Towards a Social Conception of Health in the Second Half of the Eighteenth Century: Tissot (1728–1797) and the New Preoccupation with Health and Well-Being', Ph.D. thesis, University of Rochester, 1983.

53. William Buchan, *Domestic Medicine, or the Family Physician: Being an Attempt to Render the Medical Art More Generally Useful, by Shewing*

People What Is In Their Own Power Both with Respect to the Prevention and Cure of Diseases, Chiefly Calculated to Recommend a Proper Attention to Regimen and Simple Medicines . . . (Edinburgh, 1769); *Médecine domestique, ou Traité complet des moyens de se conserver en santé, de guérir & de prévenir les maladies par le régime & les remèdes simples* . . . (Edinburgh and Paris, 1775). The best introduction to the work and the problem of its audience and influence is Charles E. Rosenberg, 'Medical Text and Social Context: Explaining William Buchan's *Domestic Medicine*', *Bulletin of the History of Medicine* 57 (1983), 22–42. See also C.J. Lawrence, 'William Buchan: Medicine Laid Open', *Medical History* 19 (1975), 20–35, and Roy Porter's essay in the present volume.

54. Tissot, *Essai sur les moyens de perfectionner les études de médecine* (Lausanne, 1785), 166.

55. *Advice to the People in General, with Regard to their Health* . . . (London, 1765, and later edns).

56. *Domestic Medicine* (Edinburgh, 1769), 'Advertisement', ix–x, xiv.

57. ibid., vii–viii; Lawrence, 'William Buchan', 22–5.

58. *Médecine domestique*, 4th edn, 7 vols (1789). Vols 6–7 were taken from the Swiss physician Johann Friedrich von Herrenschwand's *Traité des principales et des plus fréquentes maladies externes et internes: à l'usage des jeunes docteurs en médecine, des chirurgiens-médecins et des practiciens qui suppléent au défaut des médecins gradués, ainsi qu'à celui des personnes éclairées, qui, par des motifs de bienfaisance, exercent la médecine dans les campagnes, ou qui peu à portée des secours de l'art, sont obligés d'être leur propre médecin et de médicamenter ceux qui les environnent* (Berne, 1788); a 2nd separate edn of the latter carried the title *Médecine domestique* (Berne, 1795).

59. Duplanil, *Médecine du voyageur* . . . , *suivie d'un essai de médecine pratique sur les voyages, considérés comme remèdes*, 3 vols (1801).

60. Rosenberg, 'Medical Text', 24.

61. I intend to deal with the debate over self-help more extensively elsewhere, in a companion volume, now in preparation, to my *Professional and Popular Medicine in France, 1770–1830: The Social World of Medical Practice* (Cambridge, 1988).

62. On the question of self-knowledge and self-help, see Evelyne Aziza-Schuster, *Le Médecin de soi-même* (1972).

63. Philippe Pinel, 'Mémoire sur la manie périodique ou intermittente', *Mémoires de la Société Médicale d'Émulation* 1 (Year VI), 119, quoted in Mitchell, 'Rationality and Control', 101.

64. Michael Foucault, *The Birth of the Clinic: An Archaeology of Medical Perception*, trans. A.M. Sheridan Smith (New York, 1973), 35, associates the decline of self-help and regimen with the rise of a medicine based on a conception of physiological 'normality' rather than 'health'.

65. Bodin, *Bibliographie analytique de médecine, ou Journal abréviateur des meilleurs ouvrages nouveaux* . . . , 3 vols, (1799–1801), 1: xix, xxxiv–xxxv.

66. The Bibliothèque Nationale owns an 1802 edition of the Duplanil translation and a publication of 1804 combining the *Médecine*

domestique with other works by Buchan. The US *National Union Catalog* lists 39 English-language editions and reissues of Buchan published between 1800 and 1863; Rosenberg has identified an edition published in Philadelphia in 1871 ('Medical Text', p. 22).

67. The US *National Union Catalog* records 3 nineteenth-century French-language editions of the *Avis au peuple*, 2 French (1803 and 1830) and 1 Swiss (1892); the catalogue of the Bibliothèque Nationale includes none. The *NUC* lists 11 nineteenth-century French-language editions and printings of *L'Onanisme: Dissertation sur les maladies produites par la masturbation*, published between 1802 and 1870; the BN lists 22, published between 1813 and 1886, plus 1 from 1905. On the latter text, see Ludmilla Jordanova, 'The Popularization of Medicine: Tissot on Onanism', *Textual Practice*, 1 (1987), 68–79.

68. For an overview of the nineteenth-century works, see Aziza-Schuster, *Médecin de soi-même*, chap. 10, 'Médecine domestique et médecine sans médecin'.

69. See, for example, the *Semaine médicale et d'économie domestique*, which ran from 4 October 1817 to 10 January 1818.

70. Jacques Léonard, 'Les Guérisseurs en France au XIXe siècle', *Revue d'histoire moderne et contemporaine* 27 (1980), 513. The actual number, counting short-lived attempts, was almost certainly much higher.

71. Léonard, ibid., reports that in 1825, for example, 20 of 92 subscribers to the *Journal de médecine du département de la Meurthe* were not employed in medicine.

72. Marie de Saint-Ursin, *Manuel populaire de santé à l'usage des personnes intelligentes vivant à la campagne* . . . (1808), i–viii (quotation, p. iii).

73. On almanacs: see, for example, Archives nationales, F^8 156, petition from Graziani, 8 December 1814, requesting a subscription from each prefect for his enlightened almanac, *Le Trésor salutaire* (1811). For a reproduction of a broadside, see Françoise Loux, *Pratiques et savoirs populaires: le corps dans la société traditionnelle* (1979), 149, 'Le Médecin de la ville et de la campagne'.

74. Christoph Wilhelm Hufeland, *L'Art de prolonger la vie humaine* . . . (Lausanne, 1809), trans. from his *Die Kunst das menschliche Leben zu verlängern*, 2 vols (Vienna, 1797) and later edns.

75. *Hygiène domestique, ou l'Art de conserver la santé et de prolonger la vie mis à la portée des gens du monde* . . . , 2 vols (1802), trans. and adapted from Anthony Florian Madinger Willich, *Lectures on Diet and Regimen* (London, 1799).

76. [Cherfils], *Les Petits Secrets de la médecine des pauvres, contenant des remèdes choisis, faciles à préparer et sans dépense, pour la plupart des maladies internes et externes qui attaquent le corps humain*, new edn (Tournon 1831), 12–13; Elie Besnard du Château, *Le Manuel de charité: Pharmacopée, ou recueil de remèdes* . . . *mis au jour pour être distribué gratuitement aux pauvres* (Tours, 1866), cited in Jacques-Marie Rougé, *Le Folklore de la Touraine* (Tours, 1931), 210.

77. *La Médecine, la chirurgie et la pharmacie des pauvres, contenant des*

remèdes faciles à préparer et peu chers . . . par * * *, médecin de la faculté de Paris . . .* (1839), 89.

78. See, for example, the fairly traditional *Nouvelle médecine sans médecin . . . Ouvrage à l'aide duquel chacun peut se traiter soi-même . . .* trans. and adapted by Lendrain from a German work by Burckard (1828; 5th edn, 1853); and Louis Clerc (physician), *La Petite médecine sans médecin, ou l'Art de se guérir soi-même d'un grand nombre de maladies, par des moyens les plus simples et les mieux éprouvés* (Orléans, 1832). The Clerc was sufficiently current to include cholera. Charles Nisard, in his survey of popular books, sarcastically noted Lendrain's disclaimer that his work was not 'une spéculation de médecin sans clients qui veut faire du bruit pour gagner de l'argent', which is what it clearly seemed; *Histoire des livres populaires*, 2nd edn, 2 vols (1864), 1: 222.

79. See, for example, Pierre-Joseph Buc'hoz, *Nouvelle médecine domestique, tirée principalement des végétaux de la France . . .* , 2nd edn, 2 vols (1805). The works of Buc'hoz, a prolific writer on botany, popular medicine, and related subjects, take up $28^1/2$ columns in the catalogue of the Bibliothèque Nationale.

80. Dr Piquet, *Catéchisme de santé, ou Traité philosophico-médical, théorique et pratique, composé et mis à la portée de tout le monde* (Strasbourg, 1830). Cf. Faust, *Gesundheits-Katechismus zum Gebrauche in den Schulen und beym häuslichen Unterrichte* (Bückeburg, 1794); *Catechism of Health for the Use of Schools and for Domestic Instruction*, trans. J.H. Basse (Dublin, 1794). The work was also translated into several other languages, including Latvian, though never into French, despite an enthusiastic endorsement by the commission on education attached to the revolutionary National Convention's Committee of Public Safety; see Archives Nationales D XXXVIII 3, dossier 46, 'Rapport de la Commission exécutive de l'instruction publique au Comité d'instruction publique sur trois ouvrages allemands du Docteur Faust'.

81. Louis-Auguste Lesage, *La Médecine à la portée de tout le monde, ou Moyen de connaître et distinguer toutes les maladies à leur début, de prévenir ou d'empêcher leurs dangereux effets: Ouvrage utile aux pères de famille, aux gens de la campagne, et généralement à toutes personnes éloignées des premiers secours de la médecine* (1827), vii–viii.

82. Clavel, *Almanach populaire de santé: le médecin de soi-même, hygiène de la famille à la ville et à la campagne*, 2nd edn (1844). See the recommendations for treating the victim of the bite of a rabid dog, which begin with cauterizing the wound and proceed to administering Van Swieten's liquor, an alcoholic solution of mercuric chloride (49–50).

83. G.-J.-Auguste Bonhoure, *Nouvelle médecine du peuple, ou analyse succincte et claire de cette science* (1828), 5. Cf. Dr Victor Mailfert, *Almanach populaire de santé pour 1854: Ouvrage spécialement dédié aux ouvriers de la ville et des campagnes* (1854), which, without proposing to teach medical theory to the masses, argued that 'l'exemple des peuples indiens nous prouve qu'avec les médicaments de nature, on peut être, quoiqu'on en dise, son propre pharmacien et son propre médecin' (5).

84. Félix-Séverin Ratier, *Nouvelle médecine domestique*, 2 vols (1825–6), 1: 7.

85. See, for example, Marie de Saint-Ursin, *Manuel populaire*, i; Ratier, *Nouvelle médecine domestique*, 1: 2; M.-J.-F.-Alexandre Pougens, *Dictionnaire de médecine pratique et de chirurgie, mis à la portée de tout le monde, ou Moyens les plus simples, les plus modernes, et les mieux éprouvés de traiter toutes les infirmités humaines*, 2 vols (1813–14), 1: xi–xii. Pougens was also the author of a traditional health maintenance work: *L'Art de conserver la santé, de vivre longtemps et heureusement, avec une traduction, en vers français, des vers latins de l'École de Salerne* (Montpellier, 1825).

86. C. Colin, *Nouvel avis au peuple sur sa santé, ou Exposition et développement des principes modernes de la médecine, à l'usage des personnes qui n'ont pas étudié cette science* (1831); Dr Émile-Auguste Bégin, *Le Buchan français: Nouveau traité complet de médecine usuelle et domestique* (1836). The Bégin, which was to be delivered in instalments, starting with sections on anatomy, physiology, and hygiene, was never completed.

87. Audin-Rouvière, *La Médecine sans médecin* . . . 7th edn (1826), 12. The first edn appeared in 1823, the 16th in 1863.

88. *Almanach de santé, ou Étrennes d'hygie aux gens du monde* (1811), 186.

89. Caron, *Manuel de santé et d'économie domestiques, ou Exposé des découvertes modernes* . . . (1805), xvi and *passim*.

90. Amédée Massart, *Almanach populaire de la santé et de la maladie* (Luçon, 1856), 35.

91. See, for example, Bonhoure, *Nouvelle médecine du peuple*, 156–7; and see also Jordanova, 'Popularization of Medicine'.

92. See, for example, Joseph-Ch. Valpêtre, *Manuel de santé, ou Moyens simples et faciles de se traiter soi-même dans les maladies qui ne réclament pas rigoureusement la présence d'un médecin: Ouvrage utile aux pères et mères de famille; aux chefs d'établissemens où se trouvent réunis beaucoup d'individus; aux voyageurs; aux habitans de la campagne qui ne sont pas à portée des médecins, ou n'ont pas les moyens de les appeler: et généralement à quiconque veut se traiter soi-même dans les cas où cela est possible sans danger* (1824) – a work whose title says it all. For a manual exclusively limited to first aid, but whose title initially recalls the more ambitious works of vulgarization, see *Médecine populaire sur les premiers secours à donner dans les empoisonnemens et les asphyxies* (n.d. [1848]).

93. Chaponnier, *La Chirurgie sans chirurgiens* . . . *indiquant au peuple les premiers secours à porter au début de toutes les maladies* . . . , 2nd edn (1832). In case the second phrase in his title did not make his purpose sufficiently clear, the author added that 'son titre de *Chirurgie sans chirurgiens* ne veut pas dire qu'en le lisant on pourra se passer de chirurgiens' (v–vi). Chaponnier was also the editor of a short-lived popular medical journal, *Le Médecin du peuple: Journal de santé et d'économie domestique* . . . , which lasted from December 1827 until May of the following year.

94. Marie-Joseph Sambin, *Le Médecin philanthrope, ou Lettres sur la médecine, adressées au clergé des campagnes et à toutes les personnes qui, par bienfaisance, se livrent au traitement des maladies* (1827), ii.

95. Jean-Louis Michu, *Manuel de médecine et de chirurgie à l'usage du peuple* (1830), i.

96. See, for example, Valpêtre, *Manuel de santé*, and J.-M. Lambon, *Almanach de santé pour l'an XIV* . . . (Year XIV/1805–06).

97. *Gazette hebdomadaire de santé*, no. 1, Lyons, Jan. 1823.

98. This point is made explicitly in the *Gazette de santé à l'usage des gens du monde*, 1 (1833), xiii.

99. *La Santé: Journal de vulgarisation médicale et scientifique illustré*, 1, 1 Nov. 1867.

100. *La Santé: Journal d'hygiène publique et privée à l'usage des gens du monde*, 3 (1847), 1, 11–14, 33–4, 40–8, and *passim*.

101. *Hygie: Journal de santé et d'économie domestique: littérature, moeurs, théâtres: par une société de médecins et de gens de lettres*, 2 Nov. and 31 Dec. 1826. *Hygie: Recueil de médecine, d'hygiène, d'économie domestique; extraits d'ouvrages, nouvelles des sciences; mélanges critiques, historiques, et littéraires; revue générale des journaux de médecine, de pharmacie, et des sciences accessoires; bulletin de bibliographie générale*, 1 (1827), 61. Both were the work of Dr Charles-Jean-Baptiste Comet, notorious for his running battles with the Parisian medical establishment; an earlier version was begun by the prominent surgeon Pierre-François Percy in 1823.

102. See, for example, Ulysse Trélat, *De la Constitution du corps des médecins et de l'enseignement médical* . . . (1828), 27, n. 1.

103. Audin-Rouvière, *La Médecine sans médecin*.

104. Jean Giraudeau de Saint-Gervais, *Manuel de santé, ou l'Art de guérir soi-même des dartres et des maladies organiques* . . . *par le traitement végétal dépuratif du Dr Giraudeau de Saint-Gervais* . . . (1834); another, undated version has a title beginning *Le Médecin sans médecine. L'Art de guérir soi-même, ou Traitement des maladies vénériennes sans mercure* . . . (1827; at least 14 edns).

105. The Bibliothèque Nationale has a collection from ca. 1849.

106. *Gazette des malades, ou Recueil des faits pratiques de médecine, de chirurgie et de chimie*, a weekly begun in 1823 and suppressed by the government in 1824 ('Aux abonnés de la *Gazette des malades*', 31 August 1824, explaining to subscribers why they had not received no. 48).

107. Leroy, *La Médecine curative, ou la Purgation dirigée contre la cause des maladies, reconnue et analysée dans cet ouvrage*, 5th edn, 1817. The title of earlier edns differs slightly. A 19th edn was published in Brussels as late as 1852.

108. See, for example, Charles Le Maout (pharmacist), *Le Médecin de soi-même: Avis au peuple sur les moyens de conserver et de rétablir sa santé* (Saint-Brieuc, 1851).

109. See, for example, Morison, *Nouvelles vérités médicales, ou Connaissance des causes des maladies, ouvrage indispensable aux personnes qui veulent conserver leur santé* . . . (1839), and Dr V.-C. Charles de Saint-Félix, *Morisoniana français, ou Nouvelle doctrine médicale de l'hygeist Morison, président du Collège britannique de santé* (1836).

110. Goblin, *Le Médecin sans médecine, ou le Charlatanisme dévoilé; Ouvrage inverse de la médecine sans le médecin, et dont le but est de prouver que la vie des hommes est toujours exposée entre les mains de ceux qui ignorent l'art de guérir* (1830).

111. L.M.L., *Le Petit Médecin des ménages, ou Recueil des médicaments les plus efficaces, avec des réflexions sur la manière de les préparer et administrer* (1828), 15 and *passim.*

112. Morel de Rubempré, *Véritable médecine sans médecin, ou Sciences médicales mises à la portée de toutes les classes de la société* . . . (1826); a 6th edn appeared in 1829. For a list of Morel's other works, see Adolph Carl Peter Callisen, *Medicinisches Schriftsteller-Lexicon der jetzt lebenden Aerzte* . . . , 33 vols (Copenhagen, 1830–45), 30: 435–8.

113. *Véritable médecine,* vi.

114. François-Vincent Raspail, *Histoire naturelle de la santé et de la maladie chez les végétaux et chez les animaux en général, et en particulier chez l'homme; suivie du Formulaire pour une nouvelle méthode de traitement hygiénique et curatif,* 2 vols (1843).

115. *Médecine des familles, ou méthode hygiénique et curative par les cigarettes de camphre, les camphatières hygiéniques, l'eau sédative, etc., contre une foule de maux lents à guérir* . . . , 6th edn (1844).

116. *Manuel-annuaire de la santé, ou Médecine et pharmacie domestiques, contenant tous les renseignements théoriques et pratiques nécessaires pour savoir préparer et employer soi-même les médicaments, se préserver ou se guérir* . . . (1845).

117. See, for example, Dr Fl. Dubois (pseudonym of Louis-François L'Héritier], *Le Médecin de soi-même, moyen sûr et peu coûteux de se préserver et de se guérir de toutes les maladies, d'après la méthode de M.F.-V. Raspail,* 2nd edn (1844).

118. On Raspail's life and work, see Dora Weiner, *Raspail: Scientist and Reformer* (New York, 1968), and Poirier and Langlois, *Raspail.*

119. *L'Ami des peuples et du perfectionnement physique et moral de l'homme* . . . (title varied), 17 numbers, 1830. *L'Ami du peuple en 1848,* 21 numbers, 1848.

120. *Manuel-annuaire de la santé pour 1854* (1854), viii, 10.

121. *Procès et défense de F.-V. Raspail, poursuivi le 19 mai 1846, en exercice illégal de la médecine devant la 8e chambre (police correctionnelle)* . . . (1846).

122. See, for example, Henry Jacob, *L'Hygiène naturelle par le zouave Jacob, ou l'Art de conserver la santé et de se guérir soi-même* (1868), and *Charlatanisme de la médecine: son ignorance et ses dangers dévoilés par le zouave Jacob, appuyés par les assertions des célébrités médicales et scientifiques* . . . , 5th edn (1877), 6–15 on Mesmer.

123. Labarthe, *Dictionnaire populaire de médecine usuelle, d'hygiène publique et privée,* new edn, revised by Antoine de Soyre, 2 vols (n.d. [1897]), quotation: 1, ii; 1st edn, 1885. See Jacques Poirier, 'Les Discours parallèles dans le *Dictionnaire populaire de médecine usuelle, d'hygiène publique et privée* de Labarthe', *Revue internationale d'histoire de la psychiatrie,* 3 (1985), 25–36.

124. Jean de Saint-Ybault, *La Médecine populaire à l'usage de l'homme et des animaux* (Niort, 1905), 6.

125. See, for example, Henri Mangin and G. Millot, *Huit cents remèdes d'hier et de toujours, empruntés au folklore et inspirés du bon sens populaire* (1946), or Gérard Coutaret, *Le Nouveau Médecin des pauvres: 1,500 recettes pratiques* (1951).

126. Galtier-Boissière *et al.*, *Larousse médical illustré* (1912), v–vi.
127. Monin, *La Vulgarisation médicale: Allocution prononcée le 17 avril 1893* [at the 151st banquet of the Réunion amicale de la presse scientifique] (1893).
128. To stress the parallels is not to deny national differences. Nineteenth-century American works of domestic medicine form a particularly striking contrast to their French counterparts, many of them advocating drastic forms of self-help or amateur practice extending to surgery. See John B. Blake, 'From Buchan to Fishbein: The Literature of Domestic Medicine', in Guenter B. Risse *et al.*, eds, *Medicine without Doctors: Home Health Care in American History* (New York, 1977), 11–30, and Norman Gevitz's essay in this volume, which emphasizes the emergence of a distinctive American domestic medical handbook in the nineteenth century.

5

The non-naturals made easy

Antoinette Emch-Dériaz

As far as one looks into the medical past, one sees physicians concerned as much with curing diseases as with preventing illnesses. Regimen or a healthy way of life seems almost to have been the most potent arm of medicine up to the twentieth century and the discovery of antibiotics; and today a sane lifestyle is still the best investment against poor health. Thus, a large part of medical writings of the past dealt with health, hygiene, and disease prevention, rather than with cures, in order to teach ever larger numbers of the people how to keep healthy. The non-naturals (i.e. diet and exercise) were central to this tradition of popularized medicine until the nineteenth century when the term became obsolete with the complete demise of Galenic medicine.

In this chapter, I will focus on how diet and exercise were reinterpreted by eighteenth-century physicians, in particular Tissot, so as to appeal to the 'natural' mentality and drive for education propounded by the *philosophes*. But first, let me recall some medical definitions of the past. Physicians then understood that health depended on the seven naturals, the six non-naturals, and the three contra-naturals.[1]

Physiology dealt with the seven naturals:
- elements (fire, air, water, earth)
- qualities (hot, cold, dry, moist)
- humours (blood, phlegm, yellow bile, black bile)
- members
  - fundamental (brain, heart, liver)
  - subservient (nerves, arteries, veins)
  - specific (bones, membranes, muscles)

– dependent (stomach, kidneys, intestines)
- faculties (natural, spiritual, animal)
- spirits (natural, vital, animal)
- operations (hunger, digestion, retention, expulsion),

which are given by the constitution of the body.

Hygiene expounded on the use of the six non-naturals:
- air
- food and drink
- motion and rest
- sleep and waking
- retentions and evacuations, and
- the passions of the soul,

which do not depend on our nature but which profoundly affect the body.

Pathology studied the three contra-naturals:
- diseases
- their causes, and
- their sequels,

which attack the integrity of the body.

Hygiene, as well as physiology and pathology, was understood as an article of medical knowledge and as such was taught along these categories in the schools of medicine up to the end of the Old Order.[2]
Ancient physicians recognized that the body's constitution was out of reach of their art, that their remedies and treatments were too often unable to cure, and that their best hope of healthy patients lay with hygiene (or with preventive medicine in today's parlance). Hence, since Antiquity, the non-naturals have been used by the physicians of the well-to-do to inform their clients about the benefit of a healthy lifestyle. To consult a physician or a treatise of medical advice for information on how to watch over one's air, food and drink, exercise and sleep, bodily functions, and mental affections was a luxury that few could afford in Antiquity and far beyond, until a time when printing, wider literacy, and a higher standard of living allowed a larger percentage of the population to be aware of and to act upon the possibilities of bettering their health through hygiene learned from written sources. Thus, for centuries, the prevention of diseases through the practice of hygiene and under

the care of a physician remained the privilege of an élite who, however, did not always heed the advice about the proper use of the non-naturals and often preferred the quick results of purging and bleeding to correct their excesses.

Humoral physiology as elaborated by Galen from the School of Cos' Hippocratic Corpus served particularly well to explain how the non-naturals affected the balance of the humours. Pathological conditions understood in terms of plethora, depletion, and corruption of the humours were amenable to regimen, thus the preservation, conservation, and restoration of health depended on the non-naturals. Yet, by the same token, the cure of diseases provoked by unbalanced humours was thought to be achieved by means of direct action on the quantity and quality of humours through sweating, purging, vomiting, bleeding, or any other forced evacuations. In this respect, humoral medicine was no different from our own medicine, swinging over time in pendulum fashion, its emphasis shifting from curing to preventing disease with the changing intellectual premises of its practitioners. Hygiene waxed and waned, its fate linked to that of classicism.

For centuries, the Hippocratic Corpus (in particular *Diaetetica, On Airs, Waters, and Places*) and Galen's writings served as a base for much of the teaching and commentaries on hygiene. These works were adapted to new circumstances with translations into Latin (e.g. Celsus' *De re medicina*, first century AD) and Arabic (e.g. Avicenna's Canon, tenth to eleventh century), or versification for easier memorization of the material (the most famous example remains the *Regimentis Sanitatis* of the Schola Salernita, eleventh century). There were also attempts to present a successful system for personal health in a cogent form (the best known are *De triplici vita* by Marsilio Ficino (1433–99) and *Trattato de la vita sobria* by Luigi Cornaro (1475–1566)). Furthermore, these classics motivated medical writers (Laurent Joubert and George Cheyne among many) to repeat old wisdom in new ways in order to bring it to the attention of the public: 'As the ancients are not so frequently read, the advantage of modern works, which do not contain a single idea that is new, is to place before us useful truths that have been forgotten'.[3]

Consequently, in the closing decades of the eighteenth century, with literacy and affluence on the increase and faith in heroic medicine on the decrease, an opportunity appeared to widen the audience that could understand the proper use of the non-naturals; this opportunity was seized by physicians such as Samuel-Auguste Tissot (1728–97) and William Buchan (1729–1805). What the neo-hippocratic spirit of the Montpellier School of Medicine had taught its students (among them Tissot who graduated from Montpellier in 1749) was extended out of the classroom to the lay public willing to learn how to improve their health. Certainly, and not only in the field of medicine, a new awareness of the teaching and example of the Ancients as well as a ubiquitous attraction to nature and to whatever was perceived as 'natural' emerged in the eighteenth century. Artificiality in all its forms became suspicious and engaged the inquiry of cultural, medical, social, philosophical, and political critics who declared it a great perverter of human nature. A tension thus appeared between the late seventeenth-century ideal of the '*honnête homme*', polished by civilization and living in the amiable world of the city, and the mid-eighteenth-century view of the '*homme naturel*' found in the Noble Savage of far-away exotic places. A dichotomy developed in the meaning and purpose of the civilizing process: progress for some, corruption for others. However, it would lead us too far afield to explore all the ramifications of the eighteenth-century discourse on progress and corruption; its arguments have been cogently reviewed by Malcolm Jack.[4] It should be enough here to recall that urban centres, rather than rural spaces, were perceived as deleterious to one's mental, physical, and even financial equilibrium because of all the demands to keep up appearances that city or court living imposed on its participants. A marked increase in nervous disorders seemed to plague the well-to-do; some physicians, Tissot among them, thought that the corruption brought about by luxury and easy living was at the root of the problem, which could be controlled by private hygiene. Several social critics (the most famous being Rousseau[5]) perceived the élite as lost in futile pursuits which not only damaged their health but also prevented them from attending to their duties as leaders of society. This sickly traditional élite should heed the advice of physicians and *philosophes* or else risk losing their privileged position to a more sturdy and determined stock, namely the emerging élite of talents.

With a medical perspective of the problem of progress and corruption, physicians recast the traditional Galenic non-naturals, still embedded in humoral physiology, yet also refurbished in terms of the new physiology of irritability based on Albrecht von Haller's research, to fit the 'natural' mould.[6] These doctors also responded with impatience to the fatalism and inertia of the educated élite, and played on the new perception of the goodness of nature and the depravity of society, to advocate hygiene. Furthermore, they referred to new diseases (e.g. syphilis, onanism), novel treatments (e.g. Peruvian bark, digitalis), and recently learned preventive measures (e.g. inoculation) to buttress their arguments for a renewed medical approach to health.

To set the tone of any inquiry into the eighteenth-century frame of mind a look at the *Encyclopédie* is a must. Medicine had the lion's share in this monumental enterprise, and the Enlightenment was later described in terms of medicine.[7] Numerous articles in the *Encyclopédie* are devoted to medical subjects, and most relevant for our topic being '*Hygiène*' in tome VIII and '*Choses non-naturelles*' in tome XI. The author of the article on '*Hygiène*' insisted on the different roles played by patient and physician in the health of the concerned individual. Hygiene is meant for preserving health and its precepts should be followed by the patient; in contrast, therapeutics is concerned with restoring health and its tools ought to be the prerogative of the physician.[8] Clearly, here, we have the *Encyclopédie*'s didactic purpose made plain. However, only the correct use of the non-naturals is to be taught to the lay public, not the prescription of remedies, since choice of treatment ought to be the privilege of licensed doctors: 'It is with this well-considered knowledge that one can become one's own physician, not to prescribe correctly one's remedies, but to preserve oneself from diseases resulting from the lack of a proper diet'.[9]

The author went on to note that, when the six non-naturals are well used, they become the naturals, that is part of our constitution and well-being. On the contrary, when they are misused, they turn into the contra-naturals which make us sick. Thus it is of the utmost importance, the author insisted, for a health-conscious person to learn about the non-naturals and understand fully the influence they have on our well-being:

> So, when one enjoys good health and that the question is only to keep it with sobriety and moderation, one can avoid consulting a physician, and exposing oneself to be the victim of ignorance; when health fails and one is

threatened by disease, diet and water are the best remedies for preventing the danger of their sequels.[10]

In the *Encyclopédie*, its editors and contributors wanted to
appeal to the reason and common sense of their readers and
entice them to try self-help in all areas of their life, beginning
with their health, arguing that without health not much else in
life can be accomplished or enjoyed. The advice the *Encyclopédie*
had to offer on health and hygiene has been closely analysed by
the late William Coleman.[11] However, in its time, the *Encyclopédie*
was an expensive set of books to own and its *in extenso* version
took years to complete.[12]

Soon, a sense that a public wider than the wealthy subscribers
to the *Encyclopédie* was keen on self-help induced physicians and
other writers to address the challenge of popularizing medical
advice.[13] Publishers also became aware that the sale of full-folio
books was limited to a small portion of the literate public
because of their high price, while the cheaper octavo format
would find a ready market with the educated of the 'middling
set'. For them, physicians (e.g. Buchan or Tissot) wrote to
unravel the mysteries of the non-naturals, to render hygiene,
which had so far only been part of the medical school's curri-
culum, accessible to the lay public.[14]

While other chapters in this volume emphasize the 'why' of
medical popularization, my essay will address the 'how'; thus,
my title: 'The Non-Naturals Made Easy'.

Buchan's *Domestic Medicine*, published in 1769, has, in the
past decades, attracted the attention of scholars who very
cogently situated the man and the book in the context of a
secularizing urban Enlightenment and its attendant drive for
self-help and education.[15] To provide the necessary balance and
to complete the picture, I will turn my attention to the other
major popularizer of medicine: Tissot. Born in the Pays de
Vaud, a subject land of the Republic of Bern, into a family of
ministers and rural professionals, Tissot studied medicine in
Montpellier where he was a boarder of Boissier de Sauvages
(1706–67). From his mentor, he adopted not only vitalism but
also the importance of both mental and physical well-being.
Tissot acquired most of his practical skills by walking the wards
of the Montpellier hospitals as a surgeon. In that capacity, he
had numerous occasions to perform *post mortem* and later, in his
practice in Lausanne or his teaching at the University of Pavia

(1781–83), he used autopsies as often as possible to correlate symptoms with lesions, in order to learn more about pathological phenomena. Tissot wrote extensively for the lay public as well as for doctors, on subjects ranging from inoculation to the construction of the clinical ward. As head of the Lausanne College of Medicine, Tissot devoted the last years of his life to promoting public health measures and proper medical training.

Although his medical writings were avidly read and widely translated in the eighteenth century and his expertise was sought both by numerous private persons and official authorities, he received in the recent past, for reasons I have elucidated elsewhere,[16] only scant attention from medical historians, except for his *Onanisme*, published in 1760.[17] The nineteenth century saw Tissot as parochial or trite; his popularizing medical books were dismissed as elegant, yet old-fashioned, stories on a theme (the non-naturals) which was outmoded by new concepts for disease (the germs theory) as well as by the medicalization of society. Trusting medicine to the hands of the lay public was declared as dangerous as inoculating with smallpox rather than cowpox, now that nineteenth-century physicians, because of their scientific training, saw themselves as the sole dispensers of health. In spite of Tissot's success with eighteenth-century readers, for he sensed what interested them and knew how to present it in a clear and attractive fashion, Tissot has been heralded by some recent scholars as the forerunner of Victorian morality and branded as an oppressor of sexual freedom; he has also been depicted as a pompous popularizer.[18]

Yet, there is more than that in Tissot's writings, especially those directed at particular groups of individuals who shared specific habits in their way of life: *De la santé des gens de lettres* (1768) and *Essai sur les maladies des gens du monde* (1770). In these short books, Tissot focused on the relation between health and habits which, early in his career, he had singled out as a theme for research and writing the improvement of medical care.[19] *Onanisme* can be considered as the first instalment of his projected treatise on habitual diseases, since in it he repeatedly referred to the 'habit' as the cause, first of poor health, then of marasmus followed by death. And for Tissot, habits were linked to the ways in which individuals used or misused the non-naturals. Tissot also discovered that many people were attracted to *Onanisme* because of its topic, while they were not so eager to consult a treatise on hygiene. So, when he prepared its first revision, he included a long chapter of advice on regimen and exercise to prevent or cure the 'habit'.[20] In a subsequent edition, he noted: 'I have treated more fully of the regimen, because when the disease has not progressed far, the removal of the cause, and attention to regimen, may alone effect a cure, and each one may attend to it without any danger.'[21] Tissot followed Hippocrates not only in the non-naturals, but also in the motto '*primum non nocere*' (straight out of the Hippocratic Oath). Nevertheless, it seems that the book was judged more for its sexually explicit content than for its promotion of hygiene. Consequently, it was banned in France, except in its Latin version, and Tissot earned the reputation of either a pornographer or a represser of sexual fulfilment.[22]

In fact, when Tissot was consulted for cases of *tabes dorsalis* (which today is linked to syphilis), he always emphasized that the main problem was not with the 'habit', but with the patient's lifestyle. In box after box of correspondence addressed to Tissot, I found many letters discussing what was thought to be ill-health due to masturbation; Tissot had annotated them with his diagnosis and prescriptions which were most often expressed in terms of blame for indulgent living or lack of a purposeful life, to be remedied by exercise, a bland diet, and the serious occupation of one's time.[23] Tissot hired a personal secretary to answer these numerous consultations which came from large and small towns, mainly in France and the Germanies. The letters, mostly in French, some in Latin, have to do with cases of nervous illness, childhood diseases, consumption, sequels to giving birth, and chronic poor health. They ranged from requesting advice on the best way to inoculate, to thanking Tissot for the help his books provided. Some are pathetic descriptions of constant personal sufferings that neither blood-letting nor the like of blistering had relieved; others emanated from physicians and are rather technical in content.

Tissot shared the view of his century's governments when he deplored depopulation, even if hindsight tells us that this was a wrong assumption based on insufficient statistics. One culprit responsible for the decrease, identified by the political authorities as well as by physicians, including Tissot, was the medical {mis}deeds of the charlatans who supposedly cared for the people. But Tissot parted from the ruler's company when it came to the tools for fighting quackery, as the customary edicts of prohibition enacted by the Bernese or other governments only left the population helpless. He was among the first to offer something tangible to displace the quacks, the almanacs, and the traditional recipe books. His *Avis au peuple sur sa santé* (1761) was to promote and disseminate enlightened medical care. Tissot had a solid tradition of common medical advice to build on or to jettison in writing his own; however, since his correspondence is silent on the matter, we can only speculate on his real sources from the more than 2,400 different authors listed in the catalogue of his library.[24] Certainly, *Avis* differs from the discourses on popular hygiene and domestic remedies found in its predecessors; *Avis* is indeed both a private book and a public tract for improving general health and medical care.[25]

Tissot realized that the sick needed reassurance and some sort of treatment to overcome their fear and the causes of their diseases, and that the ordinances which repressed quackery did nothing to help the population in time of need. He saw that the populace clung to its healers and their folksy methods without being in a position to judge their value; for the people, the vacuum of care created by enforcing the proscription of empirics was worse than the cures they offered. While Tissot thought that, ideally, the government should promote the training of more medical practitioners,he pragmatically also realized the financial contingency of such an enterprise.[26] Thus, he settled for writing a common-sense medical book to educate the people to avoid quackery. *Avis au peuple sur sa santé* was meant for the inhabitants of the Pays de Vaud, Tissot's homeland people, whom he knew well, having grown up among them and cared for them on his return from the Montpellier Medical School. He realized that most of them were smart enough to make the right choice if only they were informed of the benefits and risks of their actions. So, he embarked on the writing of just such a book, and aimed it first at the educated segment of the rural population: the ministers and school-teachers who were to disseminate its content by dispensing proper medical advice to their charges.[27] Tissot was from a Calvinist state where ministers and school-teachers were present in every village. Next, he also perceived that the gentry could make good use of his *Avis* for themselves or their farmers.[28] Finally, he hoped that some yeomen would also read his book with profit and learn that human life is of as much economic value as that of domestic animals.[29] Tissot wanted to introduce a simple system of medicine, easily understood and easily implemented by ordinary people using common sense. He had to explain his therapy in terms that were familiar to them and build his rationale for treatment within the prevailing humoral physiology. The non-naturals fitted the purpose ideally: they carried the weight of tradition; they dovetailed nicely with humoral physiology; they were simple and easily amenable to circumstances; and more importantly they could be trusted to be almost harmless in lay hands, which was not the case for the traditional treatments (bleeding, purges, or emetics) of Galenic medicine. The proper use of the non-naturals covered both preventive and curative measures and, at the same time, was part of ordinary life for everyone.

In *Avis au peuple sur sa santé,* Tissot first described some causes of disease that were linked to poorly understood effects of the non-naturals, for example: overwork (exercise), emanations from manure piles (air), drunkenness (drink), and the mania to provoke sweating (evacuation). He limited his scope to common diseases and their treatment through proper regimen, consisting most often of plenty of drinks such as herb tea or light broth, easy-to-digest food, fresh air, and clean clothing and bedding. And when he recommended drugs, he gave the exact prescription, using few and easily available ingredients, in a table placed at the end of the book with cross-references to the numbered paragraphs in which he had prescribed them. Tissot thus aimed at reaching out to a public, disposed towards learning and often away from the cities, left alone without adequate medical care. For him, the proper and easy principles of diet and exercise were to be trusted in lay hands for medical self-help and charitable deeds, so that their observance could displace the quack's fantastic cures or the almanacs' injunctions of good days for bleeding or purging.

Tissot met with a success that greatly surpassed his expectations for the function of *Avis.* While he understood why his earlier popularizing works (i.e. *Inoculation justifiée,* 1754, and *Onanisme,* 1760), written for a wide lay audience, brought him fame, he had not suspected that his name alone would attract foreign readers to this 'local' book. He had thought to fill a gap at the regional level, when in fact no comparable recent work existed in French. *Avis au peuple sur sa santé* which, in the Hippocratic tradition, he had written for his Vaudois folks whose diseases should be treated in terms of their particular constitution and local environment, caught the attention of the whole of Europe; within six years it saw six French editions, and translations into English, German, Italian, Dutch, Flemish, and Swedish.[30] Some of the translators felt the need to adapt *Avis* to the country where it would be used.[31] Tissot was of two minds about that approach to translating his works: the Hippocrates in him applauded these adaptations, yet he was vexed by the liberties taken which altered his argument. He complained that some translators used his books as 'passports' for their own prescriptions.[32]

His success in fighting what he saw as the cause of de-population, and in promoting a healthy way of life by giving medical information in easily grasped plain terms, motivated Tissot to pursue his linking of lifestyle with health and to publish two other books aimed at different segments of society: *gens de lettres* and *gens du monde*. While Tissot wrote *Avis* with a local audience in mind, he learned from its wide acceptance that people shared some basic predicaments (scarcity of food, exhaustion, superstition) across geographical locations. He also realized that in the artificiality of modern urban life, the natural elements of climate and place were displaced by habits and customs. Therefore, he shifted his emphasis to the 'universal' artificial milieus of *gens de lettres* and *gens du monde* which he felt were above geography. Tissot first addressed his colleagues of the Lausanne Academy, on the occasion of his inaugural lecture as Professor of Medicine, on the subject of their health, a topic he thought would interest them more than the relation of medicine to law or theology. This honorary professorship encompassed no teaching duty beyond that Latin address, since the Academy was mainly a theological seminary.[33] Tissot wanted to address a personal problem which the individual concerned, namely here the cosmopolitan intellectual, had to solve in partnership with the physician. By emphasizing the importance of a person's will towards, and knowledge for, health improvement, Tissot demonstrated once more his adherence to the program of the *philosophes* so well characterized by Peter Gay as 'the recovery of nerve'.[34]

In 1766, Tissot published the text of his lecture, *Sermo inauguralis de valetudine litteratorum*; the Latin medium emphasized the academic and universal audience that Tissot aimed to reach. After the people for whom he had written *Avis*, scholars formed the group Tissot knew best, and thought deserved to be helped in matters of health. *Sermo*, translated into French, was within months published in Paris without Tissot's permission. He was so distressed by the pirated work that he decided to write his own expanded French version which he entitled *De la santé des gens de lettres*.[35] When Tissot used the expression *gens de lettres*, he meant people among whom we would today include scientists, scholars, and writers: whoever devotes long hours to intellectual endeavours.

In *De la santé des gens de lettres*, Tissot intended to instruct scholars how to interpret the physiological signs of the body in order to gain a personal understanding of their own health. So, within the framework of humoral medicine, which was the physiology predominantly understood, and adding now and then a note of modernity by citing Harvey's or Haller's discoveries, he reviewed and described the effects the non-naturals have on the health of scholars.[36] Confronting the daily behaviour and habits of the literati with the requirements for a healthy life, Tissot drew a picture of the common misuses of the non-naturals and denounced the abuses such conduct inflicted on the physical body and mental state of intellectuals. Indeed, Tissot never separated physical and mental health for any of his patients; and in the particular case of *gens de lettres*, he pointed especially to the danger of impairment of the brain provoked by long hours of intellectual tension. Taking the non-naturals one by one, Tissot first reviewed their misuse and then showed how a correct understanding of their importance and proper management brought health, happiness, and a longer productive life to the intellectual aware of the consequences of his conduct and ready to reform his ways.

Under *air*, he blamed the stuffy overheated atmosphere of the study, the windows of which the scholar hardly ever opens, for the many cases of apoplexy that strike the literati. 'Not to renew the air of one's room, is to live in the impurities of the preceding day, and yet what hard student is there who thinks of letting fresh air into his chamber every day?'[37]

Under *food and drink*, he denounced, as the cause of the too frequent stomach aches, the meals that are taken in haste without paying attention to chewing, or to what is eaten. He objected to the quantity of tea or coffee consumed by scholars; in his view, these hot drinks only weakened the digestion. He did not hesitate to transpose the political boycott of tea by the Thirteen Colonies into a wise health measure to be emulated.[38]

He disapproved of the drinking of hard liquor which either dulls or fires cerebral functions; he recommended instead the drinking of fresh cool water, and argued that: 'Water is a drink nature has given to all nations, and made it agreeable to all palates'.[39] He praised light suppers 'as those of Plato' that please on the day and the morrow.[40]

Under *motion and rest*, Tissot deplored the long periods of inactivity that writing necessitates. The immobility it entails is bad enough by itself; furthermore, the bending of the torso and the legs compounds the problem, worsening the effects on general health by preventing deep breathing and easy circulation of the blood, and congesting internal organs. The subsequent torpor is not conducive to a desire for exercise or outside activities that would counteract with exertion the stagnation of the humours. Tissot recommended physical activity that procures at the same time pleasure and sociability:

> The exercises most suitable for men of letters are such as [those that] put the whole body in motion; these are tennis, the shuttle-cock, billiards, the mall, hunting, skittles, bowling, even chuck; but these are unfortunately in such discredit in many parts, that persons who are tender of their good name would almost be ashamed to be seen playing at them, and will not be convinced that the neglect of these useful amusements, is one of the principal causes contributing to the increase of their disorders.[41]

He noted that these games ought to be played by school children of both sexes and that the value of gymnastics ought to be honoured, as it had been in ancient time. Therefore, he recommended horse-back riding, taking carriage rides, or simply walking.

Tissot was more concerned with sleep than with waking. The sleep of scholars is often agitated, light, or else too heavy to let the body replenish its strength. 'Sleep, when disturbed, is restored with more difficulty than any other of the animal functions: we lose it with cheerfulness, and regret the loss of it, almost always in vain, with sorrow.'[42] Working late and going to bed immediately afterwards is a sure way to an agitated night, and he proscribed a nap after a meal as disturbing to the digestion. To discourage the literati from working through the night, he rhetorically quipped: 'Shall the man of letters then divide the business of the night with villains and wild beast?'[43] During waking hours, Tissot advised alternating different types of work, because changing task is a distraction, and he saw distraction as the best way to rest the brain.[44] About *evacuation and retention* Tissot had many things to say. The medical philosophy of the eighteenth century regarded these functions as very important and a natural way for the body to maintain the desired balance. Tissot, however, shifted the emphasis to the balance of the body rather than that of the humours. He argued that perspiration was essential to rid the organism of acridity and waste, and thus should be kept flowing by the cleanliness of the skin. He described the sufferings induced by ignoring calls of nature for too long and drove home his point by an allusion to Rousseau's problem: 'Intense study produces also the stone and other diseases of the bladder, . . . and nobody is unacquainted with the sufferings which the illustrious antagonist of the sciences is exposed to from complaints of this nature.'[45] Too much unrelieved sitting prevents normal evacuations and this fact gave Tissot one more reason to advocate exercise.

Under the *passions of the soul*, Tissot denounced pride in, and excessive attention to, one's own intellectual pursuits. He questioned the validity and usefulness of accomplishments achieved at the price of poor health, and ultimately the incapacity to work. He concluded: 'Learning, when exchanged for health, is certainly purchased at too high a rate; and science becomes useless if it deprives us of happiness.'[46] Tissot also warned scholars to moderate intellectual activity with the passing of years: 'So that those persons who know how to moderate their application as their age advances, prevent infirmities and insure their health, those who are prudent enough to know the time when they ought to lock up their productions, certainly insure their reputation.'[47]

It seems that Tissot identified the personality of the workaholic when he railed: '[he] devours studies as gluttons cram down food, merely to glut their appetites'.[48] Far from Tissot's mind was the intention of degrading intellectual work; he thought that ignorance of any kind was shameful and led to superstition. What he wanted was to prevent or alleviate the hazards of the profession, in order to render it more enjoyable and productive. He did not wish to enter the polemic about the usefulness of the arts and sciences, yet he was ready to advocate the usefulness of medical knowledge for happiness, and to toil himself at disseminating it, albeit warning:

> The great question concerning the utility of the sciences has been much canvassed, and I am far from having any design of engaging in the contest; for even if it should be true, which is not however my opinion, that upon the whole they do not contribute to the happiness of society, it can hardly be denied, that learning adds to the happiness of the person who possesses it, provided he has acquired it without the expense of his health, or the neglect of his social duties.[49]

His cure for too much work was to spend pleasant time in the company of others: 'Men were created for each other; their mutual association is productive of advantages not to be given up without suffering for it; and it has been very properly observed, that solitude brings on a consumption. Nothing can contribute more to health than cheerfulness, which is animated by society, and damped by retirement'.[50]

Upon following his advice, the literati would banish the risk of nervous diseases – the curse of intellectuals of any time – which, Tissot thought (and in that he was not alone in his century), were on the increase because the artificiality and luxury of urban living were invading the lives of everyone. He urged *gens de lettres*, at least, to try living as close as possible to nature and he appealed to their conscience and intelligence to act responsibly and knowingly in matters of health, now that he had explained especially for them the intricacies of the non-naturals.

A few years later, when Tissot thought about the books that he and other physicians had written for particular groups of people, he came to realize that craftsmen, the literati, the poor, sailors, soldiers, even monks and nuns, had their special medical books, but up to now no physician had attempted to write for *gens du monde*. So he decided to fill the gap, even if his lack of information on court life and his position as an independent physician in a small town seemed to preclude expertise in the matter.[51] Tissot had been widely consulted by the well-to-do; hence, to address their special medical needs, he used the experience he had acquired with them, in person or by letter. His choice of title, *Essai sur les maladies des gens du monde*, for the book he directed specifically at people of fashion, immediately disclosed his disposition towards them. The wealthy had diseases to be cured, while the literati had health to preserve. The well-to-do were sick and in need of help to treat the diseases they had brought upon themselves by their lifestyle.

> My only aim is to give a general table of the Errors of Regimen, and their evil consequences. I shall speak of no remedies but what those disorders require: and finally, shall only make known to the patient what he ought to know, in order to concur in the cure, which is very often only impossible when the patient will not assist the physician.[52]

Tissot went on to state that the wealthy have all possible means to get well, but don't want to be bothered by taking care of their health regularly. They are so used to being served at their wills and whims that they think their doctor should cure them with just a few remedies taken casually. And their attitude might have discouraged any physician from writing for the well-to-do, mused Tissot.

Tissot reminded *gens du monde* that all the non-naturals were important for their health and that perhaps the single non-natural they most neglected was the one responsible for most of their health troubles; he meant the mental affections. 'The passions have a more essential influence and efficacy on the health of man than motion, aliments, or even air itself.'[53] Nevertheless, Tissot covered all the non-naturals very carefully, explaining each one for the special case of the wealthy. He reviewed the influence clothing has on the evacuations, in particular on perspiration, a function which, in Tissot's view, could not be disturbed without serious consequences for health. He also added his voice to the clamour against corsets: 'So that the very means designed to make fine shapes, are the causes of deformity'.[54]

He cited the low-cut necklines of women's dresses as the cause of many chest troubles and charged the tight breeches of men with the responsibility for poor blood circulation. He denounced make-up as much for clogging the skin as for poisoning the eyes: all too often it contained lead or mercury.[55]

While Tissot felt that, because of his privileged position, the wealthy man should have the best of life, that is health and happiness, Tissot judged him so misinformed that he wrote: 'But he is so unlucky, that he destroys the edifice of his fashionable pleasures, which is become the foundation of his pains'.[56] He urged him to realize that the more responsibility one has, the more one should take care of one's health.[57]

Returning to the subject of the passions, Tissot wrote that he would not address the practical side of the question as he had done with the other non-naturals, as this fell outside his scope: 'the politician may use, and the moralist correct, but the physician is confined to observe only their influence upon health, and to reform the pernicious effects . . .'.[58] Perhaps he thought that, as others, in particular Rousseau, had tried to reform the passions of the well-to-do to no avail, it was wiser for him to skip that subject and to insist on the physical components of hygiene. The central advice he gave to the wealthy was to use wisely the other non-naturals to build a strong body better able to withstand the bad effects of the passions. Yet he was sceptical that people of fashion would heed his advice and reform their ways: 'The reader may perhaps be terrified on finding in each article an exact regimen prescribed. I am sensible to the same, but its importance, and the little hope of success without, make it appear indispensably necessary'.[59]

Tissot concluded by hoping that his essay would change the life of a few privileged, yet languishing, readers who were destroying their health by error and not by system and who would be charmed to be disillusioned about their ways and enlightened on hygiene and the non-naturals.

The message that Tissot passed on in each of his books for special groups of individuals was that any reader was smart enough to understand the fallacies of bleeding, purging and the like as preventive measures, and was also able to grasp the truth of the influences of lifestyle on health. For these readers, Tissot recast the ancient wisdom of the non-naturals and of trusting nature in terms so very congenial to the mind and aspirations of his contemporaries that they bought his works eagerly; the numerous editions and translations are witness to their success. *Avis* was translated into seventeen languages; it was published as far west as Boston and Philadelphia and as far south as Welkom in what is today South Africa. And the letters he received tell the story of health restored, but also of resentment by doctors who found dangerous the idea of replacing their art by benevolent help guided by family medicine books.

At the same time as he was writing for the lay person, Tissot was also preparing a treatise for physicians on the influence of the non-naturals on the onset as well as on the treatment of nervous disorders. He was repeating here for the physicians what he had told the public, that the best chance of being healthy resided with:

> the labourer, who, in this respect, is superior to the mechanics, but unhappily inferior to the labourers of former times, when labour alone was his employment. Nay, at present there are nations, who, unknown to polite diseases, die only by accident, or through age . . . our labourers are not equally robust, because they do not live a life equally rural; many have been servants, others soldiers, and infected the village with the customs of the city . . . An aversion to simplicity increases among the best citizens . . . that course of life, which, having nothing useful to support it, depends upon continual dissipation . . . who, to defeat the insupportable tediousness of a life disagreeably inactive, attempt to kill time by pleasure.[60]

For him, many nervous illnesses were linked to the passions of the soul created by the demands and tensions of urbane living and it was the responsibility of doctors to identify and treat their causes accordingly. Just as he had written to educate patients to take charge of their health through a judicious use of the non-naturals, he wrote again to inform physicians of the importance of these same non-naturals in the nervous diseases they encountered in their practice and how they should develop trusting relationships conducive to the betterment of their patients. He wanted to make his colleagues more aware of their role in teaching the intricacies of the non-naturals in order to relieve or prevent all kinds of ills, including the nervous. His six-volume *Traité des nerfs et de leurs maladies* which he published over a period of ten years was meant to accomplish this task.[61] He hoped that physicians acting as advisers for the physical and mental health of their patients would displace the Catholic *directeurs de conscience* from their privileged position in the traditional culture, and that, in the newly secularized and medicalized society his books had promoted, physicians and patients would work in partnership, using the non-naturals properly to improve their life. Later, Tissot took this partnership one step further. In his unpublished *Médecine civile*, he wrote of concerned citizens, enlightened physicians, and political authorities who would work together to create a new awareness of solving social and environmental problems through better medical use of the non-naturals, not only for private hygiene but also in public health.[62]

First and foremost Tissot was a physician and, according to the Hippocratic tradition and oath to which he subscribed heartily, the physician's role is to cure, or short of this, to alleviate pain. It is in his capacity of physician that he denounced, in his writings, the ills of civilization, the shackles of tradition, the weight of fatalism, and the mischiefs of superstition which hurt people, and so he joined the ranks of *philosophes*, in particular Voltaire and Rousseau, both of whom he knew personally and appreciated in different ways.[63] In Voltaire, Tissot recognized a brilliance with words which almost magically transformed ordinary thoughts into cogent arguments, for tolerance, in particular, but he came to despise the man for his hypochondriac egocentrism and his taste for fashionable pursuits. The affinity between Tissot and Rousseau stems from a common background. Tissot's mother was from Geneva and he had studied there. Both men had been raised as Calvinists, and the Genevan spirit made them yearn for an unencumbered life and some democracy. They both loved the landscape and the country around Lake Geneva and hated the whirl of big-city living. Together with Rousseau, Tissot disliked the pretence of high society; but they departed from each other on the intensity of their attacks on civilization and its corrupting amenities. Nevertheless, Tissot might be one of the very few persons with whom Rousseau never quarrelled.

Was then Tissot a partisan of Voltaire's 'Ecrasez l'infâme'? Yes, when it meant religious intolerance, quackery, and superstition, robbing people of their health.[64] No, if it attacked any and all religious deeds. As Tissot tempered Rousseau's distrust of arts and science, he did likewise with Voltaire's assault on religion. Tissot felt much more attuned to the general spirit of the *Encyclopédie* which sought explicitly to educate, to offer to the public, in the vernacular and in simple terms, the means to escape routine and stagnation, and to embark on a road of progress and happiness, which, the Encyclopedists were quick to point out, could never be attained without health.

Publicly recognized or privately admitted, the drive to educate, to render everyone responsible for their actions, be it in terms of medicine or politics, would in the long run breed radicalism and call for deep social changes. In that sense Tissot is an elder brother to the radical physicians studied in Porter's essay.[65] By his expository and medical skills Tissot reached a large audience and prepared his readers to accept expectant and preventive medicine, weaning them from the heroic treatments described in Molière's comedies and too often used by Voltaire on himself.[66] Tissot contributed by urging his readers back to Nature. Within his area of competence, Tissot participated in the Encyclopedists' programme of education – he made the non-naturals easier.

Notes

1. *Encyclopédie ou dictionaire raisonné des arts et des sciences* (Neuchâtel, 1765); article 'non-naturelles (choses)', tome XI, 218. F.H. Garrison: *History of Medicine* (Philadelphia PA, 1929), 113.

2. G. Vigarello, *Concept of Cleanliness* (Cambridge, 1988), 168.

3. George Cheyne (1671–1743), British physician, *An Essay of Health and Long Life* (London: Strahan, 1725); *Art de conserver la santé* (Paris, 1755) and *Méthode naturelle de guérir les maladies* (Paris, 1749) are mentioned in Tissot's library catalogue; Laurent Joubert (1529–83), French physician, *Des erreurs populaires en médecine* (Paris, 1587) is also in Tissot's library catalogue. S.A. Tissot, *An Essay on the Disorders of People of Fashion* (London: Richardson and Urquhart, 1771), 96; *Essai sur les maladies des gens du monde* (Lausanne, 1770), 135: 'On lit peu les anciens livres, et l'avantage des nouveaux, lors même qu'ils ne renferment aucune idée neuve, c'est de remettre sous les yeux les vérités oubliées.' See also in this volume the chapters by Wear, Fissell, and Wilson.

4. M. Jack, *Progress and Corruption. The Eighteenth-century Debate* (New York, 1989) for a review of the problem.

5. Jean-Jacques Rousseau (1712–78), Genevan writer, in particular *Discours sur les sciences et les arts* (Paris, 1750) and *Discours sur l'origine et les fondements de l'inégalité parmi les hommes* (Amsterdam, 1755).

6. Albrecht von Haller (1708–77), Swiss physiologist, *Elementa physiologiae corporis humani* (Lausanne, 1759–66).

7. H. Zeller, *Les collaborateurs médicaux de l'Encyclopédie de Diderot et d'Alembert* (Paris, 1934); or F.A. Kafker and S.L. Kafker, *The Encyclopedists as Individuals: a Biographical Dictionary of the Authors of the Encyclopédie* (Studies on Voltaire and the Eighteenth Century 257), (Oxford, 1988); P. Gay, 'The Enlightenment as Medicine and as Cure' in W.W. Barber, ed. *The Age of Enlightenment* (London, 1967).

8. *Encyclopédie ou dictionaire raisonné des arts et des sciences* (Neuchâtel, 1765); article 'Hygiène', tome VIII, 385–8.

9. 'Non-Naturelles', 222. 'C'est d'après cette connaissance réfléchie que l'on peut devenir le médecin de soi-même, non pour s'administrer convenablement des remèdes, mais pour se garantir des maladies qui peuvent provenir du défaut de régime approprié.'

10. 'Hygiène', 387. 'Ainsi lorsque l'on jouit de la santé et qu'il s'agit que de la conserver avec la tempérance et la modération, on peut éviter d'avoir besoin de médecins, et de s'exposer à être les victimes de l'ignorance; lorsque la santé se dérange et qu'on est menacé de maladies, la diète et l'eau sont les meilleurs remèdes pour prévenir le danger des suites.'

11. W. Coleman, 'Health and Hygiene in the *Encyclopédie*' in *Journal of the History of Medicine XXIX* (1974), 399–421.

12. R. Darnton, *The Business of the Enlightenment* (Cambridge MA, 1979), part IV especially.

13. Many titles could be cited: the most representative of those by physicians are J. Ballexserd, *Dissertation sur l'éducation physique des enfants* (Yverdon, 1763); N. Brouzet, *Essai sur l'éducation des enfants* (Paris, 1754); W. Cadogan, *An Essay upon Nursing and the Management of Children* (London, 1748); and by lay writers, J.-J. Rousseau, *Emile* (Paris, 1762); J.-L. Fourcroy de Guillerville, *Les Enfants élevés dans l'ordre de la nature* (Paris, 1774); see also in this volume the chapters by Ramsey, Gevitz.

14. Samuel Auguste Tissot (1728–97), Swiss physician, *Avis au peuple sur sa santé* (Lausanne, 1761), *De la santé des gens de lettres* (Lausanne, 1768), *Essai sur les maladies des gens du monde* (Lausanne, 1770); William Buchan (1729–1805), British physician, *Domestic Medicine* (Edinburgh, 1769).

15. e.g. C. Lawrence, 'William Buchan: Medicine Laid Open' in *Medical History* 19 (1975), 20–35; C.E. Rosenberg, 'Medical text and social context: explaining William Buchan's *Domestic Medicine*' in *Bulletin of the History of Medicine* 57 (1983): 22–42.

16. A. Emch-Dériaz: *Towards a Social Conception of Health in the Second Half of the Eighteenth Century: Tissot (1728–1797) and the New Pre-occupation with Health and Well-Being*, University of Rochester Dissertation, 1983 (Ann Arbor, MI, University Microfilms International, 1984); 'Auguste Tissot (1728–1797)' in G. Saudan, ed. *L'Eveil médical vaudois* (Lausanne, 1987); *Tissot: Physician of the Enlightenment* (New York and Bern, 1992).

17. S.A. Tissot, *Onanisme* (Lausanne, 1760); 71 French editions, the last in 1991, 8 English, 21 German, 8 Italian, 16 Latin, 6 Spanish, and 1 Russian. As the literature on onanism is large, I will cite only the most recent, since often these articles contain a full bibliography on the subject: V.L. Bullough, 'Technology for the Prevention of "les maladies produites par la masturbation"' in *Technology and Society* (1987), 828–32; S. Fishman, 'The History of Childhood Sexuality' in *Journal of Contemporary History* 17 (1982), 269–83; R.P. Hudson, *Disease and its Control* (Westport, CT, 1983), 10–11; L. Jordanava, 'The Popularization of Medicine: Tissot on Onanism' in *Textual Practice* 1 (1987), 68–79; Th. Tarczylo, *Sexe et liberté au siècle des Lumières* (Paris,

1983) or his articles in *Dix-Huitième Siècle* 12 (1980), 79–96 and 15 (1983), 115–23.

18. Tarczylo, passim; G. Miller, *The Adoption of Inoculation for Smallpox in England and France* (Philadelphia, PA, 1957), 205ff.

19. Tissot to Zimmerman, letter dated 6 September 1755, in Zimmermann's Nachlass Niedersaechsischelandesbibliothek, Hanover, Germany.

20. Tissot to Zimmermann, letter dated 19 December 1759.

21. *Onanism* (New York, Collins & Hannay, 1832), 84; *Onanisme* (Lausanne, 1768), 123. 'Je me suis plus étendu sur le régime, parce que, quand le mal n'a pas fait de grands progrès, joint à la cessation de la cause, il peut seul opérer la guérison, et que chacun peut s'y astreindre sans aucun danger.'

22. Tissot to Rousseau, letter dated 8 July 1762 in Fonds Eynard, Département des manuscrits, Bibliothèque publique et universitaire, Genève; Tissot to Zimmermann, letter dated 14 November 1764.

23. Tissot's personal papers in Département des Manuscrits, Bibliothèque cantonale et universitaire, Lausanne.

24. Many of the titles of popular medical books cited in the various chapters of this volume are listed in Tissot's library catalogue.

25. E. Olivier, 'Autour de l'Avis au peuple' in *Revue historique vaudoise* XXXVI (1928), 259–94.

26. Tissot, *Des moyens de perfectionner les études de médecine* (Lausanne, 1785), 199, in particular the appendix on the education of country-surgeons, developed from his manuscript of 1765 in which he placed Buchan's *Domestic Medicine* on the same footing as *Avis* as a very useful reference book for country-surgeons. Emch-Dériaz (New York and Bern, 1992), chap. X.

27. *Avis au peuple sur sa santé* (Lausanne, 1761), 21 & 25. Editions: 46 French, 29 English, 24 German, 6 each Italian and Dutch, 9 Spanish, 4 Portuguese, 2 each Flemish, Greek, Polish, Swedish, Russian and Tagalog, 1 each Danish, Hebrew, and Hungarian. Tissot to Zimmerman, letter dated 14 March 1760: 'Navré de tristesse plus d'une fois en voyant périr misérablement dans les campagnes nos agriculteurs les plus robustes par des traitements pernicieux, j'ai pensé aux moyens de prévenir ces malheurs et mes réflexions ont fait éclore un manuscrit qui ne m'a guère peiné d'intituler *Avis au peuple sur santé* . . .'

28. *Avis au peuple sur sa santé*, 24.

29. *Avis au peuple sur sa santé*, 27 & 516.

30. The last French edition of *Avis au peuple sur sa santé* by itself came out in Paris in 1830; its last translation was in Hebrew, published in Lemberg [Lvov] in 1851.

31. See in this volume the chapters by Perdiguero and Szlatky.

32. Tissot to Zimmermann, letter dated 2 April 1763.

33. *De la santé des gens de lettres* (Lausanne, 1768), 14. The lecture took place on 9 April 1766.

34. P. Gay, *The Enlightenment* (New York, 1969), Vol. 2, chap. 1, section 1.

35. First French authorized edition Lausanne, 1768, which went through twenty-three editions, the last one in 1991. It was translated into six languages: 9 German editions, 5 English, 4 Italian and 1 each Spanish, Polish, and Greek. The Latin text had three editions.

36. William Harvey (1578–1657), English physician, *Exercitatio anatomica de motu cordis et sanguine in animalibus* (Frankfurt, 1628). For Tissot, Harvey's discovery of blood circulation marked the beginning of modern medicine.

37. *A Treatise on the Diseases Incident to Literary and Sedentary Persons* (Edinburgh: Donaldson, 1772), 51; *De la santé des gens de lettres*, 89. 'Ne pas renouveller tous les jours l'air de sa chambre c'est vivre des ordures de la veille; & quels sont les érudits qui le renouvellent tous les jours?'

38. *A Treatise on the Diseases Incident to Literary and Sedentary Persons*, 105 note +; *De la santé des gens de lettres*, 190 note n.

39. *A Treatise on the Diseases Incident to Literary and Sedentary Persons*, 100; *De la santé des gens de lettres*, 180. 'L'eau est la boisson que la Nature a donné à toutes les nations, elle l'a faite agréable pour tous les palais.'

40. *A Treatise on the Diseases Incident to Literary and Sedentary Persons*, 95; *De la santé des gens de lettres*, 172.

41. *A Treatise on the Diseases Incident to Literary and Sedentary Persons*, 77; *De la santé des gens de lettres*, 136–137. 'Les exercices dont je fais le plus de cas sont ceux qui exercent toutes les parties du corps, tels que la paulme, le volant, le billard, le mail, la chasse, les quilles, les boules, le petit palet même; mais malheureusement ils sont tombés dans un si grand discrédit que, dans plusieurs endroits, ces hommes qui s'appellent "honnêtes gens" auraient presque honte de s'en amuser, & ne veulent pas sentir que l'abandon de ces utiles plaisirs est une des causes principales de l'augmentation des maladies de langueur.'

42. *A Treatise on the Diseases Incident to Literary and Sedentary Persons*, 50; *De la santé des gens de lettres*, 87. 'De toutes les fonctions dérangées le sommeil est celle qui se rétablit le plus difficilement'; on le perd avec gaité, on le pleure avec amertume, et presque toujours inutilement.'

43. *A Treatise on the Diseases Incident to Literary and Sedentary Persons*, 49; *De la santé des gens de lettres*, 86. 'L'homme de lettres devrait-il partager l'usage de la nuit avec l'homme méchant et les bêtes féroces.'

44. *A Treatise on the Diseases Incident to Literary and Sedentary Persons*, 59; *De la santé des gens de lettres*, 103.

45. *A Treatise on the Diseases Incident to Literary and Sedentary Persons*, 42; *De la santé des gens de lettres*, 74. 'La pierre & les maladies de la vessie sont encore un fruit de l'amour des lettres; . . . & personne n'ignore les cruelles douleurs en ce genre auxquelles est fort sujet l'illustre Antagoniste des Sciences.'

46. *A Treatise on the Diseases Incident to Literary and Sedentary Persons*, 41; *De la santé des gens de lettres*, 71. 'On est trop savant quand on l'est aux dépends de sa santé; à quoi sert la science sans le bonheur?'

47. *A Treatise on the Diseases Incident to Literary and Sedentary Persons*, 67; *De la santé des gens de lettres*, 117. 'Si ceux qui savent modérer leur travail à proportion que leur âge avance préviennent par-là les

infirmités & assurent leur santé, ceux qui savent prendre à temps le parti de renfermer leurs ouvrages dans leurs bureaux assurent leur gloire.'

48. *A Treatise on the Diseases Incident to Literary and Sedentary Persons*, 71; *De la santé des gens de lettres*, 125. '& ne dévore l'étude que comme le gourmand dévore les viandes pour assouvir sa passion, . . .'

49. *A Treatise on the Diseases Incident to Literary and Sedentary Persons*, 134; *De la santé des gens de lettres*, 243–4. 'cette grande question est pendante, & je suis éloigné de vouloir entrer ce fameux procès; quand il serait vrai, ce que je ne crois pas, qu'elles ne contribuent point au bonheur de la société prise en général, on ne pourrait guère nier, il me semble, que la connaissance des Lettres n'augmente le bonheur de celui qui la possède quand il ne l'a acquise ni aux dépends de ses devoirs ni aux dépends de sa santé.'

50. *A Treatise on the Diseases Incident to Literary and Sedentary Persons*, 54–5; *De la santé des gens de lettres*, 95–6. 'Les hommes ont été créés pour les hommes; leur commerce mutuel a des avantages auxquels on ne renonce pas impunément, & l'on a remarqué avec raison que la solitude jette dans la langueur. Rien au monde ne contribue plus à la santé que la gaité que la société anime et que la retraite tue.'

51. *Essai sur les maladies des gens du monde* (Lausanne, 1770) had 18 French editions, 6 each English, German, and Italian.

Essai sur les maladies des gens du monde, VIII–X, in which Tissot cited the works of Ramazzini for the craftsmen, the monks and nuns, of Pringle, van Swieten, Monro, and Brocklesby for the soldiers, of Cockburn, Lind, and Poissonier for the sailors.

*indicates an entry in Tissot's library catalogue. Bernardino Ramazzini (1633–1714), Italian physician, *Essai sur les maladies des artisans* (Paris, 1777)*; John Pringle (1707–82), British physician, *On the Diseases of the Army* (London, 1764)*; *Observations sur les maladies des armées* (Paris 1771)*; Gerhard van Swieten (1700–72), Dutch physician at the Court of Vienna, *Kurze Beschreibung und Heilungart der Krankheiten welche am oeftesten in dem Feldlager beobachtet werden* (Vienna, 1758); Donald Monro (1727–1802), British physician, *Diseases of Military Hospitals* (London, 1764)*, *On the Means of Preserving Sailors Health* (London, 1780)*; Richard Brocklesby (1722–97), British physician, *Oeconomical and Medical Observations on Military Hospitals and Camp Diseases* (London, 1764); William Cockburn (1669–1739), British physician, *Diseases of Sailors* (London, 1736); James Lind (1716–94), British physician, *Essay on the Hygiene of Sailors* (1774)*; Antoine Poissonier-Desperrières (1722–93), French physician, *Maladies des gens de mer* (Paris, 1767)*.

52. *An Essay on the Disorders of People of Fashion*, XIV–XV; *Essai sur les maladies des gens du monde*, XIV. 'Mon seul but a été de présenter un tableau général des erreurs de régime & des maux qui en sont la suite; je n'ai parlé des remèdes que ces maux exigent, qu'afin de faire connaitre aux malades ce qu'il faut qu'ils connaissent pour concourir eux-mêmes à une guérison qui n'est souvent impossible que parce que le malade n'aide point le Médecin.'

53. *An Essay on the Disorders of People of Fashion*, 27; *Essai sur les*

maladies des gens du monde, 35–6. 'Les passions ont une influence plus marquée & plus efficace sur la santé de l'homme que le mouvement, que les aliments, que l'air même.'

54. *An Essay on the Disorders of People of Fashion*, 43; *Essai sur les maladies des gens du monde*, 58–9. 'ces moyens destinés à procurer des tailles élégantes sont sans aucun doute la cause qu'il y en beaucoup de contrefaites.'

55. *An Essay on the Disorders of People of Fashion*, 44; *Essai sur les maladies des gens du monde*, 63–4.

56. *An Essay on the Disorders of People of Fashion*, 82; *Essai sur les maladies des gens du monde*, 117. 'mais il est si maladroit qu'il a construit l'édifice de ses plaisirs de façon qu'il est devenu l'atelier de ses peines.'

57. *An Essay on the Disorders of People of Fashion*, 84; *Essai sur les maladies des gens du monde*, 119.

58. *An Essay on the Disorders of People of Fashion*, 91; *Essai sur les maladies des gens du monde*, 128–9. 'le Politique s'en sert, le Moraliste les réforme, le Médecin se borne à en observer l'influence sur la santé, & à en corriger les sinistres effets, . . .'

59. *An Essay on the Disorders of People of Fashion*, 128; *Essai sur les maladies des gens du monde*, 184. 'Les lecteurs seront peut-être ennuyés de voir revenir à chaque article le conseil d'un régime exact, je le suis presque moi-même de le rappeler sans cesse; mais il est si important, on a si peu de succès à espérer dans le traitement de toutes les maladies si on ne l'observe pas exactement, qu'il me parait absolument indispensable d'en faire sentir tout la nécessité.'

60. *An Essay on the Disorders of People of Fashion*, 9–11; *Essai sur les maladies des gens du monde*, 11–13: 'Si l'on demande quel il est, il n'y a personne qui ne réponde sans hésiter, celui du Laboureur, qui a de grands avantages, à cette égard, sur la partie du peuple qui fournit les artisans; mais qui est malheureusement bien inférieur à ce qu'il a été autrefois, dans le temps qu'il n'était que laboureur, & à ce que sont encore quelques peuplades de sauvages qui ignorent presque tous les maux, & ne meurent que d'accidents ou de décrépitude. A mesure qu'on s'éloigne de leur état, la santé semble diminuer par degrés; nos laboureurs sont moins sains qu'eux parce qu'ils ne vivent pas uniquement de la vie des champs; plusieurs ont été domestiques, d'autres soldats; ils ont affaibli leur santé dans ces deux états, & porté dans leur village quelques uns des usages de la ville . . . L'éloignement de cette vie simple augmente encore dans l'ordre supérieur . . . & leur santé diminue en proportion . . . enfin il est le plus grand possible chez les gens du monde . . . ce genre de vie, qui n'a point d'oeuvre de vocation & dont les distractions continuelles sont la base . . . qui pour tromper l'ennui insupportable d'une existence désoeuvrée, . . . ils ont dû avoir recours à des plaisirs factices . . .'

61. *Traité de l'épilepsie* (Lausanne, 1770), 7 French editions, 2 German, 3 Italian, and 1 Dutch; *Traité des nerfs et de leurs maladies* (Lausanne, 1778–80), 5 each French and German editions, 1 Italian; *Traité de la catalepsie, de l'extase, de la migraine, etc.* (Lausanne, 1780), 3 French editions.

62. Emch-Dériaz, (New York and Bern, 1992), chap. XII.
63. Emch-Dériaz (1987). François-Marie Arouet de Voltaire (1694–1778), French writer.
64. Religious intolerance, for example, in the royal decree in France which prohibited physicians from returning to the bedside of a sick person who refused the last rites.
65. See in this volume the chapter by Porter.
66. Jean-Baptiste Poquelin de Molière (1622–73), French playwright.

6

The popularization of medicine during the Spanish Enlightenment

Enrique Perdiguero

Spain began the eighteenth century with a change of dynasty which had cost a War of Succession. The country, its splendours now a thing of the past, was a second or third-rate power, turned in upon itself in its scientific development, partly as a consequence of Philip II's decree in 1559 that none of his subjects, 'of whatever state, condition or quality may leave this Kingdom to study, or teach, or learn, or be, or direct in universities, institutes or colleges beyond the frontiers of this Kingdom . . .'.[1] Although throughout the seventeenth century there had been a complex evolutionary process that had succeeded in introducing modern science to Spain, as excellently detailed by Professor López Piñero,[2] it was not until the accession of the new Bourbon dynasty that Spain felt the winds of renovation and liberalization, illustrated by the decree of Philip V of 4 July 1718 by which grants were created so that Spaniards might study abroad.[3] The country underwent important changes and, although rather late and in its own peculiar way, joined the movement of enlightenment which then dominated the European scene.[4] This incorporation became even clearer with the accession of Charles III (1759–89) and meant, as regards the sciences in general, a new impulse designed to put them at the service of the State.[5] Consequently, successive enlightened governments pursued two basic goals: to do away with, as skilfully as possible, the scholastic stagnation that reigned in the university, and to introduce new knowledge and techniques to the country in order to put them at the service of State projects. An enormous effort was therefore made to ensure, in accordance with the creed of enlightenment, 'useful knowledge', which would allow the country to improve its economy, technologically so dependent on other nations. Foreign scientists such as Bowles (1721–80), Dombey (1742–92), Proust (1754–1826), and Chabaneau (1754–1852) were brought to the country; and, at the expense of the Crown, or with grants from quasi-official institutions, many Spaniards were sent to study abroad. Institutions were set up to allow for the development of the sciences, like the Royal Library (1716), the Artillery Academy of Segovia (1763), the Natural History Laboratory (1752); and, for the improvement of medicine and surgery, the Royal Colleges of Surgery in Cadiz (1748), Barcelona (1760) and Madrid (1787). Together with these government-sponsored institutions, other privately sponsored ones were also set up, such as the Societies of Friends of the Nation, which followed the example of the one established in the Basque Country and sprang up throughout the regions, encouraged by the governments of the Enlightenment which, in general, played a dynamic role in scientific development.[6] That this enormous effort failed in the end was mainly a result of the impatience of governments, which considered the progress of scientific education too slow and its fruits too scarce; of the persistent and severe economic difficulties; and finally of the events and consequences of an unfortunate military campaign and the disastrous War of Independence (1808–14) which wasted the years and money invested.[7]

Nevertheless, from a historical perspective, what is clear is that, during the second part of the eighteenth century and above all in the final thirty years, the country lived through, at least among the enlightened élites, a dynamic period in search of knowledge to improve the conditions of life of Spanish society. This search for practical knowledge in pursuit of the peaceful transformation of society was combined with another of the main features of the Enlightenment movement: the pedagogical tendency that underlined all manifestations of Enlightenment thought.[8] Supporters of the Enlightenment believed in the transforming capacity of education and set out to spread its spirit throughout the social strata, to 'educate the people', and this zeal was revealed in some of the most particular features of the time: the erudite tendency in society which made the works of the Benedictine Feijoo[9] so successful; the great interest in travelling, a result of the Spaniards' desire to discover their own country and their past and which led to a series of works of great importance;[10] and the boom and development of journalism, stunted until then.[11] If we combine the obsession for useful information and the need to transmit this knowledge to the people in order to educate them and show them the errors of their ways, subjects on which all Enlightenment thinkers agreed, it is easy to deduce that all attempts to vulgarize or popularize knowledge received the support and encouragement of the Spanish enlightened élite. If we focus on this zeal in the field of medicine, we might suppose that the popularization of medicine was another question that attracted attention in the Spain of the Enlightenment. So it was, although, as in the case of the scientific resurgence, preference was given to imported knowledge rather than domestic production, in which little faith was placed. However, before discussing the question of what efforts were made to transmit knowledge to the Spanish people at the time of the Enlightenment so that they could take care of their health and, above all, take measures against illness, let us consider briefly the situation, in terms of their medical care, of those who inhabited the country.

Health care in the Spain of the Enlightenment

The availability of qualified medical care in the Spain of the last third of the eighteenth century was, as in other European countries,[12] very unequal, with a concentration of the more highly trained health practitioners in the cities, towns and large villages and the almost total abandonment of the rural population – especially important if we bear in mind that the rural population represented 80–90 per cent of the total.[13] This 'immense majority of the country' lived in highly precarious conditions; paying tithes, rents or local levies, duties to their lords and taxes to the Royal Treasury, they lived, more or less permanently, at the limits of subsistence.[14] Exposed to climatic variations which might cause poor harvests and with already low levels of production and commercialization, the Spanish peasants were victims, with unfailing regularity, of the famines and subsistence crises so characteristic of the Old Regime.[15] Rising prices, and salaries that did not grow at the same rate deepened this precariousness by reducing the purchasing power of those daily labourers who received their wages in money and who were affected by the surplus in the labour market.[16] The peasant's situation was therefore pitiful, as it was generally throughout Europe. So a large part of the Spanish population lived under the constant threat of food shortage, harassed by illness, with a short life expectancy – the rich had a few additional years, free from the hardship of work, exhaustion and poverty – and horribly punished by high infant mortality, a situation generally similar to that of the whole continental framework.[17]

Although there are not many statistics available, health practitioners were scarce and unevenly distributed, which meant that the population was badly cared for.[18] At the top of the health professionals pyramid, with university training, were the doctors whose numbers did not exceed 4,000 in the whole country for a population which by the end of the century was close to 11 million.[19] They too were unevenly distributed. The total number of surgeons, trained as apprentices to carry out basically manual tasks, was double that of the doctors but their distribution varied greatly between rural and urban areas. The combined total of the two groups of professionals shows significant regional differences,[20] although it must be said that the figures available are only indicative of the situation: the nature of health care in the rural villages of Spain in past centuries and its geographical distribution is one of the least known aspects of the medical history of the Spanish State, due basically to the dispersion of sources of information and the consequent difficulty of research.[21] Various orders of the time reveal a situation so precarious that healers among the rural population were excluded by law from military service because of their scarcity. The only 'qualified' health care in many villages was that offered by the barber–blood-letter and, like the doctors and surgeons, they were excluded from call-up in those places where there was no other type of professional care.[22] The barber–blood-letter's functions were limited, by law, to blood-letting; the extraction of teeth; the application of leeches and vesicatories; and the fitting and removal of cupping glasses; although, in fact, more often than not they were responsible for every type of professional health care in the rural world, taking the place of both surgeons and doctors.[23] Although differentiated by training and function, doctors, surgeons and barbers all required, in order to practise, apart from the appropriate studies for each profession, ratification by the *Protomedicato*, a longstanding body which had controlled the health practitioners of the country since its establishment by the Catholic

Monarchs,[24] or by one of its subordinate tribunals, *Protobarberato* and *Protocirujanato*. We shall return to this question below.

From the point of view of accessibility, we must bear in mind that, apart from the existence or non-existence of professionals, there was also the question of who could afford medical fees. The concentration of doctors and surgeons and even of barber–blood-letters in urban areas and large villages was due to the fact that it was precisely in these places that there were most possibilities of finding patients who could afford the treatment they required. The majority of the rural population did not have the means to pay the cost of a visit. To alleviate this situation, a regular practice was for villages to use their common funds to contract the services of a doctor or surgeon to look after the needs of the population, as is shown by the audit of these funds exercised by the Council of Castile.[25] Another means of financing health care was through the *Pósitos*, which had a decisive function in the stability of Spanish society under the Old Regime, as they were responsible for cereal supplies in times of shortage and acted as institutions of rural credit, lending grain to the farmers for sowing, which was repaid at a low interest called *crez*. Their reserves allowed them, on occasions, to contribute to the provision of health care for the rural population.[26] Care was also provided by other systems of social aid, which created a network of solidarity that helped peasants in cases of illness, death and bad harvests: for instance, the guilds of farmers, which operated in a similar way to the urban Brotherhoods. Little, however, is known about them as they were governed by custom, rarely recorded in written documents. It appears that the guilds acted as relief societies, aiding the peasant at times of illness, covering the cost of funerals and lending to farmers in times of bad harvests.[27]

In spite of these provisions, most of the population had to resort to other means to cure their ailments. Unqualified healers and empirics of all kinds were the real pillars of health care, supported by what laypeople managed to do for themselves. It is not surprising, therefore, that many works of medical popularization tackled this double angle, to resist the activities of charlatans and quacks and encourage the layperson's approach and adjust it to determined patterns.[28] In Spain there is no work on the scale of that of Ramsey for France at the end of the eighteenth and beginning of the nineteenth centuries[29] and, consequently, knowledge of Spanish irregular healers is general and vague; however, various examples provide evidence of its importance. We might begin by considering those who received a more or less formal academic training but failed to obtain a licence from the *Protomedicato* to practise. Throughout the eighteenth century various laws were introduced to enforce the obtaining of a licence,[30] the insistence upon which demonstrates the extent of the phenomenon. Faced with the shortage of registered professionals the municipal authorities consented to the practice of non-approved ones, providing them with licences to practise in the locality for periods of six or twelve months, which might be extended without difficulty,[31] as the only means of offering the residents regular health care. So, apart from the many surgeons, barbers and blood-letters who, although legally established, nevertheless performed functions for which they were neither trained nor authorized, there were others who acted as health-care givers in a totally unofficial and unauthorized capacity. Even worse was the situation of those who lacked even training but nevertheless sought to pass themselves off as professionals.[32] Many of them were forced to seek a living in this way because they had no other means of supporting themselves. This can be seen in the conscription of tramps and vagrants, which continued throughout the century, in which systematic detentions were made of people whose only occupation was that of surgeon, barber, blood-letter or even doctor.[33]

Apart from these pseudo-professionals there were many other individuals who, under different guises, acted as healers: sorcerers, quacks, charlatans, who offered various forms of treatment and relied on a long tradition in the health care of the Spanish population.[34] In some circumstances their intervention was permitted by the local authorities in order to mitigate the deficiencies of the health service which prevented the access of the popular classes to more qualified attention.[35] For instance the quack doctors who wandered across the national territory[36] specialized in the treatment of rabies.[37] Against them and other tramps, a Royal Decree was issued on 25 May 1783 which sought to find them a useful profession.[38] There were then many of these quack doctors, and records of their conduct can be found on occasions in the archives of the Inquisition as many of them were brought before the tribunal, accused of being heretics.[39] They used a wide variety of procedures – ointments, creams, religious relics, spells, incense and rituals – to cure their patients. They specialized in bizarre complaints like the evil eye; hunchbacks were cured by Galician quack doctors;[40] and children with hernias were surgically cut by quacks from Bearn in the north of the peninsula.[41] Other areas of health care were also the domain of unofficial doctors, for example in dental operations carried out by completely untrained tooth-pullers.[42] Care of women in labour was carried out by women called midwives, whose only training was to have cared for many women in the same situation. Worried by the lack of training and professionalism of many of those involved in this work, the *Protomedicato* recommended the reintroduction of an examination, suspended since the middle of the sixteenth century,[43] for all who wished to practise as midwives. Other common characters in the Spain of this time were the travelling salesmen who sold numerous types of remedies guaranteed to relieve a whole range of illnesses.[44] The economic dependency of each of these characters on their medical activities varied. It might represent their main source of income, it might be a way to earn a little extra, or it might be simply a 'gift' which they put at the service of the community in return only for presents which were considered more tokens of gratitude than payment of fees; it was, after all, a society in which community ties were stronger than the forces of individual profit-making.

The truth is that most of the population resorted to these unofficial healers, having first sought to solve their health problems themselves by resorting to their own medicines or asking advice of their family, friends or even the gentry, the clergy or teachers. Members of these local élites might offer assistance to their vassals, congregations or neighbours by giving advice culled from the many medical books which circulated and which we shall discuss below, or even by supplying them with remedies. Self-care was based fundamentally on the popular arsenal of remedies, prepared mainly from herbs, that was shared by all social classes and was the product of secular traditions which had survived through the ages and which represented the main model of popular, domestic, lay medicine.[45] So the majority of the population only rarely consulted official and properly qualified medical practitioners, and this cannot be explained only in terms of accessibility and availability.

As has been shown in the case of France,[46] attempts to spread regular health care met stiff resistance, largely because of the lack of agreement about the concepts of health and illness held by the population on the one hand and doctors and surgeons on the other. Religion was basic in the world vision of the people of the eighteenth century and therefore represented an important part of their ideas on illness. The faith of the people also included a belief in miracles that displeased supporters of the Enlightenment who considered it fanatical, erroneous and superstitious.[47] This faith, and a taste for the fantastic, resulted in the spread among the common people of tales of miracles, sorcery and spells in which illness and epidemics were caused and cured by Providence.[48] God and the Devil were, therefore, enemies in the field of health and there are many reports showing how the population turned to the saints, religious relics, shrines and pilgrimages in search of relief from illness.[49] There were even lay brothers and sisters who claimed curative powers based on their religious beliefs.[50] Other explanations of a more magical nature also recognized the existence of the supernatural in the etiology and healing of illnesses.[51] All this meant that the population's ideas on health and illness were closer to those of the unofficial quack doctors than to those of the professionals. As a result, even though official doctors were available and accessible, the common people did not usually consider consulting them, as their education placed them in a different social and cultural sphere. What all the social classes shared was the need for resources to confront accidents, consisting of self-treatment and self-medication. This need was of course met differently in different socioeconomic strata, according to the availability of different sources of information. Here it was that the different works and tracts of medical popularization entered the field to help the population, especially the literate classes, to carry out this self-care which represented the first line of defence against illness. Before entering into a description and in order to understand their diversity, we need to point out the eclectic nature of health alternatives.

Several authors have pointed out that it is not possible to draw a clear line separating the use made of professional and lay medicine by the peoples of pre-industrial Europe.[52] It has indeed been indicated that, as professional and lay medicine were complementary rather than competitive, the massive spread of orthodox and commercial medicine which began in the eighteenth century and accelerated in the nineteenth, really increased lay medical culture and self-medication.[53] This reality, which can also be applied to the Spanish case, led to the non-exclusive use of the various alternatives. Among the common people a worsening of the illness might lead the sufferer to consult the doctor as a last resort, in spite of the difficulty – perhaps impossibility – of paying the fees. The more well-to-do, who were used to consulting the professionals, surgeons or doctors, did not rule out the possibility of consulting an unofficial healer as well, who might see the patient before, during or after treatment by an official doctor, if the latter did not achieve the desired effects. There were unofficial healers, specialized in exploiting the failures of academic medicine, who could count on a good supply of clients. Patients also turned to different types of doctor for different types of illness; unofficial healers for the treatment of special ailments such as rabies, quacks for the evil eye, bone-setters and empiricists for slighter injuries like small wounds or dislocations, and the professionals when the ailment was more serious. A certain division of labour was thereby established. The possibilities were numerous and the patients and different types of doctor with their different beliefs and expectations interacted in a complex fashion, in which the economic dimension of each treatment played a role of the first order. The different alternatives competed for a limited 'medical market' and a struggle was thus established to gain the highest number of patients possible, competition in which the works of medical popularization played an important part. Let us now look at their presence in the panorama of the medical literature of the Spanish Enlightenment.

Works directed at the layperson

It is far from our intention to give an exhaustive list of all the works published in Spanish in the eighteenth century to help the population confront its health problems. We have left aside all types of journalism, although some periodicals achieved great success in eighteenth-century Spain, for example those foretelling the future. Until they were banned on 21 July 1767, together with ballads,[54] they enjoyed a wide role within the panorama of the press of the time and contained, of course, references to health and illness.[55] We shall only take into account works directed at the population in general that are, at the same time, general in content, thereby excluding works on specific subjects such as inoculation or mother–child health. Moreover, we refer only to works directed at individuals, and shall not discuss those concerning collective health which appealed for intervention by public authorities, as this question is outside the field of individual action against illness. With these parameters, the two main axes of eighteenth-century publications directed at laymen were, first, the works traditionally considered to be related to personal hygiene, in other words, those which offered advice on how to remain healthy through a correct orientation in all aspects of life; and, second, the works dedicated to remedies for the treatment of illnesses: the books of remedies. Together with these, those that won the widest presence in the Spanish publishing panorama and which most genuinely represent the characteristics of enlightened medical popularization were the translations of the works of Simon André Tissot and William Buchan, to which we shall devote the last part of this paper.

The works on personal hygiene, based on the principle of '*sex res non naturales*', sought to regulate aspects of the life of the individual in order to preserve health and prevent illness, which meant that their recommendations were only valid for the well-to-do who could afford to follow their instructions. In Spain this type of work had enjoyed a long tradition since the literary genre of the 'regimes of health'[56] had appeared in the Middle Ages. During the 1700s[57] and before the appearance at the end of the century of a new literature of public hygiene and the abandonment of the old model of individual advice, essays of this type continued to appear, based on the traditional scheme, although, evidently, brought up to date in many respects.[58] Also published in the Spain of the Enlightenment was a classic of the literature of personal hygiene which dates from the sixteenth century,[59] *La sobriedad y sus ventajas o verdadero medio de conservarse con salud perfecta hasta la más avanzada edad*[60] by Luigi Cornaro (1475–1566), which on its first edition in 1588 had begun the literary genre of life-preserving hygiene. On this occasion it was published with another treatise on hygiene by the Belgian Jesuit, Leonardo Lessius.[61] In this same tradition of personal hygiene, but limiting themselves to aspects related to diet, many other treatises also appeared.[62]

As for the prescription books – the presence of which in the Spanish panorama may be described in parallel form to the description given by Ramsey in this volume of the situation in

France – they were characterized by a series of remedies for specific illnesses, and usually explained the ingredients and means of preparing them. The peak of this literary genre is to be found in the sixteenth century, within the vast charitable movement which accompanied the Catholic Reformation.[63] Their aim, as well as to advise, was often to reveal secret remedies for the benefit of the poor, acting as a vehicle of charity opposed to the appropriation of knowledge. They also sought to put in writing popular empirical knowledge confirmed by experience and so in reality took over from the oral tradition. Usually directing their works to the peasants, the authors encouraged the search in nature for all that was necessary to cure illness. Of those we find in eighteenth-century Spain, some are not originals but rather later editions of works of the previous century or even of the fifteenth or sixteenth centuries, as is the case with the highly popular *Tesoro de Pobres*, published for the first time in Spanish in 1519, as a translation of the famous *Thesaurus Pauperum*, attributed to the Portuguese Pedro Hispano, usually identified with the man who would later become Pope John XXI.[64] Editions of this work, a classic of popular medical literature, appeared in 1705, 1722, 1727, 1734, 1764, 1765, 1791 and 1795 and, together with the publications of Buchan and Tissot, which we shall discuss below, represented the greatest success in its field of medical popularization. In the 1765 and 1795 editions the *Tesoro de Pobres* was published with another book of remedies by Antonio Bandinelli, *Experiencias y Remedios de Pobres*. Other works of the same type included *Medicina y Cirugía Racional y Espagírica*, published for the first time in 1691[65] and with new editions in 1709, 1720, 1722 and 1732,[66] and *Tratado del méthodo y orden de curar las enfermedades de los niños* by Gerónimo Soriano[67] and *Medicina Doméstica* by Felipe Borbón, published first in 1686 and again in 1705.[68] Members of the Church with charitable motives also published several remedy books.[69] Furthermore, works were published in eighteenth-century Spain which had been widely used in the colonies the previous century, together with others which appeared in the peninsula throughout the century.[70] Also worthy of mention is a whole series of publications which sought to defend one remedy as a panacea against all types of illness and which shared with the remedy books the aim of making known easy and inexpensive methods for self-treatment of illness. The remedy which caused the most ink to flow and created

170

the most controversy was, without doubt, water. We do not refer, of course, to the growing prestige which mineral water enjoyed in the course of the eighteenth century as a therapeutic resource, but rather to the curative virtues of natural water as a remedy or universal medicine. The purgative powders of Doctor Aylhaud of Aix (Provence) also received attention until their import into Spain was banned by the Royal Decree of 15 May 1750.[72] Other works sought to point out that the advantages of various 'secret medicines'; the works that gained greatest reknown in eighteenth-century Spain were those by the Portuguese Curbo Semmedo[73] and the Salamanca doctor Francisco Suárez de Rivera, whose remedies are distinguished by the high complexity of their ingredients.[74]

This rapid survey should also mention that translations into Spanish were made of some of the works of the philanthropic movement, the 'Médecine des pauvres', which, as Ramsey describes in his chapter, had so many exponents in the France of the seventeenth and eighteenth centuries.[75] In this way was published one of the most widely used remedy books in seventeenth-century France, by Marie de Mampeou, known as Mme Foucquet.[76] A joint translation also appeared of two works by Paul Dube,[77] which shared the characteristics of the remedy books but, unlike most of them, succinctly set out the symptoms of the illnesses to help with their diagnosis; this was an addition to the first editions of the works, according to the author, in response to the demands of the readers.[78]

However, in all this panorama, what stand out for their tremendous success are the translations in Spanish of the work of Tissot, which appeared under the title *Aviso al pueblo sobre su salud o Tratado de las enfermedades más frecuentes de las gentes del campo* and that of William Buchan, *Medicina Doméstica*. In the short space of time from 1773, the year in which the first edition of Tissot's work appeared, until 1808, the year of the invasion by Napoleon which marks the end of the Enlightenment in Spain,[79] these works out-published any other medical work of the period. Tissot's *Avis* was published in 1773, 1774, 1776, 1778, 1781, 1790, and 1795, and Buchan's *Domestic Medicine* appeared in three editions in 1785, by different translators, and other editions appeared in 1786, 1792 and 1798. Other works by the same authors appeared, also devoted to advice to laypeople, although they had considerably less success than the *Avis* or *Domestic Medicine*.

Tissot's work on inoculation was never published, although the ideas expressed in it circulated widely throughout Spain thanks to the Catalan doctor Francisco Salvá y Campillo, who described them in his own works.[80] A translation of *De la santé des gens des lettres* did appear, published in 1771,[81] and became the first work of the Swiss to be published in Spanish. Years later it was translated again and published together with a translation of the *Essai sur les maladies des gens du monde* and other minor works.[82] As regards *L'Onanisme*, during the period of the Enlightenment, there were repeated attempts to publish the work, which were blocked by the health and government authorities as they considered that the book might spread the habit of masturbation rather than put an end to it;[83] it finally appeared in 1807[84] but, as its publication had not been authorized, the Council of Castille ordered the immediate withdrawal of all the copies in circulation through a series of meticulous searches.[85] We do know that the work was read, at least in French, as the prohibition did not extend to that language, and numerous copies of *L'Onanisme* and all the other works of Tissot can be found in the stocks and catalogues of libraries today.[86] This shows, as pointed out by Maria Szlatky in her chapter on Hungary, the wide readership obtained by the works of the author of the *Avis*.

As regards Buchan, his only other work to appear translated into Spanish was *Advice to mothers on the subject of their own health and the means of promoting the health, strength and beauty of their offspring*, but as this occurred in 1808,[87] the year of the Napoleonic invasion, its influence was limited and it did not reach a second edition.

Between 1771, the year in which the first edition of a translation of Tissot's work appeared, and 1808 there were eighteen editions of the works of these authors, which represents, if only from the numerical point of view, a highly relevant statistic in the Spanish medical panorama. From the point of view of the assimilation of European tendencies, in which Spanish supporters of the Enlightenment had worked so hard, the works of Tissot and Buchan represented a vital link in the diffusion of European medicine in the Spain of the Enlightenment,[88] above all as regards the ideas relating to health education,[89] an effort equalled only by that made in the field of surgery.[90] This is not surprising as these same works were those that excited by far the most interest in the whole European scene[91] and even, in the case of Buchan, as shown by Gevitz in his contribution, in North America.[92] What does attract attention is the great success in Spain of these works considering their price which, as in other countries,[93] was higher than others of less volume.[94] Perhaps the rural (Tissot) and urban (Buchan) local élites at whom these works were aimed were the only groups with the purchasing power necessary to acquire this type of book and the only ones that could read them, given the low level of literacy in the country.[95] In any case it does not seem exaggerated to say that to talk of popularization of medicine in the Spain of the Enlightenment is to talk of Tissot and Buchan. It was the accurate descriptions that these works included, their therapeutic advice, their denial of all that the unofficial practitioners stood for, and their delimitation of what laypeople could do for themselves against illness – more critical of popular ideas in the case of Tissot, more tolerant in the case of Buchan, who, as shown by Porter in his chapter, was the one who supported a greater 'democratization' of medical knowledge among laymen – which captivated the Spanish reader interested in medical questions and in having a useful and practical guide to self-treatment. Several authors[96] have pointed out the importance of studying this type of work in order to understand in depth the process of exchange of medical knowledge between professionals and laypeople, in a context where, as we have seen above, no clear line could be drawn between the two worlds. From this point of view the works of Tissot and Buchan have been the main focus of attention in recent decades[97] and the nature of their work is consequently well known. But how were these works presented to the Spanish reader? We shall devote the last part of this paper to the clarification of these peculiarities which, we can say in advance, were not excessive.

Tissot's *Avis au Peuple* and Buchan's *Domestic Medicine*

The *Avis au Peuple sur sa Santé* was first published in Spanish in 1773, in Pamplona,[98] following the translation made by an obscure provincial clergyman, Joseph Fernández Rubio, from the Paris edition of 1767[99] to which he added only an insignificant prologue. This translation was not reprinted and it was the translation of 1774[100] by Juan Galisteo y Xiorro which was published in 1776, 1778, 1781, 1790 and 1795. Juan Galisteo y Xiorro, together with his brother Félix, was one of the professional practitioners who did most work in terms of the translation of medical works in the Spain of the Enlightenment, although the scant attention paid to them by medical history means we know very little about their professional careers: they were trained in those Madrid surgical circles of the middle of the century which took shape in the creation of the Royal College of Surgery of San Carlos,[101] one of the most innovative of the health institutions of the Enlightenment, together with the Royal Colleges of Surgery of Cadiz and Barcelona; and apart from the above-mentioned translation of the works of Tissot they carried out important work in the translation of medical and surgical texts, among which we can mention the works of Georges La Faye (1699–1781), Johannes Gorter (1689–1762), Herman Boerhaave (1668–1738), John Pringle (1707–82), Jean Astruc (1684–1766), Henri François Le Dran (1685–1770), Jean Louis Petit (1674–1750) and André Levret (1703–80).[102] Together with Iberti, one of the translators of Buchan's *Domestic Medicine*, the Galisteo brothers were the main exponents of the health professionals who took up the ideas of the Enlightenment and directed their efforts at bringing within reach of Spanish readers those works of medical popularization successful in Europe.

The 1774 edition of the *Avis* was also based on the original third Paris edition of 1767 but the translator affirms that he includes additions which appear in the second original edition of the work;[103] these consist of the 'Prologue to Mr. Hirzel on the Nature of the Real and False Doctor', attributed to the author of the German translation of the work and appearing first in French in the Lyon edition of 1763;[104] and a whole new chapter, 'Additions on different common and frequent illnesses', which appeared in the Paris editions of 1762 and 1763, but which Tissot did not approve as it deviated from the field of acute illnesses; so it did not appear in the following French edition.[105] Juan Galisteo did, however, keep this chapter with slight amendments in all the Spanish editions, although he always noted that it was an additional chapter. This addition also meant, as in the case of the French edition, the extension of the chapter devoted to 'Questions one must be able to answer when one consults a Doctor', and 'Table of remedies' and a series of appendices with explanations of how to prepare them, in which Galisteo introduced the names of many of them in vulgar Spanish.[106] The translator added, as well as a prologue,[107] some 'Tables of the main Baths and sulphurous and iron Springs in Spain of the type proposed by Mr Tissot', for which he used contemporary European and Spanish treatises on hydrotherapy.[108] Likewise, Galisteo y Xiorro was required, according to his own criteria, to add sections on stings and bites by vipers, scorpions, spiders and toads, because of their frequency in Spain.[109] Another short addition is a description and diagram of a machine to introduce tobacco smoke into the intestines in order to revive drowning victims, which was included as an alternative method to that proposed by Tissot.[110] Juan Galisteo y Xiorro also includes a limited series of translator's notes and it is worth drawing attention to those which point out special circumstances in Spain and which serve as clarification of Tissot's comments about the Pays de Vaud or Lausanne; also of interest are those that refer to surgical conditions and external illnesses prompted by the translator's own experience in this field, although, as Philip Wilson points out in his contribution to this book, only with difficulty can these be considered a true attempt to popularize surgery.

With these additions, which we can see make only minor adjustments to the work of the Swiss writer for the benefit of Spanish readers, and which also occurred with the Hungarian translation that Maria Szlatky describes in this volume, the remaining editions of *Avis* were published unamended except on two subjects: that of apparent death, so popular among followers of the Enlightenment,[111] and that of venereal disease. In the 1776 edition the chapter on drownings was replaced by one on sudden and apparent deaths[112] which sets out the procedure to follow in cases of asphyxia and how to operate a machine for introducing tobacco smoke into the intestines. Likewise a chapter was included devoted to venereal diseases which included a description of their symptoms and treatment.[113] Both additions were the work of the French doctor Joseph Jacques Gardane, an important contributor on questions of public health.[114] The translator further added a new appendix in which he offered instructions on the method of testing mineral waters;[115] this, together with Gardane's chapters, was published separately in a 95-page booklet.[116]

There were other small differences between the editions of 1774 and 1776, which appear above all in the translator's notes, among which it is worth drawing attention to a denial of the harmful effects of the ingestion of horned-rye grains,[117] a note on the legislative prohibition of the removal of hernia sufferers' testicles by charlatans and quacks;[118] other differences occur in the chapter on inoculation which defends the practice and recommends the Sutton method.[119]

The next edition, in 1778,[120] showed no changes. In the 1781[121] edition the differences are minimal, although there is a new prologue by Tissot, dated in 1778 in Lausanne,[122] an article devoted to malignant dysentery[123] which appears to be the work of the translator; and the description, method of use and diagram of 'Mr Mudge's Breathing Aid',[124] an apparatus to relieve coughing. Nine years later, in 1790,[125] a new edition appeared in which the most important change was the replacement of the chapter on asphyxia by a new work by Gardane on the same subject which had been first published separately in 1784,[126] also translated by Juan Galisteo y Xiorro. The work was written in the form of a catechism to make it easier to understand.[127] New descriptions and diagrams illustrate the operation of other machines.[128] There is also a new appendix on the precautions that should be taken when exhuming bodies, also structured in the form of a catechism,[129] written by Dr Maret[130] and published with the work of Gardane in the 1784 edition. The 1795[131] and 1815[132] editions, published outside the period to which we have limited ourselves, include virtually no changes.

As regards the position of *Domestic Medicine* by William Buchan in the Spanish publishing panorama of the Enlightenment, the most notable thing is that in the year of its first edition, 1785, three publishing concerns coincided in their plans to make the work available to Spanish readers. One of these was under the auspices of the Crown, as it was an important figure in government circles, the Count of Floridablanca, then attorney of the Council of Castile, who commissioned José Iberti, a royal physician and one of the outstanding medical figures of the Spanish Enlightenment,[133] to translate the work. This was done and a first volume appeared, printed on the Royal Press.[134] It contained the first part of Buchan's work, devoted to the general causes of illnesses, together with a supplement designed '. . . to corroborate some of the author's doctrines, add some omitted articles which seemed to me useful and adapt the medical precepts to the particular climate and way of life of this Kingdom . . .'[135] and some of the additions made by the French translator, Mr Duplanil.[136] This was the only volume to appear, as the royal project was abandoned in the face of private initiatives.

The other translations were undertaken by Pedro Sinnot, an Irish clergyman who was put in charge of the task as a result of his knowledge of the English language,[137] and by Antonio de Alcedo, military officer and historian,[138] who had this one contact with the task of translating medical texts as a result of his role as officer during the seige of Gibraltar when he had had access to Buchan's work.[139] We can conclude, therefore, that except in the case of the Galisteo brothers and of José Iberti, true representatives of the renewal of and introduction to European trends in the Enlightenment in Spain, the other translators of the works of popularization which concern us had only an occasional and chance part to play in the task.

Sinnot undertook the publication of Buchan's work based on M. Duplanil's French translation,[140] which was full of additions and appendices and meant that five volumes appeared between 1785 and 1786.[141] Alcedo on the other hand translated the work directly from the original English and published it in a single quarto volume.[142] Their simultaneous appearance led both authors to become involved in a lawsuit over the rights of publication in Spanish, which can be followed through the printing applications for the works.[143] All authors and translators were obliged to go through this process in order to obtain permission for publication,[144] a permission which was usually accompanied by exclusive rights of sale for five or ten years and which might be renewed. After many hearings, the publication of both translations was permitted and both Sinnot and Alcedo were granted rights, from which, as in the case of Buchan himself,[145] they gained only minimal benefit. Sinnot acted on behalf of Pedro Kearney,[146] to whom the rights of the translation really belonged, and Alcedo sold his rights and 785 copies of the work to Valentin Francés[147] for 17,500 reales, a substantial sum which would nevertheless be far exceeded by the sale of successive editions of the translation.

As we have said, it was Alcedo who most faithfully followed Buchan's text; according to the translator himself, '. . . I have only put notes of things I have experienced and which prove, in our country, the opinion of the author, and modifications of some remedies made necessary by the climatic differences between our country and England . . .'[148] This single-volume translation was the most successful and with hardly any changes was republished in 1786, 1792 and 1798[149] and then later in 1818.[150]

Sinnot, as mentioned above, did not translate into Spanish Buchan's *Domestic Medicine*, but rather the *Médecine Domestique* of Buchan and Duplanil, which contains numerous additions in every chapter of the Scotsman's work. This work had been approved by Buchan himself,[151] although he criticized its excessive length. For his own part, Duplanil had included a prologue in which he criticized Tissot's *L'Avis au Peuple* – despite quoting widely from it throughout his translation – for failing to include chronic illnesses.[152] As well as the additions, this edition included summaries intended to make the work easier to understand.[153] It also included a list of '. . . simple and compound medicines which one should always have at hand especially in the country'[154] and a 'Glossary'[155] which set out in alphabetical order remedies, general medical terms, wounds, symptoms and surgical terms. Each entry in the glossary included a reference to where the item appeared in the book, a genuine effort to provide an easier and more practical guide.

This edition was reported to the Inquisition,[156] which, although languishing in the eighteenth century, had still made trouble for Jorge Juan (1713–73) in 1748 when he published his *Astronomy Observations* in which he defended heliocentrism.[157] The fact that prior censorship existed in Spain, so that no work could be published in the realm without the prior authorization of the government,[158] meant that those books published in Spain that were liable to be banned by the Inquisition were exceptional cases. The Inquisition was concerned above all with books written in French and occasionally in German and English, whose entry into Spain was prohibited.[159] These works were mainly on philosophical subjects and related to the *Encyclopédie* movement, but also included works on public and private law, theology, the history of the Church, canon law, antireligious and anticlerical literature, history, memoirs, geography, travel, the history of the revolution and also romantic and erotic novels.[160] In general, very few books connected with medicine were submitted to the Inquisition during the eighteenth century,[161] and of those that were it was the result, in some cases, of their ideas on astrology.[162] In the case of books published in Spain, such as Buchan's *Medicina Doméstica*, the only ones condemned were those that defended 'royal prerogatives' and were censored by the Inquisition because they attacked the rights and immunity of the Church; and Spanish translations of foreign works that included 'errors of faith' and attracted the attention of the Inquisition because they thus reached a wider public.[163] The latter seems to have been the case with Buchan's work, as the reason given in the findings of the Inquisition's report was that this book described the custom of ringing church bells when someone died as superstitious, and furthermore suggested that it might cause shock and death in women in labour.[164] Although the reference was to England, the Inquisition considered it '. . . false doctrine, rash, impious, scandalous, offensive and verging on heresy . . .'[165] and demanded the suppression of these paragraphs. After various deliberations and pleas this finding was published in an edict on censored books on 24 May 1789.[166] The book continued to cause problems but this did not prevent a new edition appearing,[167] also by Sinnot and based on the ninth English edition – London, 1786[168] – and Duplanil's last French edition – Paris 1788.[169] The changes to the 1785/6 edition included new prologues by Duplanil, Sinnot and Buchan and a reordering of the chapters, and Volume V was devoted entirely to a list of remedies and the glossary, both of which were reorganized and extended. Two appendices were added, one with the 'Remedies of the Pharmacopoeias of London and Edinburgh'[170] and another which, as in the work of Tissot, made reference to the mineral waters of the different Spanish regions and methods of testing them.[171]

In conclusion, therefore, we can say that the works of Tissot and Buchan, which by embodying so well the spirit of the time had been so successful in Europe and North America, had the same effect in the Spain of the Enlightenment. A few changes, especially as regards the remedies – although slighter than claimed by the authors – were enough for them to take command of the panorama of medical popularization in Spain, pushing aside the rather limited domestic productions, their position only slightly threatened by the remedy books. The educated élites at which Tissot and Buchan aimed their works also found them useful guides to explain the omnipresent layman's responsibility in questions of health and illness, at a time when the professionals did not exercise the strict hegemony that they would later achieve. The books' influence spread during the first decades of the nineteenth century, when, as we have seen,[172] the last editions of the works appeared, coinciding with a greater presence of Spanish works of this type such as Francisco Javier Rivera y Aravigt's *El médico y cirujano de valde*.[173] Halfway through the century, the field of popularization became dominated in Spain by the works of representatives of the hygienic movement like Pedro Felipe Monlau whose *Nociones de Higiene Doméstica*, published for the first time in 1860, was widely reprinted.[174] This author was also responsible for various popular medical periodicals[175] which initiated the long list of works of popularization that flooded the Spanish publishing world at the end of the nineteenth century.[176]

Acknowledgement

I would like to thank Jonathan Ch. Whitehead for his translation of the Spanish version of this paper.

Notes

1. E. Balaguer, 'La ciencia y la técnica', in *Historia general de España y América* (Madrid, 1983), vol. X–1, 177.

2. J.M. López, *La introducción de la ciencia moderna en España* (Barcelona, 1969); J.M. López, *Ciencia y técnica en la sociedad españa de los siglos XVI y XVII* (Barcelona, 1979).

3. Balaguer, 'La ciencia y la técnica', 177.

4. A. Mestre, *Despotismo e ilustración en España* (Barcelona, 1976).

5. J. Fernández, I. González (eds), *Cienca, técnica y estado en la España ilustrada* (Madrid, 1990); M. Sellés, J.L. Peset, A. Lafuente (eds), *Carlos Ill y la ciencia de la ilustración* (Madrid, 1988).

6. F. Aguilar, *La Real Sociedad economica matritense de amigos del pais* (Madrid, 1972); P. Demerson, J. Demerson, F. Aguilar, *Las sociedades económicas de amigos del pais en el siglo XVIII. Guía del investigador* (San Sebastián, 1974).

7. Balaguer, 'La ciencia y la técnica', 193–4.

8. J.L. Abellán, 'La ilustración', in *Historia critica del pensamiento español. 3. Del Barroco a la ilustración (siglos XVII–XVIII)* (Madrid, 1981), 486–7.

9. The benedictine B.J. Feijoo wrote *Teatro Crítico Universal*, published for the first time between 1726 and 1740, and *Cartas eruditas y curiosas* (1742–60). He achieved overwhelming success. See the bibliography on Feijoo in A.R. Fernández González 'Introduction' and 'Bibliografia', in B.J. Feijoo, *Teatro Crítico Universal*, 2nd edn (Madrid, 1983), 11–69.

10. See the compilations J. Garcia, *Viajes por España* (Madrid, 1972); G. Gómez, *Los viajeros de la ilustración* (Madrid, 1974).

11. M.D. Saiz, *Historia del periodismo en España, I. Los origenes: el siglo XVIII*, 3rd edn (Madrid, 1990).

Medicine during the Spanish Enlightenment

12. See, for example, M. Ramsay, *Professional and Popular Medicine in France, 1770–1830. The Social World of Medical Practice* (Cambridge, 1988).
13. Abellán, *Historia crítica del pensamiento español. 3. Del Barroco a la ilustración (siglos XVII–XVII)*, 468–70; G. Anes, *El Antiguo Régimen: los Borbones.* 5th edn (Madrid, 1981), 92; A. Domínguez, *Sociedad y estado en el siglo XVIII español* (Barcelona, 1976), 197; P. Saavedra; R. Villares, 'Galicia en el antiguo régimen: la fortaleza de una sociedad tradicional', in R. Fernández (ed.), *España en el siglo XVIII* (Barcelona: 1985), 474.
14. A. Dominguez, 'La sociedad española en el tránsito del siglo XVIII al XIX', in G. Anes *et al. España a finales del siglo XVIII* (Tarragona, 1982), 51–2.
15. V. Pérez Moreda, *Las crisis de mortalidad en la España interior (siglos XVI–XIX)* (Madrid, 1980); J.S. Bernat, M.A. Badenes, 'Cronologia, intensidad y extensión de las crisis demográficas en el Pais Valencià', in C. Pérez, *Estudis sobre la població Valenciana* (Valencia/Alicante, 1988), 537–60; M. Lázaro, P.A. Gurria, *Las crisis de mortalidad en La Rioja (siglos XVI–XVIII)* (Logroño, 1989); A. Rodríguez, 'Las crisis de mortalidad en la Alta Extremadura durante el siglo XVII', *Boletín de la Asociación de Demografía Histórica* (1989), 3: 37–54.
16. G. Anes, 'Obstáculos para el crecimiento agrario en la España del siglo XVIII', in Anes, *España a finales del siglo XVIII*, 39–40; G. Anes, 'La Asturias preindustrial', in Fernández (ed.) *España en el siglo XVIII*, 530; Dominguez, *Sociedad y estado en el siglo XVIII español,* 180, 209–10; A. García, 'El interior peninsular en el siglo XVIII: un crecimiento moderado y tradicional', in Fernández (ed.) *España en el siglo XVIII*, 651–2; G. Lemeunier, 'El reino de Murcia en el siglo XVIII: realidad y contradicciones del crecimiento', in Fernández (ed.) *España en el siglo XVIII*, 322; C. Martínez, 'La Cataluña del siglo XVIII bajo el signo de la expansión', in Fernández (ed.) *España en el siglo XVIII*, 100; I. Moll, J. Suau, 'Memoria explicativa del estado de la isla de Mallorca en el siglo XVIII', in Fernández (ed.) *España en el siglo XVIII*, 270–1; J. Sarrailh, *La España ilustrada de la segunda mitad del siglo XVIII* (Mexico, 1957), 20–36.
17. F. Braudel, *Civilización material, economía y capitalismo. Siglos XV–XVIII: 1. Las estructuras de lo cotidiano: lo posible y lo imposible* (Madrid, 1984), 63–4, 238.
18. A. Lafuente, J. Puerto, M.C. Calleja, 'Los profesionales de la sanidad tras su identidad en la Ilustración española', in J.M. Sánchez (ed.) *Ciencia y sociedad en España* (Madrid, 1988), 73–4.
19. Dominguez, *Sociedad y estado en el siglo XVIII español,* 383–5; A. Eiras, 'Problemas demográficos del siglo XVIII', in Anes, *España a finales del siglo XVIII*, 20–1; M. Martín, *Pensamiento económico español sobre la población* (Madrid, 1984), 34–5; V. Pérez, 'La población española', in M. Artola (ed.) *Enciclopedia de historia de España* (Madrid, 1988), 384–5.
20. R. Muñoz, *Ejercicio legal de la Medicina en España (siglos XV al XVIII)* (Salamanca, 1967), 17.
21. A. Domínguez, 'Algunos datos sobre médicos rurales en la España del siglo XVIII' in *Hechos y figuras del siglo XVIII español* (Madrid,

181

1973), 143; Domínguez, *Sociedad y estado en el siglo XVIII español,* 249–51; J. Ramos, *La salud pública y el hospital general de la ciudad de Pamplona en el Antiguo Régimen (1700 a 1815), Doctoral thesis* (Pamplona, 1988), 58–9; J.M. López, 'Contribución al estudio de la sanidad rural en la provincia de Valladolid durante el siglo XVIII', *VII Congreso Nacional de Historia de la Medicina* (Alicante, 1983), unpublished manuscript.

22. J.M. Massons, 'Los cirujanos madrileños del siglo XVIII ante el Servicio Militar', *Actas del XXVII Congreso Internacional de Historia de la Medicina* (Barcelona, 1981), vol. II, 578–9.

23. A. Carreras, 'Las actividades de los barberos durante los siglo XVI al XVIII', *Cuad.Hist.Med.Esp.* (1974) XIII: 208.

24. P. Iborra, 'Memoria sobre la Institución del Real Proto-Medicato', *Anales de la Real Academia Nacional de Medicina* (1885) VI: 183–307, 387–418, 496–522, 571–94; M. Parrilla, 'Apuntes históricos sobre el protomedicato. Antecedentes y organismos herederos', *Anales de la Real Academia Nacional de Medicina* (1977) XCIV: 475–515; M.C. Calleja, 'Centralización y unificación de la administración sanitaria española durante el siglo XVIII', *Boletín Sociedad Española Historia de la Farmacia* (1986) 147: 189–210; M.C. Calleja, 'El protomedicato y su proyecto de renovación de la sanidad española durante el siglo XVIII', in M. Esteban *et al.* (eds), *Estudios sobre historia de la ciencia y de la técnica. I* (Valladolid, 1988), 495–504; M.C. Calleja, *La reform sanitaria de la España ilustrada,* doctoral thesis (Madrid, 1989).

25. Domínguez, *Hechos y figuras del siglo XVIII español,* 251–4. Domínguez, *Sociedad y estado en el siglo XVIII español,* 189, 395, 463 and 465–6.

26. G. Anes, *Economía e 'Ilustración' en la España del siglo XVIII,* 3rd edn (Barcelona, 1981); P. Trinidad, 'Asistencia y previsión social en el siglo XVIII', in C. López (ed.) *4 siglos de acción social: de la beneficencia al bienestar social* (Madrid, 1985), 111–12.

27. Trinidad, 'Asistencia y previsión social en el siglo XVIII', 110; J. Pereira, 'La religiosidad y la sociabilidad popular como aspectos del conflicto social en el Madrid de la segunda mitad del siglo XVIII', in Equipo Madrid, *Carlos III, Madrid y la ilustración* (Madrid, 1988), 223–54; J.L. De los Reyes, 'Carlos III, padre de los vasallos', in Equipo Madrid, *Carlos III, Madrid y la ilustración,* 360–2.

28. See chap. 6.2 of my doctoral thesis, E. Perdiguero, 'El ámbito de la medicina doméstica', in *Los tratados de medicina doméstica en la España de la ilustración* (Alicante, 1989), vol. II, 328–52.

29. Ramsey, *Professional and popular medicine in France, 1770–1830.* See also T. Gelfand, 'Medical Professionals and Charlatans. The Comité de Salubrité enquête', *Histoire Sociale/Social History* (1978) XI: 62–97.

30. R. Muñoz, C. Muñiz, *Fuentes legales de la medicina española (siglos XIII–XIX)* (Salamanca, 1969), 64, 69–72, 72–3, 75, 89–91; Iborra, 'Memoria sobre la institución del Real-Protomedicato', 266; Muñoz *Ejercicio legal de la medicina en España (Siglos XV al XVIII),* 141–2; J. Alvarez, *Carlos III y la higiene pública* (Madrid, 1956), 27–8; Lafuente,

Puerto, Calleja, 'Los profesionales de la sanidad tras su identidad en la Ilustración española', 75–80.

31. Iborra, 'Memoria sobre la Institución del Real Proto-Medicato', 266; Perez, *Las crisis de mortalidad en la España interior (siglos XVI–XIX)*, 441–2.

32. A. Fernández *et al.* 'Intrusismo profesional sanitario y ejercicio legal de la medicina y otros menesteres curadores durante el siglo XVIII en el reino de Córdoba', *VII Congreso Nacional de Historia de la Medicina* (Alicante, 1983). Unpublished manuscript, J.L. Valverde, *La farmacia y las ciencias farmacéuticas en las obras de Suárez de Ribera* (Salamanca, 1970), 69.

33. R.M. Pérez, *El problema de los vagos en la España del siglo XVIII* (Madrid, 1976), 124–5, 147–9.

34. L.S. Granjel, *La medicina española antigua y medieval* (Salamanca, 1981), 150–60; L.S. Granjel, *La medicina española renacentista* (Salamanca, 1980), 133–50; L.S. Granjel, *La medicina española del siglo XVII* (Salamanca, 1978), 113–25.

35. F. Guillén, *La introducción de la salud pública en la medicina española del siglo XVIII*, doctoral thesis (Murcia, 1987), vol. I, 126.

36. Perez, *El problema de los vagos en la España del siglo XVIII*, 62–3.

37. L.S. Granjel, 'El pensamiento médico del Padre Antonio José Rodriguez', in *Humanismo y medicina* (Salamanca, 1968), 216–17; S. Muñoz, *Inquisición y ciencia en la España moderna* (Madrid, 1977), 174.

38. L.M. Enciso, 'Prólogo', in Pérez, *El problema de los vagos en la España del siglo XVIII*, 15–16; Anes, *El Antiguo Régimen: los Borbones*, 154.

39. See, as examples: Muñoz, *Inquisición y ciencia en la España moderna*, 150–2, 162, 182–3; G. Folch, A.M. Gil, 'La inquisición y el Curanderismo en Canarias durante el siglo XVIII', *Anales de la Real Academia de Farmacia* (1971) 37: 71–85; J. Diaz, *Conflicto social, marginación y mentalidades en la Mancha (siglo XVIII)* (Ciudad Real, 1987), 196–201.

40. P. Marset, 'El "Arte de conocer" de Francisco Rubio. El empirismo médico en la España del siglo XVIII', *Medicina Española* (1974), 72, 189.

41. Anes, *El Antiguo Régimen: los Borbones*, 144.

42. J.M. López, J.M. Pastor, 'La posición del "Tratado" de Félix Pérez de Arroyo en la odontología española del siglo XVIII', in J.M. Pérez de Arroyo, *Tratado de las operaciones que deben practicarse en la Dentadura* (Valencia, 1985), 7–26 (1799); M. Irigoyen, *La odontología española del siglo XVIII* (Salamanca, 1967), 52.

43. Pérez, *Las crisis de mortalidad en la España interior (siglos XVI–XIX)*, 442–3.

44. J.L. Valverde, J.A. Pérez, 'Intrusismo profesional médico farmacéutico en España (siglo XVIII): el curandero Cristobal Martinez', in G. Folch, F.J. Puerto (eds), *Medicamento, historia y sociedad* (Madrid, 1982), 621–32.

45. B. Gebhard, 'Historical Relationship between Scientific and Lay Medicine for Present Day Education', *Bull.Hist.Med.* (1958), 32: 226–7.

46. J.P. Goubert, 'The Medicalization of French Society at the End of the Ancien Régime', in Ll.G. Stevenson (ed.), *A Celebration of Medical History* (Baltimore, 1982), 157–72; H. Mitchell, 'Rationality and Control in French Eighteenth-Century Medical Views of the Peasantry', *Comp.Stud.Soc.Hist.* (1979) 21: 82–112; J.P. Peter, 'Disease and the Sick at the End of the Eighteenth Century', in R. Forster, O. Ranum, *Biology of Man in History* (Baltimore, 1975), 81–124.

47. A. Castillo de Lucas, 'El Padre Feijoo y la medicina popular', *Bol.Soc.Esp.Hist.Med.* (1960–67) V: 1–7, 7–19; Granjel, 'El pensamiento médico del Padre Antonio José Rodriguez', 226–7.

48. J. Caro, *Ensayo sobre la literatura de cordel* (Madrid, 1969), 22–3; Sarrailh, *La España ilustrada de la segunda mitad del siglo XVIII*, 59.

49. See J.R. Zaragoza, J.L. Peset, 'Medicina y sociedad en la España del siglo XVIII según el viaje de Townsed', *Medicina española* (1970) 63: 308; Sarrailh, *La España ilustrada de la segunda mitad del siglo XVIII*, 612, 656–9, 661–5, 672; R. Herr, *España y la Revolución del siglo XVIII* (Madrid, 1975), 26–7; L.S. Granjel, *La medicina española del siglo XVIII* (Salamanca, Universidad), 112.

50. Granjel, *La medicina española del siglo XVIII*, 112.

51. J.R. Zaragoza, 'Medicina, ciencia y técnica en la España ilustrada según el "viaje" de Peyron', *Cuad.Hist.Med.Esp.* (1967) VI: 140–1; Zaragoza, Peset, 'Medicina y sociedad en la España del siglo XVIII según el viaje de Townsend', 309; Sarrailh, *La España ilustrada de la segunda mitad del siglo XVIII*, 108; Herr, *España y la Revolución del siglo XVIII*, 34, 127.

52. R. Porter, 'Introduction' in R. Porter (ed.), *Patients and Practitioners. Lay Perceptions of Medicine in Pre-industrial Society* (Cambridge, 1985), 15–16; Ramsey, *Professional and Popular Medicine in France*, 2–4.

53. Porter, 'The Patient in Eighteenth-Century England', 46.

54. F. Aguilar, *La prensa española en el siglo XVIII. Diarios, revistas y pronósticos* (Madrid, 1978), XIX.

55. Aguilar, *La prensa española en el siglo XVIII*, XIII.

56. J.M. López, 'Breve historia de la medicina española', in Ch. Singer, E.A. Underwood, *Breve historia de la medicina* (Madrid, 1966), 727.

57. We consider 1808 as the limit of our study, when the Independence War ended the Enlightenment in Spain.

58. A.G. Begue de Presle, *El conservador de la salud* (Madrid, 1776); G. Rowley, *Obras* (Madrid, 1796–98); J.B. Pressavin, *Arte de conservar la salud y prolongar la vida o tratado de higiene* (Salamanca, 1800), (Madrid, 1804); E. Tourtelle, *Elementos de hygiene* (Madrid, 1806), (Madrid, 1818).

59. G.J. Gruman, 'The Rise and Fall of Prolongevity Hygiene (1558–1873)', *Bull.Hist.Med.* (1961) 35: 221–9; A. Palau, *Manual del librero hispanoamericano* (Barcelona, 1948–77), vol. IV, 106; H. Sigerist, 'La búsqueda de una larga vida en el Renacimiento' in *Hitos en la historia de la salud pública* (Mexico, 1981), 58–9.

60. L. Cornaro, *La sobriedad y sus ventajas o verdadero medio de conservarse con salud perfecta hasta la más avanzada edad* (Madrid, 1782).

61. L. Lessius, *Hygisticon sue vera ratio valetudinis bonae et vitae una*

cumsensuum, judici et memoriae integritate ad extreman senectutem conservandae, in Cornaro, *La sobriedad y sus ventajas.*

62. G. Arias, *Tratado físico-médico de las virtudes, cualidades, provechos, uso y abuso del cafe, del the, del chocolate y del tabaco* (Madrid, 1752); A. Lavedan, *Tratado de los usos, abusos, propiedades y virtudes del café, te y chocolate* (Madrid, 1796).

63. M. Laget, 'Les livrets de santé pour les pauvres aux XVIIé et XVIIIé siècles', *Histoire, Economie et Societé* (1984) 3: 567–8.

64. A. Hernández Morejón, *Historia bibliográfica de la medicina española* (New York–London, 1967), vol. I, 235–6; Palau, *Manual del librero hispanoamericano,* vol. XII, 180–4; J.A. Paniagua, *El maravilloso regimiento y orden de vivir de Arnau de Vilanova* (Zaragoza, Universidad), 84–6; M.H. Rocha, *Obras médicas de Pedro Hispano* (Coimbra, 1973).

65. J. Vidos y Miró, *Medicina y cirugia racional y espagírica* (Zaragoza, 1691). About this work see also Granjel, *La medicina española del siglo XVII,* 113–14.

66. J. Vidos y Miró, *Medicina y cirugia racional y espagírica* (Zaragoza, 1709), (Zaragoza, 1720), (Sevilla, 1722), (Madrid, 1732).

67. Work first published in Zaragoza in 1600.

68. F. Borbon, *Medicina y cirugía doméstica* (Valencia, 1705).

69. D. Bercebal, *Recetario medicinal y espagírico* (Zaragoza, 1713), (Zaragoza, 1734): Gil de Villalón, *Tesoro de medicina sacado de los aphorismos de la charidad, según la práctica de los enfermeros capuchinos* (Madrid, 1731), (Madrid, 1750); Agustín del Buen Suceso, *Introducción de enfermeros y modo de aplicar los remedios a todo género de enfermedades y acudir a los accidentes que sobrevienen en ausencia de los médicos* (Madrid, 1728),

70. For remedy books in the colonies see: G. López, *Tesoro de medicinas* (Madrid, 1708), (Madrid, 1727); about this work see F. Guerra, *El tesoro de medicinas de Gregorio López 1542–1596* (Madrid, 1982); J. Steinhoffer, *Florilegio medicinal* (Madrid, 1730), (Madrid, 1755).

For other peninsular remedy books see: I.F. Ameller, *Preventivo saludable particular o Botiquín para sí mismo con el cual se provee de ciertos medicamentos* (Barcelona, 1777); P. Biureta, *Libro de medicina y remedios de las enfermedades* (Madrid, 1703); A. Sánchez, *Despertador médico con su botica de pobres* (Madrid, 1729).

For a complete list of remedy books, see Perdiguero, 'Los tratados de medicina doméstica entre otras obras dirigidas a profanos en la España del siglo XVIII', in *Los tratados de medicina doméstica en la España de la Ilustración,* 59–112.

71. Granjel, *La medicina española del siglo XVIII,* 247–51. See also A. Hernández Morejón, *Historia bibliográfica de la medicina española,* vol. III, 197–234; A. Chinchilla, *Apuntes históricos de la medicina en general y biográfico-bibliográficos de la española en particular* (New York–London, 1967), vol. III, 233–59.

72. Hernández Morejón, *Historia bibliográfica de la medicina española,* vol. III, 188.

73. T. Cortijo, *Los secretos médicos y quirúrgicos del Dr. D. Juan Curvo Semedo* (Madrid, 1730), (Madrid, 1735); F. Suárez de Rivera, *Ilustración*

y publicación de los diez y siete secretos del Dr. Juan Curvo Semmedo confirmadas sus virtudes con maravillosas observaciones (Madrid, 1732); F. Suérez de Rivera, *Manifestación de cien secretos del Dr. Juan Curvo Semmedo esperimentados e ilustrados por el Dr. Rivera* (Madrid, 1732); *Declaración de los verdaderos diez y siete secretos de Curvo, de la incertidumbre de los publicados por el Dr. Rivera y de algunos errores que sobre otro secreto de Curvo, cometió el Dr. Cortijo* (Madrid, 1735). The original work of Juan Curbo Semmedo was called *Polyanthea medicinal* and was published in Lisbon in 1704, 1716 and 1727: L.S. Granjel, *Francisco Suarez de Rivera. Médico salmantino del siglo XVIII* (Salamanca, 1967), 48.

74. F. Suárez de Rivera, *Remedios de deplorados, probados en la piedra lidio de la esperiencia* (Madrid, 1732); F. Suárez de Rivera, *Secretos médicos estraordinarios descubiertos en la escuela de la esperiencia* (Madrid, 1733); F. Suárez de Rivera, *Colectánea de selectísimos secretos médicos chirúrgicos* (Madrid, 1737); F. Suárez de Rivera, *Breviario médico y quirúrgico de nuevos y raros secretos* (Madrid, 1740).

75. W. Coleman, 'The People's Health: Medical Themes in 18th Century French Popular Literature', *Bull.Hist.Med.* (1977) 51: 55–74; Laget, 'Les livrets de santé pour les pauvres aux XVIIe et XVIIIe siècles', 571–2; F. Mayor, 'Sobre el libro "Obras Medico-Chirurgicas" de Madama Fouquet', *Bol.Soc.Esp.Hist.Farm.* (1959) 10: 62–76.

76. Mme Foucquet, *Obras médico-quirúrgicas* (Valladolid, 1748), (Valladolid, 1750), (Salamanca, 1750), (Valencia, 1771).

77. P. Dube, *El médico y cirujano de los pobres* (Madrid, 1755). The translation was done from the French edition of 1678: Coleman, 'The people's health: medical themes in 18th century French popular literature', 60.

78. Dube, *El médico y cirujano de los pobres*, 14.

79. M.L. López, *Libros y folletos científicos en la Valencia de la ilustración (1700–1808)* (Valencia-Alicante, 1987), 11.

80. F. Salvá y Campillo, *Proceso de la inoculación presentado al Tribunal de los Sabios para que la juzguen* (Barcelona, 1777); F. Salvá y Campillo, *Respuesta a la primera pieza que publico contra la inoculación Antonio de Haen . . . Van añadidas dos disertaciones de el autor, una sobre el influjo del clima . . . y otra sobre los saludables efectos de los frutos* (Barcelona, 1777).

81. S.A. Tissot, *Aviso a los literatos, y a las personas de vida sedentaria, sobre su salud* (Zaragoza, 1771).

82. S.A. Tissot, *Aviso a los literatos y poderosos acerca de su salud o tratados de las enfermedades mas comunes a esta clase de personas* (Madrid, 1786).

83. About these troubles, see E. Perdiguero, A. González, 'Los valores morales de la higiene. El concepto de onanismo como enfermedad según Tissot y su tardía penetración en España', *Dynamis* (1990) 10: 131–62.

84. S.A. Tissot, *Enfermedades de nervios, producidas por el abuso de los placeres del amor y excesos del onanismo* (Madrid, 1807).

85. Perdiguero, Gonzalez, 'Los valores morales de la higiene. El concepto de onanismo como enfermedad según Tissot y su tardía penetración en España', 156–8.

86. Perdiguero, *Los tratados de medicina doméstica en la España de la Ilustración*, 541–5.

87. W. Buchan, *El conservador de la salud de las madres y de los niños* (Madrid, 1808).

88. Guillén, *La introducción de la salud pública en la medicina española del siglo XVIII*, 164–7; J.M. López, 'Social and Economic Factors in the Translation of Medical Texts in Spain (16th–19th centuries), *Rev.Esp.Doc.Cient.* (1981) 4: 49–59.

89. Guillén, *La introducción de la salud pública en la medicina española del siglo XVIII*, 217–18, 224, 274, 286 and 328–38.

90. J. Riera, *Cirugía española ilustrada y su comunación con Europa* (Salamanca, 1976).

91. About the life and works of S.A. Tissot, see old studies such as Ch.Eynard, *Essai sur la vie de Tissot (1728–1797)* (Lausanne, 1839); R. Cochet, *Etudes sur S.A. Tissot (1728–1797)* (Paris, 1902); A. Guisan, 'Le livre de malades du Dr. Tissot', *Rev.Med. Suisse Romande* (1911) 11: 711–22; F. Olivier, 'Autor de l'Avis au Peuple', *Revue Historique Vaudoise* (1928) 36: 259–94; and many recent works: L. Benaroyo, 'La médecine éclairée vue par un médecine du 18e siècle, Samuel Auguste Tissot (1728)', *Praxis* (1987) 76: 308–10; L. Benaroyo, *"L'avis au peuple sur sa santé": La voie vers une médecine éclairée* (Zurich, 1988); V. Boschung, 'Médecine et santé publique au XVIIIe siècle à travers la correspondance d'Albert de Haller et d'Auguste Tissot', *Rev.Med.Suisse Romande* (1986) 106: 34–5; E. Bozzi, 'Avvertimenti al popolo sopra la sua salute del Sig. Tissot . . .', *Minerva med.* (1970) 61: 1324–6; H.W. Bucher, *Tissot und sein "Traite des nerfs" ein Beitrag zur Medizingeschichte der schweizerischen Aufklärung* (Zurich, 1958); A.S. Emch-Dériaz, *Towards a Social Conception of Health in the Second Half of the Eighteenth Century: Tissot (1728–1797) and the New Preoccupation with Health and Well-Being*, PhD dissertation (Rochester, 1984); A.S. Emch-Dériaz 'Auguste Tissot (1728–1797)' in G. Saudan (ed.), *L'eveil medical vaudois (1750–1850)* (Lausanne, 1987), 9–49; F. Giordani, 'La teoria dell'inoculazione di S.A. Tissot vista alla luce delle recenti scoperte nel campo dell' immunologia', *Riv.Stor.Med.* (1973) 17: 59–67; E. Harms, 'Simon André Tissot (1728–1797), the Freudian before Freud', *Amer.J.Psychiat.* (1956) 112: 744; C. Imbrosio, 'Tissot e il suo tempo', *Atti Accad.Sci.Ist. Bologna Cl.Sci.mor.Ser.Rc.* (1979) 67: 323–43; M.L. Portmann, 'Relations d'Auguste Tissot (1728–1797) médecin à Lausanne, avec le patriciat bernois', *Gesnerus* (1980) 37, 21–7; T. Vieira de Faria, 'Simon André Tissot. Sôbre a saude dos intelectuais', *Rev.Med.Rio Grande do Sul* (1955) 11: 201–15; 12: 37–42.

92. About the life and works of Buchan, see L. Stephen, S. Lee (eds), *Dictionary of National Biography* (London, 1908), vol. III, 180–1; J.B. Blake, 'From Buchan to Fishbein: The Literature of Domestic Medicine', in G.B. Risse, R.L. Numbers, J.W. Leavitt (eds), *Medicine without Doctors. Home Health Care in American History* (New York, 1977), 11–30; J.P. Bishop, 'References to Consumption in William Buchan's Domestic Medicine – 1812', *Tubercle* (1966) 47: 297–301; M. Geshwind, 'Buchan's Domestic Medicine', *Bull.Hist.Dent.* (1989) 37: 139–42; L.S. King, 'Do-It Yourself Medicine', *JAMA* (1967) 200: 129–35; A.

Labensky, 'Dr. William Buchan and his Domestic Medicine', *Conn.St.Med.J.* (1975) 91: 222–3; C.J. Lawrence, 'William Buchan: Medicine Laid Open', *Med.Hist.* (1975) 19: 20–35; Ch.E. Rosenberg, 'Medical Text and Social Context: Explaining William Buchan's "Domestic Medicine", *Bull.Hist.Med.* (1983) 57: 22–42.

93. G. Smith, 'Prescribing the Rules of Health: Self-help and Advice in the Late Eighteenth-Century', in Porter (ed.), *Patients and Practitioners*, 249–82.

94. El "Aviso" of Tissot, for example, had a price of 22–26 reales, very expensive.

95. R.L. Kagan, *Universidad y sociedad en la España moderna* (Madrid, 1981), 64–6; Sarrailh, *La España ilustrada de la segunda mitad del siglo XVIII*, 55, 57 and 77; J. Soubeyroux, 'Niveles de alfabetización en la España del siglo XVIII', *Revista de Historia Moderna. Anales de la Universidad de Alicante* (1985) 5: 159–72; A. Viñao, 'Del analfabetismo a la alfabetización. Analísis de una mutación antropológica e historiográfica', *Historia de la educación* (1984) 3: 151–89; (1985) 4: 209–26.

96. See, among others, W.F. Bynum, 'Health, Disease and Medical Care', in G.S. Rousseau, R. Porter (eds), *The Ferment of Knowledge* (Cambridge, 1980), 227–8; L. Jordanova, 'The Popularization of Medicine: Tissot on Onanism', *Textual Practice* (1987) 1, 68–79; L. Jordanova, 'The Culture of Health', *Seminaire sur la medecine et le declin de la mortalité*, Annecy (France), 22–25 juin 1988, Foundation Marcel Marieux/I.U.S.S.P.; R. Porter, 'Lay Medical Knowledge in the Eighteenth Century: the Evidence of the "Gentleman's Magazine"', *Med. Hist.* (1985) 29: 138–68; R. Porter, 'Introduction' in Porter, *Patients and Practitioners*, 1–22; R. Porter, 'The Patient's View. Doing Medical History from Below', *Theory and Society* (1985) 14, 175–98. For a theoretical discussion on popularization, see: T. Shinn, R. Whitle (eds), *Expository Science: Forms and Functions of Popularization* (Dordrecht, 1985); S. Hilgartner, 'The Dominant View of Popularization: Conceptual Problems, Political Uses', *Social Studies of Science* (1990) 20: 519–39.

97. See notes 91 and 92.

98. S.A. Tissot, *Avisos al pueblo sobre su salud* (Pamplona, 1973).

99. S.A. Tissot, *Avis au peuple sur sa santé*, 3rd edn (Paris, 1767).

100. S.A. Tissot, *Tratado de las enfermedades mas frequentes de las gentes del campo* (Madrid, 1774).

101. M.E. Burke, *The Royal College of San Carlos. Surgery and Spanish Medical Reform in the Late Eighteenth Century* (Durham, NC, 1977).

102. About Juan y Felix Galisteo y Xiorro, see: F. Aguilar, *Bibliografía de autores españoles del siglo XVIII* (Madrid, 1986), vol. IV, 19–23; J. Galisteo, 'Prólogo del Traductor', in H. Boerhaave, *Aphorismos de Cirugía de Herman Boerhaave . . . comentados por Gerardo Van-Swieten, y traducidos al castellano con las notas de Mr. Luis y varias memorias de la Real Academia de Cirugía de Paris* (Madrid, 1786), vol. I; Riera, Cirugía española ilustrada y su comunicación con Europa, 28–30 and 227–33; J. Riera, *Medicina y ciencia en la España ilustrada. Epistolario y documentos I.* (Valladolid, 1981), 15; J. Riera, 'La creación del Colegio de

Profesores Cirujanos de Madrid', in *Anatomia y cirugía española del siglo XVIII (Notas y estudios)* (Valladolid, 1982), 13–34; Riera, 'Los precedentes ilustrados del Real Colegio de Cirugía de San Carlos', in *Anatomia y cirugía española del siglo XVIII (Notas y Estudios)*, 37–54; Riera 'Médicos y cirujanos en la Corte', in *Anatomia y cirugía española del siglo XVIII (Notas y Estudios)*, 68–75; J. Riera, 'Los comienzos de la inoculación de la viruela en la España ilustrada', *Medicina e historia* (1985) 8: VI–X; J. Riera, J. Granda, *La inoculación de la viruela en la España ilustrada* (Valladolid, 1987), 15–20. Among translations, we can quote G. La Faye, *Principios de cirugía* (Madrid, 1760, 1761, 1771, 1777, 1781 and 1789); J. Gorter, *Cirugía expurgada* (Madrid, 1780 and 1795); H. Boerhaave, *Aphorismos de cirugía de Herman Boerhaave*... *Comentados por Gerardo Van Swieten* (Madrid, 1774–79, 1786 and 1788–90); H. Boerhaave, *Tratado de las enfermedades de los niños, traducido al francés de los Aphorismos de Boerhaave, comentados por el Barón de Van Swieten* (Madrid, 1787); J. Astruc, *Tratado de las enfermedades venéreas* (Madrid, 1772 and 1791); H.F. Ledran, *Tratado de reflexiones sacadas de la práctica, acerca de las heridas de armas de fuego* (Madrid, 1774 and 1789; Barcelona), H.F. Ledran, *Observaciones de cirugía* (Madrid, 1780); H.F. Ledran, *Tratado de operaciones de cirugía*... *Aumentado con las operaciones que se hacen en el hombre muerto* (Madrid, 1784); J.L. Petit, *Tratado de las enfermedades de los huesos, en el que se trata de los aparatos y máquinas más útiles para curarlas* (Madrid, 1774, 1789 and 1802); A. Levret, *Tratado de partos, demostrado por principios de phísica y mecánica* (Madrid, 1778).

103. S.A. Tissot, *Avis au peuple sur sa santé* (Paris, 1763).

104. See S.A. Tissot, 'Prefaction...', in *Tratado de las enfermedades mas frequentes de las gentes del campo* (Madrid, 1781).

105. S.A. Tissot, *Avis au peuple sur sa santé* (Paris, 1770) and S.A. Tissot, *Avis au peuple sur sa santé* (Lyon, 1769).

106. See, for example: Tissot, *Tratado de las enfermedades mas frequentes de las gentes del campo* (Madrid, 1774), 566.

107. J. Galisteo, 'Al lector', in Tissot, *Tratado de las enfermedades mas frequentes de las gentes del campo* (Madrid, 1774).

108. On Spanish hydrotherapy in the XVIII century, see: S. Málaga, 'La hidrología española del siglo XVIII', *Cuad.Hist.Med.Esp.* (1969) 8: 169–218. Galisteo quoted the treatises of Charles Le Roy (1726–79), Pierre Joseph Macquer (1718–84) and Antoine Grimoald Monnet (1734–1817).

109. Tissot, *Tratado de las enfermedades mas frequentes de las gentes del campo* (Madrid, 1774), 187–93.

110. *Idem*, 257–63.

111. Porter, 'Lay Medical Knowledge in the Eighteenth Century: the Evidence of the "Gentleman's Magazine"', 155. About the Spanish concern on the theme, see *Memorias de la Sociedad Economica* (Madrid, 1780), vol. II, N.VIII.

112. J.J. Gardane, 'De las muertes aparentes y repentinas', in S.A. Tissot, *Tratado de las enfermedades mas frequentes de las gentes del campo* (Madrid, 1776), 260–307. This work is the translation of *Avis au peuple*

sur les asphyxies ou morts apparentes et subites, contenant les moyens de les prévenir et d'y remédier avec la description d'une nouvelle boite fumigatoire portative (Paris, 1774).

113. J.J. Gardane, 'De las enfermedades venereas', in Tissot, *Tratado de las enfermedades mas frequentes de las gentes del campo* (Madrid, 1776), 438–68. This work is the translation of *Manière sure et facile de guérir les maladies vénériennes* (Paris, 1773).

114. N.F.C. Eloy, *Dictionnaire historique de la médécine ancienne et moderne* (Bruxelles, 1973), vol. II, 303–4 (1778); W. Haberling *et al.* *Biographisches Lexikon der hervorragenden Arzte aller Zeiten und Völker* (München-Berlin, 1962), vol. II, 638; A. Dechambre, L. Lereboullet, *Dictionaire encyclopédique des sciences médicales* (Paris, 1880), vol. VI, 725–6; J.Fr. Michaud, *Biographie universelle ancienne et moderne* (Graz, 1967), vol. XV, 562–4.

115. Tissot, *Tratado de las enfermedades mas frequentes de las gentes del campo* (Madrid, 1776), 577–81.

116. J.J. Gardane, *Aviso al pueblo sobre las asfixias o muertes aparentes . . . a que va añadido un método seguro y fácil de curar las enfermedades venéreas . . .* (Madrid, 1776).

117. Tissot, *Tratado de las enfermedades mas frequentes de las gentes del campo* (Madrid, 1774), 377–8 (Madrid, 1776), 426.

118. *Idem*, (Madrid, 1776), 349–51.

119. *Idem*, 485, 488, 491 and 493–4.

120. S.A. Tissot, *Tratado de las enfermedades mas frequentes de las gentes del campo* (Madrid, 1778).

121. S.A. Tissot, *Tratado de las enfermedades mas frequentes de las gentes del campo* (Madrid, 1781).

122. Tissot, 'Prefacion', in *Tratado de las enfermedades mas frequentes de las gentes del campo* (Madrid, 1781).

123. *Idem*, 231–7.

124. John Mudge (1721–93) wrote *A Radical and Expeditious Cure for a Recent Catarrhous Cough* (London, 1778). See the description in Tissot, *Tratado de las enfermedades mas frequentes de las gentes del campo* (Madrid, 1781), 605 and onwards.

125. S.A. Tissot, *Aviso al pueblo acerca de su salud* (Madrid, 1790).

126. J.J. Gardane, *Catecismo sobre las muertes aparentes llamadas asfixias o instrucción acerca del modo de remediar las diferentes especies de muertes aparentes fundada en la experiencia y ordenada por preguntas y respuestas, de suerte que todos la entiendan* (Madrid, 1784).

127. Tissot, *Aviso al pueblo acerca de su salud* (Madrid, 1790), 511–605.

128. See the machine of Phillipe Nicolas Pia (1721–99) who wrote *Détail des succès de l'establissement que la ville de Paris a fait en faveur des personnes noyees* (Amsterdam, 1773) and some supplements: J.B. Blake, *A Short Title Catalogue of Eighteenth Century Printed Books in the National Library of Medicine* (Bethesda, 1979), 352.

129. Mr Maret, 'Aviso sobre las precauciones que deberán tomarse en caso de ser preciso desenterrar cadáveres' in Tissot, *Aviso al pueblo acerca de su salud* (Madrid, 1790), 618–30.

130. Hughes Maret (1726–86) wrote a *Mémoire sur l'usage où l'on est*

d'enterrer les morts dans les eglises (Dijon, 1733) and a *Nota a ajoteur au mémoire de M. Maret, sur l'abus des enterrements* (Dijon, 1774).

131. S.A. Tissot, *Aviso al pueblo acerca de su salud* (Madrid, 1795).

132. S.A. Tissot, *Aviso al pueblo acerca de su salud* (Madrid, 1815).

133. Chinchilla, *Anales históricos de la medicina en general y Biográfico-Bibliográficos de la española en particular*, vol. IV, 186–90; Guillén, *La introducción de la salud pública en la medicina española del siglo XVIII*, vol. III, 761–3; J.L. Morales, *El niño en la cultura española. I. Biografías* (Madrid, 1960), 241. He wrote *Método artificial de criar a los niños recién nacidos y de darles una buena educación física* (Madrid, 1795).

134. W. Buchan, *Medicina doméstica* (Madrid, 1785).

135. *Idem*, XLV–XLVIII.

136. About J.D. Duplanil, see Michaud, *Biographie universelle ancienne et moderne*, vol. XII, 10.

137. About Sinnot, see Archivo Histórico Nacional (A.H.N.) Councils, Bundle 5548, Expedient 41.

138. About Antonio de Alcedo, see Th.F. Glick, 'Alcedo y Bejarano, Antonio de' in J.M. López *et al.* (eds), *Diccionario histórico de la ciencia moderna en España* (Barcelona, 1983), vol. I, 36–7; C. Pérez, 'Estudio Preliminar' in A. Alcedo, *Diccionario geográfico de las Indias Occidentales o América* (Madrid, 1967), I–XXXIX; C. Pérez, *Antonio de Alcedo y su "Memoria" para la continuación de las "Décadas" de Herrera* (Madrid, 1968).

139. A. Alcedo, 'Prólogo del traductor' in W. Buchan, *Medicina doméstica* (Madrid, 1798), VI.

140. Duplanil published his translation in Paris in 1775.

141. W. Buchan, *Medicina doméstica, o tratado completo sobre los medios de conservar la salud, precaver y curar las enfermedades por el régimen y remedios simples. Obra tan útil para toda clase de gentes, como fácil la práctica de sus reglas* (Madrid, 1785–86), 5 vols.

142. W. Buchan, *Medicina doméstica, o tratado completo sobre los medios de conservar la salud, precaver y curar las enfermedades con el régimen y medicinas simples, y un apendice que contiene la farmacopea necesaria para el uso de un particular* (Madrid, 1785).

143. A.H.N. Councils, Bundle 5540, Expedient 21; Bundle 5548, Expedient 41; Bundle 11277, Expedient 8.

144. On censorship in the eighteenth century, see A. Rumeu, *Historia de la censura gubernartiva en España* (Madrid, 1940), 55–66; L. Gil, *Panorama social del humanismo español (1500–1800)* (Madrid, 1981), 632–5; *Novísima recopilación de las leyes de España* (Madrid, 1805) Book VIII, Title XVI, Laws XXIII, XXIV, XXVI, XXVII, XXXIV and XL.

145. Lawrence, 'William Buchan: Medicine Laid Open', 22–4.

146. A.H.N. Councils, Bundle 5548, Expedient 41.

147. A.H.N. Councils, Bundle 5550, Expedient 21.

148. A. Alcedo, 'Prólogo del traductor' in Buchan, *Medicina Doméstica*, (Madrid, 1785), VIII.

149. W. Buchan, *Medicina doméstica, o tratado completo del método de precaver y curar las enfermedades con el régimen y medicinas simples, y un apéndice que contiene la farmacopea necesearia para el uso de un particular . . .* (Madrid, 1786), (Madrid, 1792), (Madrid, 1798).

150. W. Buchan, *Medicina doméstica, o tratado completo del método de precaver y curar las enfermedades con régimen y medicinas simples, y un apéndice que contiene la farmacopea necesaria para el uso de un particular* (Madrid, 1818).

151. See W. Buchan, *Medicina doméstica, o tratado completo sobre los medios de conservar la salud, precaver y curar las enfermedades por un régimen y remedios simples* . . . (Madrid, 1792) vol. I, XXXVII and W. Buchan, *Médecine Domestique*, 4ème ed. (Paris, 1788) VI I, lvij.

152. J.D. Duplanil, 'Aviso del Traductor' in Buchan, *Medicina doméstica* (Madrid, 1785–86) vol. I.

153. J.D. Duplanil, in Buchan, *Medicina doméstica* (Madrid, 1785) vol. I, 169–208 and 209–326.

154. Buchan, *Medicina doméstica* (Madrid, 1785–86) vol. V, XXV, XXXI.

155. *Idem*, XXXII and 1–157.

156. A.H.N. Inquisition, Bundle 4500, Expedient 3.

157. Balaguer, 'La ciencia y la técnica' 179, about the Inquisition during the Enlightenment. See also A. Alvarez de Morales, *Inquisición e ilustración (1700–1834)* (Madrid, 1982); M. Deforneaux, *Inquisición y censura de libros en la España del siglo XVIII* (Madrid, 1973); L. Domergue, *Tres calas en la censura dieciochesca* (Toulouse, 1981).

158. See note 144 and A. Sierra Corella, *La censura de libros y papeles en España y los indices y catálogos españoles de libros prohibidos* (Madrid, 1947).

159. Deforneaux, *Inquisición y censura de libros en la España del siglo XVIII*, 59.

160. For a complete list of the French books forbidden by the Inquisition, see Deforneaux, *Inquisición y censura de libros en la España del siglo XVIII*, 217–68.

161. See S. Muñoz, *Inquisición y ciencia en la España Moderna* (Madrid, 1977), 188–210. For a general view of the interplay between Inquisition and science, see J. Pardo, *Ciencia europea y censura inquisitorial española (1599–1707)*, doctoral thesis (Valencia, 1986).

162. For example, J. Cortés, *Lunario y pronóstico perpetuo general y particular* (Madrid, 1759).

163. Deforneaux, *Inquisición y censura de libros en la España del siglo XVIII*, 52–3.

164. Buchan, *Medicina doméstica* (Madrid, 1785-6), vol. I, 142–3.

165. A.H.N. Inquisition, Bundle 4500, Expedient 3.

166. Deforneaux, *Inquisición y censura de libros en la España del siglo XVIII*, 89.

167. Buchan, *Medicina doméstica* (Madrid, 1792), 5 vols.

168. W. Buchan, *Domestic Medicine* (London, 1786).

169. W. Buchan, *Médecine domestique* (Paris, 1788), 5 vols.

170. Buchan, *Medicina doméstica* (Madrid, 1792), vol. V, 345–52.

171. Buchan, *Medicina doméstica* (Madrid, 1792), vol. V, 353–62.

172. See notes 132 and 150.

173. F.J. Rivera y Aravigt, *El médico y cirujano de valde* (Barcelona, 1838).

174. About Monlau, see M. Granjel, *Pedro Felipe Monlau y la higiene española del siglo XIX* (Salamanca, 1983). Monlau's work *Nociones de higiene doméstica y gobierno de la casa* was published in 1860, 1867, 1875 and 1897.

175. P.F. Monlau (ed.), *El médico de las familias* (Madrid, 1851); P.F. Monlau (ed.), *El monitor de la salud y de la salubridad de los pueblos* (Madrid, 1858–64).

176. About this literature, see E. Balaguer, R. Ballester, J. Bernabeu, E. Perdiguero, 'La utilización de fuentes antropológicas en la historiografía médica española contemporánea', *Dynamis* (1990) 10, 193–208; E. Perdiguero, E. Balaguer, R. Ballester, J. Bernabeu, 'La literatura de divulgación higiénico-sanitaria y su importancia para la historia de la Antropología española', *V Congreso de Antropología*, Granada, December 1990.

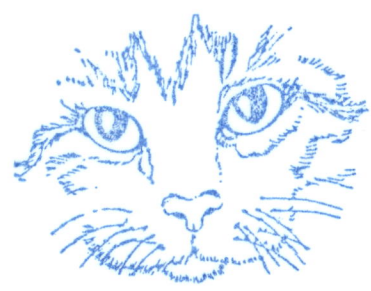

7

Tissot as part of the medical Enlightenment in Hungary

Maria Szlatky

The Enlightenment, whatever we mean by it, was imported from Western Europe into Hungary during the eighteenth century. The reception of the new ideas and values was a slow and contradictory process. A few learned individuals, moved by a somewhat missionary zeal, played a mediatory role, but their efforts were often wrecked by the backward social and political conditions. On the other hand, some enlightened ideas were introduced to, and occasionally forced on, society by the absolutist government.[1]

The Habsburg absolutism in Central Europe reached its zenith in the eighteenth century. The policies of the absolutist government implied economical and political oppression, aggressive Catholicism in Hungary, and the overshadowing of Hungarian national interests in favour of those of the Empire. Yet, in spite of its restrictive tendencies and sometimes against its will, the absolutist government and the Habsburg Court contributed a lot to the spread of enlightened ideas in Hungary.[2]

The Court of Vienna, like, indeed, almost the entire Continent, was under the influence of French culture. Court society looked to France as the model of taste in literature, art and architecture, as well as in the new refinement of social behaviour, dress and cuisine. Young Hungarian noblemen were attracted to the Court to form the bodyguard of Maria-Theresa, who wanted to 'tame' her rebellious subjects. French was generally spoken and French books and thoughts widely discussed in educated circles by the *habitués* of the salons. It is hardly surprising, then, that the leaders of the later cultural and political movements, starting in the 1770s, were mostly noblemen who had spent years at the Viennese Court.[3]

In a roundabout way, Catholicism also contributed to the spread of the Enlightenment.[4] As universities were strictly Catholic within the Empire, the non-Catholic students – mainly from Transylvania and the north-eastern parts of the country – had no other choice than to go abroad to continue their studies. These young men attended, therefore, the most famous European universities of the time and, in these places, met all the new ideas that influenced European thought and science. After their return, they became, of course, the most devoted protagonists of the Enlightenment in Hungary.[5]

The Habsburg sovereigns, ruling in the name of the '*raison d'État*', pursued a conservative reform policy.[6] *Raison d'État* demanded money, and getting more money demanded changes. Both Charles III and Maria-Theresa, as well as her son Joseph II, were eager to rationalize the administration of their scattered territories. The Hungarian Governors' Council was formed in 1727 and, within its particular sphere of competence, the Public Health Commission of 1738 was charged with the affairs of '*medizinische Polizey*'.[7] The sovereigns' constant struggle against the conservative opposition of the national nobility led them to deliver fierce attacks on tradition and superstitions in the name of scientific government.[8] The central laws and orders issued by them were warmly welcomed by members of the bourgeoisie, who found support in them against the power of the local nobility. Reforms were needed badly and, particularly after losing the prosperous lands of Silezia, efforts were made by the government to ameliorate conditions in the remaining provinces. Influenced by the cameralist ideas of J.H. Gottlob von Justi, Joseph von Sonnenfels and others, the government of Maria-Theresa tried to make the provinces richer, healthier and more solvent.[9] Indeed, several reforms were introduced during this period, but those of most lasting value were in the fields of education and health (Ratio Educationis, 1777, Generale Normativum in Re Sanitatis, 1770).

The establishment of an elementary school system was perhaps the greatest achievement of the reforms in education. The institution of a strict quarantine zone along the border, the decree for the compulsory appointment of district medical officers (county-, town- and mine-physicians), the definition of their duties and rights, and the government's clear recognition of those who made efforts in popularizing medicine were, among others, the outstanding points of reform in public health.[10]

In eighteenth-century Hungary, the urgent need to improve the health of the population was widely recognized.[11] Poverty and ignorance were considered to be the root of sickness, much before the time of Johann Peter Frank's famous lecture '*De populorum miseria morborum genetrice*' held on 7 May 1790 in Padua, then under Austrian rule. Social reforms would have been too risky. The less risky way which still promised some progress in health, and which was probably the only means within reach for the individuals who wanted to help, was popularizing medicine by publishing books on health and disease. The fight against Ignorance and Darkness seemed to be easier than the fight against Poverty. The Enlightenment's belief that the advancement of knowledge must make its contribution to the progress of health and well-being was held by all educated men. The number of medical publications increased tenfold during the century. Latin works, however, could not reach the wider audience. Only books written in or translated into the vernacular could convey essential knowledge on health and disease to the people.[12] As the '*Bevölkerungsvermehrung*', the '*Erhaltung der Lebensprozesse*' or the '*Körperliche Sicherheit der Bürger*' belonged to the main concerns of the absolutist government, the State's interest met the intention of the authors in this field.[13] As these texts did not deal with overt political ideas, the government encouraged their publication. Indeed, this was one of the few fields where the enlightenment–humanistic initiatives of individuals and the conservative reform policy of the absolutist government luckily coincided.[14]

There are approximately eighty titles in the vernacular medical literature published during the eighteenth century in Hungary. As some of these were published more than once, there were about 120 publications in all during this period. They formed about 9 per cent of all medical publications and about 1 per cent of all eighteenth-century publications. These figures may seem extremely small in comparison to the enormous output of some Western European countries, but it represents a considerable growth when compared with figures from previous periods in Hungary. It is also worth pointing out that in the first half of the eighteenth century there was hardly any increase in vernacular medical publication compared to the previous period. In the second half of the century, however, there was a sudden growth both in the number of publications and in the subjects they dealt with. More than half of the so-called 'useful' (non-fiction, non-religious) publications in the vernacular dealt with medical subjects. They formed only 2 per cent of the whole vernacular output in the first half of the century, but more than 10 per cent in the second half. By that time, every twentieth book in the vernacular dealt with questions of health and disease.[15] The most frequently discussed subjects were epidemics, diet, midwifery, childcare and the so-called common diseases. While the plague was mostly a thing of the past in Western Europe, it was still causing devastation in Hungary until the end of the eighteenth century. Numbers of books have been published on the subject. Strangely enough, it was the vernacular books on plague that first presented, in Hungary, the enlightened attitude of learned physicians towards the lay patient, when the authors called directly upon individuals to protect their own health. As the titles indicate, their intention was to teach the laity 'how to be his own physician'. Ignoring the actual remedy of the disease, they focused on preventive measures, and gave general and useful advice concerning hygiene and diet. County-physician David Gömöri's *Advice against plague* (1739) was, for example, an excellent manual of diet.[16] Vernacular works on midwifery, childcare and children's diseases as well as modern handbooks on regimes of health began to be published in greater numbers from about the 1760s, and the process reached its full flowering only in the last quarter of the century.

Whatever their subject, these books shared the optimism concerning the prospects of teaching the laity to protect their own health. They declared the right of everyone to a healthy life. The Enlightenment paradox, so well-known in England, as to whether it was useful or harmful (if indeed possible at all) to make fundamental medical knowledge accessible to non-professionals did not seem to occur to the Hungarian authors. At least, there is no sign of any sceptical view in these documents. Many of these books were openly addressed to the poor or to the learned members of illiterate communities. Denying any but natural causes for the diseases, and basing their teaching on the Healing Power of Nature, they advised simple treatments and medicaments in therapy, and revealed first of all the importance of prevention. The authors recognized the correlation between life conditions and diseases and demanded – although in an indirect way – social reforms. Fighting against all kinds of superstitions and charlatans, these books conveyed, in short, the basic ideas of medical Enlightenment. The use of the vernacular and the popular appeal of these books also justifies identifying them as Enlightenment texts, since the Enlightenment in Hungary – as in other Central European countries – was connected closely with the fight for the right to use the mother tongue. In this respect, too, medical books were ahead of the political and ideological literature and prepared the way for the Enlightenment in Hungary.

The Hungarian version of Tissot:
Avis au peuple sur sa santé

The Hungarian version of Tissot's *Avis au peuple sur sa santé* held a distinguished place among the vernacular medical publications. First published in Lausanne in 1761, Tissot's work soon became one of the most popular medical books of eighteenth-century Europe. Containing essential information on the most common diseases, and written in a clear and distinct manner, this book had an enormous success all over Europe. It was translated into several languages (German, Dutch, Italian, English, etc.) and was reprinted a number of times within a few years.[17]

The Hungarian version was published in Nagykároly in 1772, under the title *A néphez való tudósítás miképpen kellyen a' maga egésségére vigyázni*. The translator of the book, Márton Marikowzki, was a doctor himself.[18] The gifted son of a Lutheran family, he studied for years in Wittenberg, Halle and Erlangen and became a Doctor of Medicine in 1755. In the next two years he travelled Europe, visiting France, Belgium, the Netherlands and England. Soon after his return, he was converted to the Catholic faith, obviously for the sake of his career. He worked as a physician for a while for the Brothers of Mercy at Pozsony (today called Bratislava, in Czechoslovakia) then for the Bishop of Vác. Later, he became senior physician in several counties. The only medical book he wrote, the *Ephemerides Syrmiensis, seu Observationes Physico-medicae . . . methodo Hippocratico-Sydenhaimiana practica . . .* was published in 1767 in Vienna. The observations show him to be an enlightened physician. Nevertheless, he was better known for his deep interest in the philosophy of Leibnitz and Wolff than for his knowledge of medicine. In the last three years of his life, he worked as senior physician of Szathmár County under the chief-lieutenant Count Antal Károlyi. The two men did not get along well, yet the translation of Tissot's book was the result of their ambivalent relation. Soon after finishing this work, Marikowzki had to leave his job. He went to Pest, where he died in the same year, 1773. To all appearances, the good doctor was not very eager to translate the book. As he remarks in the Preface, the Count 'almost forced him' to do the job.[19] Thus, in this case, we can speak about neither an initiative coming from below, nor an action backed by the government. It was the Count alone who insisted on publishing the *Avis au peuple* in Hungarian, and the book was printed at his own expense, by his own private press.

A member of one of the oldest Hungarian families, Count Antal Károlyi was a rich and illustrious aristocrat, who held various high positions and gained the greatest distinctions from the Habsburg sovereigns. He was famous for his country-planning projects such as river control, swamp draining, settlement of new villages, building of new schools and churches. He was also noted for his charity, and the support of poor students and scholars. Count Antal Károlyi was, in short, one of the very few enlightened aristocrats who, fired by a patriotic zeal, spared no trouble in the cause of his nation's rise.[20]

The press of Nagykároly was founded by his father in 1753, and started production in 1755 with the privilege granted by the Queen. Count Antal Károlyi used the press in carrying out his popular culture programme. The brightest period of the press was during the 1770s, when the Hungarian version of Tissot's book was also published. One third of the publications of Nagykároly were in the vernacular. Among the books in Hungarian – grammars, alphabets, geographies, cathecisms, stories from the Bible, etc. – there were three medical books, too. The first one, written by József Csapó, town-physician of Debrecen, covered children's diseases and came out in 1771. The second was Tissot's work in 1772. The third one, published in 1783, was written by János Lalangue, county-physician, on Hungarian mineral waters, and was translated from Latin into Hungarian on the Count's orders.[21] All these three books aimed at popularizing medicine among the people. Two of them were written by Hungarian authors, but why did the Count choose Tissot's work to publish? The answer is obvious. As an aristocrat and a frequent visitor to the Court of Vienna, he knew the French language and culture well. As an enlightened reformer, he was familiar with the latest European cultural trends. Tissot's name was well-known in Vienna, anyway. His public debate on inoculation with Anton de Haen (1759), his works and his public correspondence with Zimmerman, Haller, etc. were all known in educated and progressive circles.[22] The *Avis au peuple* was very famous, and it was addressed to the friends of the poor, so there was nothing unusual in that the Count knew this book well. He had both the French and the German version of it in his library.[23] When it turned out that the new county-physician, Marikowzki, spoke French, the Count's plan was ready, and his impatience knew no bounds. The book's aim corresponded to his reform endeavours, and he wanted to give it into the hands of his own people as soon as possible. That is why he urged, even forced, the doctor to do the translation.

As the Preface, written by Marikowzki, says, the translation was made directly from French. He used the text of the fourth, improved and enlarged edition published in Lausanne in 1769.[24] The Hungarian version also contains Tissot's Preface dated 21 April 1769, and the two additional chapters on inoculation and long-lasting diseases, which formed part of the book from the third edition onward (Paris, 1767). It seems, however, that Marikowzki also used the German version made by Hirzel, parallel to the French text. For example, on page 89, he writes that the German translator could not find the right word for the 'abcès au poulmon', and when rachitis is discussed, on page 386, he calls it the English disease, giving the German version 'Englische Krankheit' between brackets. Further examples could also be listed proving the parallel use of the German text.

According to the title page, Marikowzki did not only translate Tissot's work, but also adapted it to Hungarian conditions. To what extent, if at all, had the original text been changed or enlarged by him? Well, the Hungarian and the French versions differ from each other only to a very small extent. Marikowzki departed from the original text eleven times, to allow a place for shorter or longer remarks. Most of them were related to some special feature of Szathmár County, such as its famous spas (on pages 181, 283, 355). The longest remark was related to the dangerous drinking habits of the Hungarians. 'The abuse of strong drinks is so common among the people that it became the first cause of several illnesses', Marikowzki writes.[25] Twice he criticized Tissot's standpoint. When Tissot expressed his sceptical view on balms, Marikowzki was eager to remark that he knew no better means of treating phthisis, for example, than balms, namely the Peru-balm of Sydenham.[26] In connection with small-pox, he again agreed with Sydenham rather than with Tissot, who opposed the use of painkillers and narcotics during the illness.[27] These remarks show Marikowzki's slight conservatism, his 'fidelity' to Sydenham, whom he accepted as the highest authority.[28] Two of his further remarks are worth mentioning. When talking about fevers, he emphasized the health hazard of uncontrolled rivers among the causes.[29] By adding this, he probably wanted to please the Count who made serious efforts to control rivers in his county. Finally, in the chapter on charlatans and quacks, Marikowzki felt the need to express his own worries about the activities of these 'people-killers'. 'They must be banned and seriously punished since there are so many other causes which diminuate the population that one can scarcely find a real Hungarian in Hungary nowadays.'[30] He must have been referring to the mass settlement of Germans into Hungary, supported by the government in this period.

Apart from these additions, Marikowzki followed the original text closely, yet his book does not belong among the best Hungarian medical texts of the age. The nicety, the clarity and the distinctness of the original text disappeared somehow from the Hungarian version, which lacks the forceful and colourful prose of some other contemporary medical writers, such as István Mátyus, István Weszprémi, Sámuel Benk and others. In 1781, in his medical biography, István Weszprémi greeted warmly the publication of Tissot's work in Hungarian, but at the same time he expressed his hope that a better and 'more precise Hungarian version' of the book would soon be published.[31] This hope has not been realized so far.

In the Preface, however, Marikowzki praised the values of the translated book. 'As it offers help in sudden diseases, when there is no doctor at hand, and teaches the people to help themselves in sickness, this book is useful not only for the sick, but for the whole society', he said, and continued with a typical cameralist argument: 'The happiness of the society hinges un-separably upon the health and growth of the population'.[32] The same thought was expressed by other Hungarian medical authors, too. It can be found in the works of Daniel Perliczy, István Mátyus, István Weszprémi, Samuel Rácz and others.

Tissot also started his book with a demographical argument. Calculus, statistics and demographical arguments entered the arsenal of medical reasoning with the Enlightenment.[33] Marikowzki did not mention his targeted audience, but we know from the famous paragraphs of Tissot's book that it was addressed to poor peasants through the intermediation of their superiors or learned members: through the priests, landowners, schoolmasters, barbers, literate women, etc.[34] The Hungarian version must have been addressed to the same circles. Unfortunately, we have no data about the exact number of copies, but it could hardly exceed a few hundred.[35] The question of how a few hundred copies of a book could play any role in the spread of the Enlightenment in Hungary arises. Especially, if it was – as Marikowzki stated – the only book in the Hungarian language in its genre. It is also questionable whether it actually reached the peasants that it was addressed to.

In the event, the Hungarian version, important as it was, was far from being the only means of making Tissot's views and advice known to a Hungarian audience. The French and the German versions of the *Avis au peuple sur sa santé* were known and used by doctors and by educated laity alike. According to the evidence provided by contemporary library catalogues, Tissot's book in foreign versions was collected by most library-owners of the time. Some of his other works were also possessed by them.[36] His work on inoculation (*L'inoculation justifiée*, 1754) and, above all, the public debate on the same subject between himself and Anton de Haen (Wien, 1759) made him famous at least among the professionals.[37]

The spread of inoculation for smallpox was rather slow on the Continent, compared to England. It was even slower in the Habsburg Empire, where the new practice was opposed by leading physicians such as van Swieten and Anton de Haen.[38] Thus, inoculation has never become officially accepted in its territories. In spite of that, there were some advocates of the method among Hungarian doctors.[39] Among its supporters, István Weszprémi was, indeed, a firm advocate of inoculation. In the introductory essay of his book on child care (1760), he advised strongly the introduction of the new practice, and demanded the foundation of smallpox hospitals.[40] Although he referred only to his experience in England, he was obviously inspired and encouraged to make his 'rebellious' opinion public by the above-mentioned debate. His correspondence

with van Swieten, published by Weszprémi in 1787, gives sufficient evidence of that.[41]

The *Avis au peuple sur sa santé* in Hungarian was an important
book not just because it made known some new ideas, but
because it showed how to extend this knowledge to a wider
audience. And now, we come back to the second part of our
question: is it really true that Tissot's book was the only advice
manual in Hungarian in that period?

The Hungarian context of Tissot's advice manual

When Tissot mentioned in the introduction the works of van
Swieten and Nils Rosen as the most similar ones to his own
book, Marikowzki added that he knew only one similar book in
Hungarian.[42] That was the *Pax Corporis*, written by Ferenc Pápai
Páriz, first published in 1690 and republished six times during
the eighteenth century. It dealt with the most common diseases
of the people, arranging the diseases according to the structure
of the human body, from the head to the feet. From its third
edition (1695), the book was enlarged with chapters on the
diseases of women and children. Both the author's declared
intention 'to help the poor', and the content of the book show
the *Pax Corporis* to be, *par excellence*, an enlightened work of its
time. By the second half of the eighteenth century, however, it
had become more or less obsolete. That is why Marikowzki
partly disapproved of it. 'This book,' he continued, 'although it
has merits, can also be dangerous to the ignorant people
because of its conciseness in the description of the diseases and
because of its eclectic advices.'[43] Marikowzki was right in this
respect. Apart from the *Pax Corporis*, there was no printed book
in the Hungarian language which discussed so systematically a
certain – probably the most important – group of diseases as
Tissot's book did. But, if we consider the authors' intention,
their knowledge and medical ideas, as well as the nature of their
advice, we can find some good Hungarian precedents. I do not
mean recipe books or herbals in the vernacular, nor the books
on plague and other epidemics, although lots of them went far
beyond the subject indicated by their title. I think of books
which corresponded to what Foucault defined as 'the main
characteristics of eighteenth-century noso-politics: the privilege
of the child and the medicalisation of the family, and the

privilege of hygiene and the function of medicine as instance of social control'.[44] There are various works on diet, child care, midwifery, etc. They, indeed, conveyed the same ideas as Tissot's book did.

Not only these works but also their authors had some qualities in common. All of them came from Protestant (Lutheran or Presbyterian) families. While two-thirds of the population was Catholic, there was no Catholic – except a few converted ones – among the authors or translators of medical books in the vernacular. This shows what an important pioneer role the Protestant bourgeoisie played in the spread of the Enlightenment in Hungary. All these authors were well-trained, learned physicians who had obtained their degrees at foreign universities. Because there was no medical faculty in Hungary until 1770, Hungarian students were forced to study medicine abroad. The nearest university was that of Vienna, but it was useless to the majority because it refused to graduate Protestant students. For similar religious reasons, they also kept away from the other universities in the Empire (Prague, Pavia, Freiburg, Innsbruck, etc.). The universities most frequented by Hungarian medical students in the eighteenth century were those of Leyden, Halle, Jena, Basel, Erlangen, Fraenecker and Utrecht.[45] This trend had changed by the last two decades of the century, when the universities of Vienna and Buda (from 1777) took first place. It is also characteristic of the Hungarian medical authors that, after their return, they worked as medical officers: as county-physicians or town-physicians.[46] These posts made it possible for them to gain wide experience of the common diseases of the people, their backward social conditions and their most urgent health needs. The physicians were moved by the poor people's suffering to write their books, and the introductory essays prove their philanthropic and national feelings. Many of them used almost the same words: they wanted to help, and to raise the Hungarian nation to the level of the more developed countries from where they had returned.[47]

I should perhaps mention first Daniel Perliczy, senior physician of Nógrád County, who published three works in the vernacular in 1740. One of them was a special advice and recipe book for the poor.[48] Then István Weszprémi, town-physician of Debrecen, should be mentioned. He studied medicine at Zurich and Utrecht and spent two years in England, where, among others, he attended the midwifery course of William

Smellie, and regularly visited hospitals such as the London Hospital, St Thomas Hospital, St George Hospital and smallpox hospitals.[49] After his return, he published two works in the vernacular in 1760. One was on child care, and was a translation of William Cadogan's *An Essay upon Nursing and Management of Children* (London, 1748).[50] The other was a set of rules for health and long life, translated from George Cheyne's *Essay of Health and Long Life* (London, 1724).[51] István Weszprémi, however, failed to mention that these works were translations. He also failed to refer to the English authors. He left out or changed those sections which might have given a clue to their origin. It is beyond the limits of this paper to investigate what possible reasons he might have had to act like that. His trick was so successful that, until recently, these books were considered his own work.[52] Whatever the reason, with the publication of these important works of the European medical Enlightenment, Weszprémi introduced a new approach to child and health care into Hungary.

In 1766 he published another work in the vernacular, this time on midwifery. It was a translation of Johann Nepomuk Crantz's *Einleitung in eine wahre und gegrundete Hebammenkunst* (Vienna, 1756).[53] It proved to be a good choice, as Maria-Theresa made Crantz's work a compulsory textbook on midwifery all over the Habsburg Empire in 1770, and the sovereign honoured Weszprémi with a beautiful medal for his translation.

Succeeding works on midwifery were mostly translations from authors who belonged to the school of Crantz in Vienna. Károly Szeli, for example, translated and published Johann Steidele's *Lehrbuch von der Hebammenkunst* (Vienna, 1775) in 1777.[54] The original Hungarian works, such as county-physician Samuel Dombi's *Art of Midwifery* (1772), also showed the influence of the Viennese midwifery texts.[55] At the end of the 1760s, Weszprémi's younger colleague, Joseph Csapó, town-physician of Debrecen, wrote a comprehensive book on children's diseases.[56] It was published in 1771 by the same press that put out Tissot's work. Csapó's book is a compilation. He often referred to foreign authors, to Petit, Mauriceau, Sydenham, Harris and others. Until the publication of Rosen's books in Hungarian (1785, 1794) this work was the only manual on the diseases of children.[57]

The above-mentioned books show clearly that, from the second half of the eighteenth century, in conformity with the general trend of the age, the main concern of practical medicine had been to raise the level of obstetrics and paediatrics. The other main concern of practical medicine was undoubtedly the preservation of health. István Mátyus, town-physician of Marosvásárhely in Transylvania, produced a two-volume book on the subject of diet and regimen, the *Diaetetica* of 1762–64.[58] Mátyus made a systematic inquiry into the means of preserving health. He began with a chapter on the temperaments, and went on to explain and examine the traditional categories of the non-naturals. In the second volume he dealt with what might be translated as the 'medicine of interference', where he dealt with the diseases and regimen appropriate to women, children, and the aged. He detailed the management of pregnancy and childbirth, and the nursing and management of children. He also dealt with disorders of the young, writing about students and soldiers. He described the most common diseases and the most frequently used therapies. Although the book is full of references to various authors, it can rightly be considered one of the earliest and most original modern works on the subject. The authors most frequently quoted by Mátyus were undoubtedly Sydenham, Boerhaave, G.E. Stahl, Hoffmann, and Ettmüller, but he also referred often to John Allen's *Synopsis Universae Medicinae Practicae* of 1719, and to Thomas Fuller's three collections of prescriptions, which were very popular works in Europe in the first half of the eighteenth century.[59] Mátyus's book, in fact, is a thesaurus of medical opinions on health and diseases, on diet and regimen. Although it required a certain amount of education to understand this text, the *Diaetetica* can be considered the nearest relative to the *Avis au peuple* from among its Hungarian precedents.

All these books were, pre-eminently, enlightened works on health and disease, if we interpret the Enlightenment as a way of thinking rather than as new facts and discoveries in science. From this point of view, the Hungarian version of Tissot's *Avis au peuple sur sa santé* was no more than one among the others. It was undoubtedly one of the best, and it was soon followed by other books on exactly the same subject.

The *Avis au peuple* served most probably as a model to *Medical Teaching*, first published anonymously in 1776 and republished in 1778, by this time under the name of its author, Sámuel Rácz. At the time of the first edition of the book, Rácz worked as town-physician of Nagybánya, a royal borough very near to Nagykároly, where Tissot's work had been published. The *Avis au peuple* was certainly still in circulation in the town in 1774, when Rácz arrived there. In the epilogue to the second edition of the book, Rácz says: 'Everything that I wrote here was approved by myself, but I learnt a lot from the works of some famous and successful doctors'.[51] Although he mentioned only 'Baron Anton von Störck' by name, Tissot must have been among the others. The grouping of the diseases and the advised treatments are very much alike in Tissot's and Rácz's work. Rácz's book, however, is much shorter. It lacks the chapters on smallpox, long-lasting diseases and charlatans, but it has a separate chapter on Colica Metallica, quite understandably as Nagybánya was a mining town. In spite of these slight differences, the two books are very similar.

Medical Teaching brought success to its author. Samuel Rácz was appointed as professor at the Medical Faculty of Buda in 1777, and the second edition of his book (1778) was directly supported by the sovereign. From that time on, Samuel Rácz did not cease to work on popularizing medicine, and he became the most zealous fighter for the use of the mother tongue both in medical teaching and in medical literature.[62] He has translated several works from German and Latin into Hungarian. Among his first translations was the two-volume book by Anton von Störck: *Medizinische-praktische Unterricht für die Feld- und Landwundärzte der österreichischen Staaten* (Vienna 1776), published in Hungarian in 1778.[63] (Störck's book, however, was published in another Hungarian translation, made by József Milesz, in the same year.)[64]

Rácz's *Medical Teaching* and Störck's *Medical Instruction* in Hungarian – are very close to each other. This is not surprising, as Anton von Störck used to be Rácz's teacher at the University of Vienna, where Rácz, as a converted Catholic, obtained his degree in 1773. He obviously used his notes made during his university years, and he referred to Störck as his master. But Störck's *Unterricht* is also very close to the *Avis au peuple*. As Tissot's book was well-known in Vienna, the possibility of a direct influence cannot be excluded. The only essential difference between the two works is, in fact, that Störck wrote his advice manual as a textbook for the barbers. He avoided Tissot's 'naivety' and did not turn directly to the people, but addressed his teaching to the lowest-level professionals. Sámuel Rácz followed Störck's example when he addressed the second edition of his own book to the same group. By that time it was recognized that, in the absence of doctors, the practice of curing was best left in the hands of midwives and barbers. They had to be addressed first, their knowledge had to be improved for the sake of a healthier population, and in order to help the peasants. Anton von Störck also organized the higher training of the barbers, launching a compulsory two-year course for them. These courses at the University of Buda were conducted by Sámuel Rácz, who later published several translations as well as his own texts on the subject.

Most of the vernacular books on health and disease, published before 1778, were addressed directly to the people, but we must be sceptical about their ever reaching the audience they were intended for. The peasantry accounted in that period for about 80 per cent of the population. According to recent research, some 17 to 20 per cent of the higher peasant strata were literate around 1769 in Hungary. Hence, no more than about 2 or 3 per cent of the peasants could read.[65] Thus, the efficiency of the vernacular literature in popularizing medicine is more than questionable as far as the peasants are concerned. Only the higher strata of society could be reached by these books. The readers came from members of the aristocracy, nobility and bourgeoisie, from among priests and professionals. The fact that almost every medical book in the vernacular, published after 1772, mentioned Tissot's work with honour proves that, although the book was not intended for them, it did first reach the professionals.[66] Hungarian doctors were deeply impressed by the usefulness, rationality and straightforward approach of the book. One of them said a few years later that 'there has never been anybody among the doctors, who found better the way to the people than Tissot did'. We have no evidence for the use of Tissot's book by midwives, barbers or learned peasants, but Tissot had followers among the physicians. In Hungary, as in so many other European countries, the idea of the Enlightenment failed to penetrate to the peasant masses. This fact, however, does not justify disdain for the merits of those who played the role of pioneer. And Tissot belonged to them.

By the last two decades of the century, popularizing medicine had become an official program led, and partly carried out, by university professors. By that time, German influence was dominant in Hungary. The popular works of the Austrian professors, Joseph Plenck, Johann Steidele, Johann Schosulan, Rudolph Becker, Martin Lange and others, had all been translated into Hungarian, and some of them published more than once within a short time. The *Gesundheits-Katechismus* of Cristoph Bernard Faust had been published twice in Hungarian (1794, 1796).[68] The famous *Die Kunst das menschliche Leben zu verlängern* of Christoph Wilhelm Hufeland had been re-issued three times in two years (1798, 1799).[69] Beside the translations from German there were, of course, numbers of original Hungarian publications, as well as translations from other European languages. From English, for example, William Grant's work on gout (1780) was translated and published by Samuel Benkó in 1791.[70] Nils Rosen's books should also be mentioned – they were translated from German into Hungarian in 1785 and 1794.[71]

By the turn of the century a really wide range of vernacular books popularizing medicine was at the Hungarian readers' disposal. This trend continued without interruption during the nineteenth century. But popular medical literature itself could not and did not result in any measurable improvement in the health of the poor. Only modern public health, shaped in the second half of the nineteenth century, brought some results in this respect.

Notes

1. From the enormous literature on the Enlightenment, see P. Chaunu, *La civilisation de l'Europe des lumières* (Paris, 1971); P. Gay, *The Enlightenment*, 2 vols (New York, 1967–69); L.E. Wangermann, *The Austrian Achievement, 1700–1800* (London, 1973); R. Porter and M. Teich (eds), *The Enlightenment in National Context* (Cambridge, 1981); N. Hampson, *The Enlightenment. An Evaluation of its Assumptions, Attitudes and Values* (Middlesex, 1968); R. Mandrou, *La France au XVIIe et XVIIIe siècles* (Paris, 1967); W.H. Bruford, *Germany in the XVIIIth Century* (Cambridge, 1962); R. Porter, *English Society in the Eighteenth Century* (Harmondsworth, 1982); V.L. Tapié, *L'Europe de Marie-Therese. Du baroque aux Lumières* (Paris, 1973).
2. For eighteenth-century history of the Habsburg Empire and Hungary, see C.A. Macartney, *The Habsburg Empire* (London, 1968) and *The New Cambridge Modern History*, vol. III (Cambridge, 1965); W. Andreas, *Das theresianische Österreich und das 18. Jahrhundert* (München, 1930); L.E. Wangermann, op.cit. (1. note); V.L. Tapié, op.cit. (1. note); H. Marczali, *Hungary in the Eighteenth Century* (Cambridge, 1910); D. Kosáry, *Culture and Society in Eighteenth Century Hungary* (Budapest, 1987).

3. For French influence, see L. Réau, *L'Europe français au siècle des lumières* (Paris, 1938, 1951); H. Wagner, '*Der Höhepunkt des französischen Kultureinflusses in Österreich*' in *Österreich in Geschichte und Literatur* (Wien, 1961); Z. Baranyai, *A francia nyelv és müveltség Magyarországon* (French Language and Culture in Hungary), (Budapest, 1920).

4. Reform Catholicism is discussed in E. Winter, *Der Josefinismus. Die Geschichte des österreichischen Reformkatholizismus, 1740–1848* (Berlin, 1962) and L.E. Wangermann, 'Reform Catholicism and Political Radicalism in the Austrian Enlightenment' in R. Porter and M. Teich (eds), *The Enlightenment in National Context* (Cambridge, 1981).

5. Unfortunately, we have no general work on Hungarian students who studied abroad during the eighteenth century, but lots of data can be found in I. Weszprémi, *Succincta medicorum Hungariae et Transilvaniae biographia*, vols 1–4 (Leipzig, 1774–87). D. Kosáry estimates their number at about 2000. See D. Kosáry, *Müvelódés a XVIII. századi Magyarországon* (Culture in Eighteenth Century Hungary), (Budapest, 1980) 128–9.

6. For enlightened absolutism and especially for its contradiction in terms, see R.W. Harris, *Absolutism and Enlightenment* (London, 1967); Ch. Morazé, 'Essai sur les despotes éclairés' in *Annales historique de la Revolution Française* (1948) 279–96; G. Lefebvre, 'Le déspotisme éclairé' in *Annales historique de la Révolution Française* (1949) 97–115.

7. The basic eighteenth-century works on 'medizinische Polizey' were: J.P. Frank, *System einer vollständigen medicinischen Polizey*, Bd. 1–4 (Mannheim, 1779–88) and G.Z. Huszty, *Diskurs über medizinischen Polizei* (Pressburg, 1786).

8. A pamphlet, *Vexatio dat intellectum* (Pressburg, 1764), shows clearly the nobility's stand against any reform. See also D. Gerhard, (hrsg), *Standische Vertretungen in Europa im 17. und 18. Jahrhundert* (Göttingen, 1969).

9. For cameralism, see W. Small, *The Camerialists* (Chicago, 1909); L. Sommer, *Die österreichischen Kameralisten*, Bd. 1–2 (Wien, 1920–25); G. Rosen, 'Camerialism and the Concept of Medical Police' in *Bulletin of the History of Medicine* 27 (1953) 21–42; E. Lesky, 'Osterreichisches Gesundheitswesen im Zeitalter das aufklärten Absolutismus' in *Archiv für österreichische Geschichte*, 122. Bd (1959).

10. See D. Kosáry, 'Die ungarische Unterrichtsreform von 1777' in *Ungarn und Osterreich unter Maria Theresia und Joseph II* (Wien, 1982) 21–100. The text of the Generale Normativum in Re Sanitatis can be found in X.F. Linzbauer, *Codex Sanitario-Medicinalis Hungariae*, Tom. II (Buda, 1852) 535–71. Also see A. Szállási, 'Vor zweihundert Jahren war das Generale Normativum in Re Sanitatis herausgegeben werden' in *Communicationes de Historia Artis Medicinae*, Supp. 4 (1970) 103–10.

11. For health conditions and medical life in eighteenth-century Hungary, see (in foreign language) Gy. Magyary-Kossa, *Ungarische medizinische Erinnerungen* (Budapest, 1935).

12. For eighteenth-century Hungarian medical literature, see general bibliographies: I. Weszprémi, *Succincta medicorum Hungariae et Transilvaniae biographia*, Tom. 1–4 (Lipsiae, 1774–87); G. Petrik, *Magyarország bibliográfiája 1712–1860* (Bibliography of Hungary,

1712–1860), (Budapest, 1888–92); J. Szinnyei, *Magyar írók élete és munkái* (The life and works of Hungarian authors) vols 1–14 (Budapest, 1891–1914); and T. Győry, *Magyarország orvosi bibliográfiája, 1472–1899* (Medical bibliography of Hungary, 1472–1899), (Budapest, 1900). Apart from these bibliographies there are only two studies on the subject, both in Hungarian and both unpublished: the manuscript of I. Friedrich, *18th-century Popular Medical Books* (1978) and the manuscript of M. Szlatky, *Vernacular Medical Literature in Eighteenth Century Hungary* (1987).

13. These expressions derive from the basic works of the camerialists, from C. Wolff, *Vernünftige Gedanken von dem Gesellschaftlichen Leben der Menschen* (Halle, 1721). G. von Justi, *Grundsätzen der Polizey-Wissenschaft* (1756) and J. von Sonnenfels, *Grundsätzen der Polizey, Handlung und Finanzwissenschaft* (1765).

14. Several Hungarian medical authors, such as I. Weszprémi, I. Mátyus, D. Gömöri and others, were awarded or raised to noble rank by Maria-Theresa for their literary activity.

15. These figures derive partly from Cs. Csapodi, 'Könyvtermelésünk a XVIII. században' (Publishing in the 18th century) in *Magyar Könyvszemle* (Hungarian Book Review) 4 (1942) 392–8 and from M. Szlatky's yet unpublished study (see note 12).

16. David Gömöri, *A pestisről való orvosi tanácslás* (Győr, 1739).

17. For Tissot, see H. Buess and M.L. Portmann, 'A. Tissot' in *Médecine et Hygiène* 37 (1979) 3909–10; E.K. Barnum, 'S.A.D. Tissot' in *The Swiss Monthly* 7 (1928) 182–7; A. Guisan, 'Le livre de malades du Dr. Tissot' in *Revue Médicale de la Suisse Romande* 31 (1911) 713–21; H.M. Koelbing, 'Que devons-nous en médecine a la Suisse Romande?' in *Gesnerus* 32 (1975) 123–8; M.L. Portmann, 'Relations d'Auguste Tissot (1728–1797) médecin à Lausanne, avec le patriciat bernois' in *Gesnerus* 37 (1980) 21–7; E. Olivier, *Médecine et santé dans le Pays de Vaud au XVIIIᵉ siècle*, 1675–1798, 2 vols (Lausanne, 1939); A. Emch-Dériaz, *Towards a Social Conception of Health in the Second Half of the Eighteenth Century: Tissot (1728–1797) and the New Pre-occupation with Health and Well-being* (Dissertation, Rochester, 1983); L. Benaroyo, *L'Avis au peuple sur sa santé de Samuel-Auguste Tissot (1728–1797): la voie vers une médecine éclairée* (Zurich, 1988).

18. For M. Marikowzki (1728–72), see I. Weszprémi, *Succincta medicorum Hungariae et Transilvanie biographia*, Tom. II (Wien, 1781) 525–41; J. Szinnyei, *Magyar írók élete és munkái* (The life and works of Hungarian authors) vol. 8 (Budapest, 1902) 593–4.

19. A. Tissot, *A néphez való tudósítás miképpen kellyen a maga egésségére vigyázni* trans. by M. Marikowzki (Nagykároly, 1772) 3.

20. For Count Antal Károlyi (1732–91), see I. Nagy, *Magyarország családai* (Families of Hungary) vol. 6 (Pest, 1860) 107–88; J. Szinnyei, *Magyar írók élete és munkái* (The life and works of Hungarian authors) vol. 6 (Budapest, 1901) 1073–4; A. Szirmay, *Szathmár vármegye* (Szathmár County) vols 2 (Buda, 1810).

21. On the press of Nagykároly, see G. Eble, *Egy magyar nyomda a XVIII. században* (A Hungarian Press in the 18th C.), (Budapest, 1891).

22. The debate has been published in one volume: M. Tissot, *Lettre*

à M. de Haen . . . en réponse à ses questions sur l'inoculation and A. de Haen, *Refutation de l'inoculation* (Vienna, 1759). Tissot's essays were often written in letter form and addressed to one of his colleagues: to Zimmermann in 1760, 1765, 1766; to Haller in 1760, etc. For the medical life of Vienna, see E. Lesky and A. Wandruszka (eds), *Gerard van Swieten und seine Zeit* (Vienna, 1973).

23. See note 20, A. Szirmay, op.cit. 119–20.
24. A. Tissot, *A néphez való tudósitás* (Nagykároly, 1772) 5–6.
25. *Idem*, 34–6.
26. *Idem*, 89.
27. *Idem*, 22.
28. His own work, the *Ephemerides Syrmiensis* (1767) has also been written in 'methodo Hippocratico-Sydenhaimiana'.
29. A. Tissot, 'A néphez való tudósitás (Nagykároly, 1772) 261.
30. *Idem*, 581.
31. I. Weszprémi, *Succincta medicorum Hungariae et Transilvaniae biographia*, Tom 2 (Vienna, 1781) 541.
32. A. Tissot, *A néphez való tudósitás* (Nagykároly, 1772) 4–6.
33. See G. Rosen, 'Problems in the Application of Statistical Analysis to Questions of Health' in *Bulletin of the History of Medicine* 29 (1955) 27–45, and E.A. Underwood, 'The History of the Quantitative Approach in Medicine' in *British Medical Bulletin* 7 (1951) 265–74.
34. A. Tissot, *A néphez való tudósitás* (Nagykároly, 1772) 13.
35. See A. Gárdonyi, 'Magyarországi könyvnyomdák a 18. században' (Hungarian Presses in the 18th Century) in *Irodalom és Felvilágosodás* (Enlightenment and Literature), (Budapest, 1974) 283–333, and K. Benda and K. Irinyi, *A négyszáz éves debreceni nyomda* (the 400-year-old Press of Debrecen), (Budapest, 1961).
36. See M. Szarvasi, *Magánkönyvtáraink a XVIII. században* (Private Libraries in the XVIIIth Century), (Budapest, 1939).
37. See note 22.
38. In spite of the opposition of these physicians, the royal family of Maria-Theresa was successfully inoculated in 1768 by a Dutch physician, Ingenhous. For the spread of the inoculation, see G. Miller, *The Adoption of Inoculation for Small-pox in England and France* (London, 1957).
39. The first successful inoculation took place in 1721 in Hungary, when J.A. Raimann, town-physician of Eperjes, inoculated his two-and-a-half-year-old daughter when his son had smallpox during an epidemic. He published his experience in the *Sammlung der Natur- und Medizin-Geschichten* Versuch XVII (1723) 254–74.
40. I. Weszprémi, *A kisded gyermekeknek nevelésekről való rövid oktatás* (Kolozsvár, 1760).
41. Weszprémi published these letters in his *Succincta*, vol. 4 (Vienna, 1787) 930–9.
42. A. Tissot, *A néphez való tudósitás* (Nagykároly, 1772) 11.
43. *Idem*, 12.
44. M. Foucault, 'The Politics of Health in the Eighteenth Century, in *Power and Knowledge, Selected Interviews and other Writings of M. Foucault* (The Harvester Press, 1980) 166–82.

45. See note 5, and, for the universities of Jena and Halle, see O. Feyl, 'Die führende Stellung der Ungerländer in der internationalen Geistegeschichte der Universität Jena' in *Wissenschaftliche Zeitschrift der Friedrich Schiller Universität Jena* (1953–54) 399–445; H. Peukert, *Die Slawen der Dunaumonarchie und die Universität Jena 1700–1848* (Berlin, 1958); G. Mende, 'Die Universität Halle als Zentrum der deutschen Aufklärung' in *450 Jahre Martin Luther Universität Halle-Wittenberg*, vols 2 (Halle, 1952).

46. See N. Duka Zolyomi, 'The Development of the District Medical Officer in Hungary from the Middle-Ages to the 18th Century' in A.W. Russell (ed), *The Town and State Physician in Europe from the Middle Ages to the Enlightenment* (Wolfenbüttel, 1974) 131–40.

47. This kind of argument can be found in the introductions of the works of Gömöri, Perliczy, Weszprémi, Szeli, Dombi, Csapó, Mátyus, and Rácz; see notes 16, 48, 50, 53, 54, 55, 56, 58, 60.

48. D. Perliczy, *Consilium Medicum* (Buda, 1740); *idem, Medicina pauperum* (Buda, 1740); *idem, Testi békességre vezető utitárs* (Buda, 1740).

49. For Weszprémi, see T. Vida, 'British Contacts of the Hungarian István Weszprémi' in *Orvostörténeti Közlemények* (Medical Historical Quarterly) Suppl. 6 (1972) 119–37.

50. I. Weszprémi, *A kisded gyermekeknek nevelésekről való rövid oktatás* (Kolozsvár, 1760).

51. I. Weszprémi, *Az egésségnek fenntartására és a hosszu életnek megnyerésére szükséges regulák* (Kolozsvár, 1760).

52. See M. Szlatky, 'Wesprémi magyar nyelvü orvosi müveinek angol gyökerei' (The English origins of Weszprémi's Hungarian Works) in *Orvosi Hetilap* (Medical Weekly) (1987) 1931–2.

53. I. Weszprémi, *Bába mesterségre tanitó könyv* (Debrecen, 1766).

54. J. Steidele, *Magyar bábamesterség* trans. by K. Szeli (Bécs, 1777).

55. S. Dombi, *Bábamesterség* (Pozsony, 1772).

56. J. Csapó, *Kisgyermekek isputálja* (Nagykároly, 1771).

57. M. Rosen, *Az hójagos és veres himlőnek gyógyitására és beoltására való utmutatás* trans. from German by J. Báti (Kolozsvár, 1785); M. Rosen, *Orvos-tanitás a gyermekek nyavalyáinak megeséméréseikről és orvoslásokról* trans. from German by S. Dombi (Pest, 1794).

58. I. Mátyus, *Diaetetica, az az a jó egészség megtartásának módját elé adó könyv* vols 2 (Kolozsvár, 1762–67).

For Mátyus and the Hungarian books on diet and regimen, see M. Szlatky, *A jó egészség megtartásának módjáról* (Preservation of Good Health), (Budapest, 1989).

59. T. Fuller, *Pharmacopoea Extemporanea* (1702), *Pharmacopoea Bateana* (1718), *Pharmacopoea Domestica* (1723).

60. *Orvosioktatás* (Buda, 1776) and S. Rácz, *Orvosi oktatás* (Buda, 1778).

61. S. Rácz, *Orvosi oktatás* (Buda, 1778) 243.

62. For Rácz, see T. Győry, *Az Orvostudományi Kar története, 1770–1935* (History of Medical Faculty, 1770–1935), (Budapest, 1936).

63. A. Störck, *Orvosi tanitás* trans. by S. Rácz (Buda, 1778).

64. A. Störck, *Orvos-könyv* trans. by J. Milesz (Vienna, 1778).

65. See D. Kosáry, *Culture and Society in Eighteenth Century Hungary* (Budapest, 1987) 24.

66. Tissot is mentioned by I. Mátyus (1787), S. Rácz (1782), J. Csapó (1791), S. Benkó (1791), J. Kiss (1794, 1796), S. Dombi (1794), M. Kováts (1798).

67. In the introduction to C.W. Hufeland, *Az emberi élet meghosszabbitásának mestersége* vols 2, trans. and enlarged by M. Kováts (Pest, 1798).

68. J. Kiss, *Egésséget tárgyazó katekésis* (Sorpon, 1794, 1796). Kiss referred to C.B. Faust, but he did not consider the book a translation, and published it under his own name.

69. C.W. Hufeland, *Az emberi élet meghosszabbitásának mestersége* trans. by M. Kováts, vols 2 (Pest, 1798), and in one volume (Kolozsvár, 1798), and again in two volumes (Pest, 1799).

70. W. Grant, *Some Observations on the Origin, Progress, and Method of Treating the Atrabilious Temperament and Gout* (London, 1780) and S. Benkó, *A fekete epés mértékletnek . . . leirása* trans. from W. Grant and enlarged by S. Benkó (Pest, 1791).

71. See note 57.

8

Spreading medical Enlightenment

The popularization of medicine in Georgian England, and its paradoxes

Roy Porter

Georgian England experienced a boom in 'popularized medicine', taking that phrase to mean advice works purveying regular medical information in simplified language to a broad public.[1] Various cultural currents promoted this development, including populist radicalism and Enlightenment faith in the diffusion of knowledge; the drive to reform popular culture; and the birth of a consumer society.

The first of these leaps off the pages of many 'Every Man His Own Physician' texts. The empire of disease and death, readers are routinely told, has been prolonged by popular ignorance and perhaps professional mystification. Now, thanks to printing and the liberty of the press, a new age of practical help is dawning; medical enlightenment will take its place alongside improvements in the arts and sciences and the securing of basic political rights.[2]

A completely different mode of explanation is possible. High culture (it has been argued) was bent on distancing itself from 'plebeian' outlooks.[3] The élite aimed to 'reform' popular beliefs, thereby reinforcing social control and cultural hegemony. Grass-roots healing certainly caused unease. It smacked of magic, witchcraft and astrology, and the village wise woman was often suspected of involvement with abortion and infanticide.[4] Hence instructional texts would denounce folk cures as grossly superstitious, and seek to sanitize dangers by inculcating moral ideals like cleanliness. 'Medicalization' of this kind – the propagation of élite medicine among the masses – was, it may be suggested, only one of many normalizing 'invasions' aimed at neutralizing demotic culture.[5]

215

Third, the inflation of popular medical texts might be read as an expression less of ideology than of economics. It was a commercial age. Marketing and distribution were improving with the spread of turnpikes, newspapers, and shops; surplus income grew, authorship expanded. In what may be called an emergent consumer society, more people were consuming more knowledge, not least medical knowledge, alongside a diet or drugs and medications.[6]

By no means mutually exclusive, these varied explanations of the spread of popularized medicine should alert us to a diversity of aims and postures among their authors. It was axiomatic that ignorance and error must be combated, and proper attitudes propagated towards health, disease, treatments, and doctors. But what should those attitudes be? Indeed, to put it in a nutshell, how far was it desirable that the common man be encouraged to be his own physician?

Here I shall examine three doctors, prominent in the late eighteenth century for their contributions to this didactic genre: William Buchan, Thomas Beddoes, and James Parkinson, men whose views are of special interest, because all were belligerent sociopolitical radicals no less than medical enlighteners. What, then, were the ties, but also the tensions, between political and medical radicalism?[7]

William Buchan, a Scots-born Edinburgh graduate who settled first in Sheffield and then in London, was the author of the evergreen *Domestic Medicine,* first published in 1769, and reprinted well into the nineteenth century, and also of *Observations Concerning the Prevention and Cure of the Venereal Disease* (1796). Sympathetic to both the American and the French revolutions, Buchan became a bitter critic of the medical establishment.[8]

Thomas Beddoes was so ardent a supporter of the French Revolution, and opponent of Pitt, that he felt obliged in 1793 to quit his position as Reader in Chemistry at Oxford University, retiring to private practice in the fashionable Bristol suburb of Clifton, where he opened his Pneumatic Institution in 1799. Beddoes wrote health-care books for the well-to-do, above all *Hygëia: or Essays Moral and Medical, on the Causes Affecting the Personal State of our Middling and Affluent Classes* (1802), and the *Manual of Health: or, the Invalid Conducted Safely Through the Seasons* (1806). But he mainly targeted his tracts at the lower orders, in particular his much-reprinted *The History of Isaac*

Jenkins, and of the Sickness of Sarah his Wife, and Their Three Children (1792), *A Guide for Self Preservation, and Parental Affection; or Plain Directions for Enabling People to Keep Themselves and their Children Free from Several Common Disorders* (1793), and *Good Advice for the Husbandman in Harvest* (1808).[9]

James Parkinson, a talented scientific polymath, general practitioner and parish doctor in London's East End, was a political radical of real stature. In the 1790s he was active in the pro-Jacobin London Corresponding Society – the Privy Council quizzed him on his involvement in the so-called 'pop-gun plot' – and a fiery political pamphleteer. He also wrote numerous health advice books, including *The Budget of the People* (1793), *Medical Admonitions to Families, Respecting the Preservation of Health, and the Treatment of the Sick* (1801), *The Town and Country Friend and Physician* (1803), and *The Villager's Friend and Physician* (1802) – this last also being condensed into a handbill, entitled *The Way to Health* (1802).[10]

All three railed against Old Corruption, denouncing despotism, oligarchy and aristocracy, and parading their contempt for grandee corruption. They embraced the cause of the people, and propounded an Enlightenment faith in human betterment, to be achieved by the defeat of vested interests, the progress of science, and the diffusion of useful knowledge. Each diagnosed ill-health as symptomatic of the evils of the *ancien régime* body politic,[11] tolerated by the nepotism, toadyism, and incompetence of a medical profession moved by love, not of health, but of wealth. All believed the rights of man included the right to health, indeed, the right to its self-management. Beyond such consensus, however, their views notably diverged, in ways significant for the future politics of health. I shall examine the three in turn.

Buchan's *Domestic Medicine* (1769) was the age's best-selling text written by a medical regular, reputedly partnering the Bible by the bedside of every Scottish crofter.[12] Unlike John Wesley's *Primitive Physick* (1747),[13] *Domestic Medicine* went beyond bare recipes and 'do's and don'ts', expounding a broad philosophy of health to be achieved through temperance, hygiene, and obedience to Nature's laws.

Especially in his *Observations Concerning . . . Venereal Disease*, Buchan embraced a democratic late Enlightenment populism, aimed at 'rendering medicine more extensively beneficial to mankind'.[14] Medically speaking, the people were childlike: 'this credulity of mankind in regard to medicine is truly astonishing'.[15] Hence sickness crises left them 'the easy dupes of every pretender to a secret medicine'.[16] Sufferers thus needed to be safeguarded against quackery, and those 'not able to employ' regular doctors, for reasons of cost or inaccessibility, required instruction in self-help.

Buchan had no rose-tinted Rousseauvian faith in folksy wisdom or habits. Often dirty, slovenly and feckless, the masses also held bizarre medical prejudices, some of which – for example, sex with a virgin as a syphilis cure – boggled the understanding (was it more 'wicked or absurd'?).[17] Not least, they failed to obey doctors. 'He will seldom tell the truth, and perhaps never the whole truth' – thus began Buchan's unflattering portrait of the venereal patient:[18]

> but what is still worse, he seldom implicitly follows the doctor's directions, with regard, either to regimen or medicines . . . Some patients think it is the business of the doctor to find out their disorders, without being told any thing about them. They treat physicians as conjurors, and think they need no information.

Yet their ignorance deserved pity not blame. The real cause of this benightedness was that 'Physic is still engrossed by the faculty'.[19] Physicians had too long cynically monopolized medicine as a mystery, a closed shop whose shop-talk was a dead tongue, all to gratify the sordid greed of those who would 'make a trade of it'.[20] Popery had reduced religion to mumbo-jumbo and priestcraft; physicians had similarly sought to 'disguise and conceal the art', and had set up doctorcraft.[21]

'While men are kept in the dark, and told that they are not to use their own understanding, in matters that concern their health', Buchan explained, *à propos* of venereal disorders:[22]

> they will be the dupes of designing knaves; and a disease the most tractable in its nature, and almost the only one for which we possess a specific remedy [i.e. mercury], will be suffered to commit its ravages on the human race, and to embitter the most delicious draught that Heaven has bestowed for the solace of human life.

Monopoly perpetuated ignorance. Quoting Benjamin Rush[23] – a man holding 'the same liberal sentiments concerning medicine as I entertain' – Buchan vented his anger that

> for a long while, air, water, and even the light of the sun, were dealt out by physicians to their patients with a sparing hand. They possessed for several centuries the same monopoly over many artificial remedies. But a new order of things is rising in medicine, as well as in government. Air, water, and light are taken without the advice of a physician, and Bark and Laudanum are now prescribed every where by nurses and mistresses of families, with safety and advantage.

So there were grounds, at least, for optimism: 'The time must, and will come, when, in addition to the above remedies, the general use of Calomel, Jalap, and the lancet, shall be considered among the most essential articles of the knowledge and rights of men'.[24]

An age of democratic revolution thus demanded the democratization of medicine, and that meant openness and education.[25] 'It is no more necessary', he writes, again approvingly quoting Rush, 'that a patient should be ignorant of the medicine he takes to be cured by it, than that the business of government should be conducted with secrecy in order to insure obedience to just laws. Much less is it necessary that the means of life should be prescribed in a dead language, or dictated with the solemn pomp of a Necromancer'.[26] The goal? 'To bring medicine out of the schools, to lay open its hidden treasures'. The means? 'A code of laws for the preservation of health'. 'Properly digested, and duly executed', this would 'be of more use to mankind than all the efforts of the faculty'.[27] Above all, medical terms should be tailored to popular minds. The incomparable Thomas Sydenham had made notable medical breakthroughs, but, writing in Latin, it had proved easy for the faculty to impede the diffusion of his works. Buchan by contrast prided himself upon having 'addressed my publications to the people'.[28] He would be a medical missionary to the people. 'I shall never cease to give them all the information in my power, both with regard to the prevention and cure of diseases'.[29]

Progress would necessarily be a struggle, however, because of sinister vested interests. He had himself, he claimed, been persecuted by 'the faculty' for his popularizing pains. Publications of his *Observations* would, he predicted, inevitably draw 'fresh torrents of abuse from the faculty'[30] – especially from that 'sordid part' . . . 'who think their trade in danger' if medical mysteries are exposed.[31] For medical monopolists abhorred open minds and free thought: 'whoever has dared to think for himself, in matters relating to health, and was not of the faculty, has been looked upon as an intruder, and held up to ridicule'.[32] Such a vile 'spirit of persecution' was sure to persist, till medicine's 'doctrines are laid open, and candidly submitted to the examination of all men' – until then, 'medicine will be little better than a piece of mummery'.[33] Of course, such plain speaking was 'not likely to lessen their malice', and persecution would continue, but 'I am prepared for the worst they can do', Buchan confided to his readers, for, 'While the rest of mankind are on my side, I can laugh at the malice, and despise the resentment of the faculty'.[34]

So what future did Buchan foresee? He urged not the abolition of professional medicine but its reform. He had no desire to 'supersede the physician', he insisted, for 'to talk of making all men physicians, is the extreme of folly'. But he did want the people to be well-informed judges of medicine – the sure way to spike corporate mystification and knavish quackery. And he was confident that most disorders could be self-treated. A reader of *Domestic Medicine* would conclude that few clinical problems, from diarrhoea to dislocated necks, lay beyond the capacities of a sensible layman or woman. Nature would cure many disorders; nothing would cure others; and most of the rest could at least be relieved by a simple regimen – above all, the use of fresh air, cleanliness, and plain diet – and a handful of drugs. Even with venereal disease, 'in nineteen out of twenty cases, where this disease occurs, the patient may be his own physician'.[35] In Buchan, the Enlightenment ideal of 'committing the care of . . . diseases to the people' – medicine for the people, by the people – appears with its most triumphant fanfare.

Thomas Beddoes, too, believed that health reform mattered no less than political change – the two must go hand in hand. And, like Buchan, he deprecated the poisoning of medicine by Mammon and detested quackery. People ought to be caretakers of their own health.[36]

The folly and prejudices of the laity appalled Beddoes no less than Buchan. 'Vulgar errors' and 'erroneous domestic opinion' were epidemic[37] – though it was a contagion, he insisted, quoting the great German hygienist, Struve, by no means confined to the masses: 'Medical superstition is to be sought, not only in the peasant's hut, but in the city and in the palace; beside the toilette of the lady of first fashion, and in the cabinet of the philosopher'.[38] No end of erroneous conceptions were entertained. 'Some philosopher remarks', Beddoes commented, 'that a life would hardly suffice to enumerate the vain fantasies of mankind. No title in the list would, perhaps be more copious than that of supposititious and exaggerated diseases'.[39]

There was thus no solid foundation of popular wisdom to build upon. People had to 'unlearn' their mistakes – to have their minds reduced 'to that *blank* state in which, according to Locke, it originally exists'.[40] But the knowledge which they ought then to acquire was emphatically not the principles and practice of medicine. In lay hands, Beddoes never tired of insisting, medicine was a menace. Clinical treatment was an art so intricate, requiring such vast experience and refined judgement, that only the trained physician should tackle it. Lay physic was bad physic.

Here Beddoes, of course, departed root-and-branch from Buchan's Jacobin dictum that medicine was essentially a simple art accessible to anyone (complexity was a professional smokescreen), and from the Buchanite pledge to impart 'all the information in my power, both with regard to the prevention and cure of diseases'.[47] Indeed, Beddoes probably believed Buchan himself had done the people's health grave disservice. For he condemned the torrent of 'Every Man His Own Physician' volumes – *Domestic Medicine* and its brood – as little better than a sewer. Most were wrong-headed. They were bound to be misunderstood. And they would give readers false confidence in their right to pop pills and wield the lancet. 'No such treatise', Beddoes pointedly concluded, 'has been attempted by any experienced physician, whose judgement had been approved by other productions'.[42]

Ever radical, Beddoes naturally did not see the perpetuation of popular ignorance as the panacea. But the desideratum must be to teach the people, not the arts of self-medication – physic must be left to experts! – but skills in cultivating and preserving health. Above all, he wished to promote the application of 'physiological knowledge to domestic use'[43] – it would be desirable, he argued, if 'physiology will come to be considered as the domestic science *par excellence*'.[44]

Passionately committed to the practical, sense-oriented peda-gogics championed by Rousseau and his own father-in-law, Richard Lovell Edgeworth, Beddoes thought it best to start with 'teaching children accurately to distinguish the parts of the body. Such information will lead them to observe many impor-tant changes, which as they take place slowly, are apt to proceed unobserved'.[45] And not only youngsters: 'The ignorant of all denominations, and the poor and the young among the rest, were perpetually unable to fix, with any tolerable accuracy, the seat of their maladies'.[46]

Crucial to Beddoes's strategy was health education by pamphlets and public lectures: general courses in anatomy and physiology, but also, dearer to his heart, clinical lectures too. 'It must be', he insisted,[47]

their aim to make fully sensible the mischiefs arising from systematic irregularity; from injudicious management after exposure to the inclemencies of the weather, and from the other innumerable ordinary errors of individual conduct. They must explain the origin and conduct, much more minutely than the treatment of diseases. They may be conveniently undertaken wherever there exists an infirmary.

Such lectures would benefit posterity 'in the most effectual manner'.[48] Elementary physiological education became, as Roger Cooter has shown, central to the self-improvement campaigns of nineteenth-century petty bourgeois and artisan radicals.[49]

If Beddoes thus felt constrained to be less epistemologically egalitarian than Buchan – for their own good, people must defer to expert authority – he nevertheless believed the circum-stances of the labouring poor remained, in one respect, highly eligible. For their lifestyle was, perforce, more robust, more manly, less vitiated, than that of their betters. Through idleness and fashion, anxiety and luxury, the rich ruined their natural constitutional vivacity. Worse still, genteel vices – sickly sensi-bility, faddish diet, sedentary occupations, morbid introspec-tion – induced class-specific diseases like nervous hypochondria and gout. Upper-class effeteness turned unhealthiness into style: 'no mortal would ever have thought of making apathy the mode, but a worn out beau'.[50] Even worse, top people had money to squander on fashionable physicians, spa treatments, and other dire health hazards! By contrast, necessity, labour, exposure to the elements, and plain food – all these hardened the labouring poor, reinforcing resistance. 'If you would do well', Beddoes instructed the *bon ton*, 'you must eat and digest like a ploughman'.[51] Beddoes's was a radicalism which valued – even romanticized – the robust health and salutary rude strength he identified with plebeian habits.

This is plain in Beddoes's most popular tract for the times, *The History of Isaac Jenkins, and of the Sickness of Sarah his Wife, and Their Three Children* (1792), a moral tale of a lower-class household that fell into destitution and disease, once, beset by misfortunes, the husband took to drink. Fortunately, the intervention of a wise and worthy surgeon helped to restore both the morale and the health of the family. The homily ends with a heart-warming vignette of the simple but honest Jenkins household, toiling hard to maintain its dignity, but, thanks to its distance from fashionable vices, well on the road to recovery.[52]

This sentimental picturing of simple swain and doctors who are the people's friends also looms large in the tracts of James Parkinson, whose main practical experience lay in treating the Shoreditch poor.[53] Was lay medical activity desirable? On this, Parkinson was a pragmatist, midway between Buchan and Beddoes. Like a ship without a pilot, self-medication was hazardous. Expert help was best. Hence *The Villager's Friend and Physician* instructed readers when sick to 'apply directly to the man of judgement and experience'.[54] If a regular doctor could not be afforded, try a hospital, but never a quack or the neighbourly amateur who 'possesses a medicine chest and the small share of skill which is derived from the perusal of some treatise on domestic medicine'.[55] Parkinson specifically condemned Buchan for the irresponsibility of advising self-care in cases of dysentery and so forth.

Yet Parkinson was a realist, who knew people would inevitably undertake self-medication. So if some ships inevitably lacked a pilot, they should at least carry good charts. And it was in this light that Parkinson regarded his own popularizing publications like *Medical Admonitions to Families Respecting the Preservation of Health and the Treatment of the Sick*[56] which, 'convinced that many lives are lost by neglecting to apply sufficiently soon for medical aid, and by improper treatment of disease by domestic practitioners', was designed to enable readers to judge, from self-scanning of symptoms, which disorders required professional aid, and which could safely be handled by domestic first aid.

Parkinson's most substantial popular appeal was *The Way to Health*,[57] a body maintenance guide for manual labourers that was also published as a handbill. In it, Parkinson paints a pastoral picture of manual work: thanks to their routines of honest toil, labourers are potentially blessed with sound constitutional health. If the doctor's day involved endless anxiety, their labour, by contrast, should be a joy. 'The All Wise Disposer of all things has decreed the due exercise of our powers to be an inexhaustible source of pleasure; so that man returns to his daily toil with cheerful alacrity'.[58] Labourers must, however, he warns, avoid dissipating their strength through the temptation to overwork, for 'all violent and long continued exertions, even in your wonted labours, may not only prove a serious injury to your health, but will also lessen, rather than increase, the weekly provision for your family'. Not least, overwork would encourage boozing, and by that fatal road, 'industry may become the mother of drunkenness',[59] and the alehouse 'the house of misery and disease'. 'He who being engaged in works of labour, flies to liquor for a spur, whenever nature droops from too great exertion, makes terrible havoc with himself', bringing on 'tremblings, sinking of the spirits' and, finally, some 'deadly malady'.[60]

As pernicious as liquor were the perils of the table. Avoid fancy, spicy fare – it causes indigestion and ruins the stomach.[61] Eat plain instead: 'he that breakfasts on milk, dines one day on animal food, and the other on pudding etc., and sups lightly on milk, pottage, &c. may with reason hope for health'.[62] Furthermore, labourers should cultivate the mind – though, even here, 'moderation in the enjoyment of pleasure' was needed.[63] Workmen should pass their evenings instructing their families in the 'advantages of industry, civility and sobriety; let them see the necessity and advantage of rendering themselves useful to those around them. Place before them particularly the policy of such conduct towards their employers'.

Medicine thus afforded Parkinson an idiom for imparting to the poor a homespun moralism that valued conformist personal responsibility. The reward of regular work habits was health. Idleness, or the overwork that greed induced, would dissipate God's gifts by producing alcoholism and debility. Parkinson's individualist medical perspective enabled him to sidestep any consideration of the actual conditions of labour and the labouring poor in the early nineteenth-century city. The economy of health and the sanctions of disease were invoked to promote moral reformation in his readers. If the unlettered poor were the authors of their own misfortunes, with instruction they could become guardians of their own health. In Parkinson's account, responsibility for health disorders rested ultimately neither with society, nor with the medical profession, but in the individual's own hands.

My rapid survey of this triumvirate of radicals has revealed certain ambiguities, paradoxes even. Buchan, Beddoes and Parkinson all criticized the *status quo* in society and medicine alike. They lambasted enforced ignorance, and believed injustice and oppression undermined the people's health. In pamphlet after pamphlet, Beddoes accused Pitt's warmongering policies[64] of depleting the health of the labouring poor.[65] Parkinson damned the callous rich prepared to stand by while the poor starved.[66] Buchan and Beddoes judged medicine seduced by commerce and fashion. Such indictments came easily to men steeped in radical Enlightenment ideologies.

All embraced the people's health and sought emancipation from the corruptions of 'the sick trade'.[67] Yet Beddoes and, to a lesser degree, Parkinson were convinced that the population would cease to be sick only when it ceased to medicate itself, and trusted instead in the enlightened, expert practitioner.

For, in the name of preventive medicine and doctors' orders, they also felt obliged to protect the people from their own vices. Ordinary people did not, and could not, know their own best medical interests. Only with guidance, or even coercion, would they reach the promised land of health. The altruistic, paternalist physician would be the tutor of the new common man, who must adopt the habits of sobriety and cleanliness.[68] Herein lies the classic radical doctor's dilemma: might not the people, to echo Rousseau, also need to be forced to be healthy?

Notes

1. An excellent survey of this popular literature is afforded by Ginnie Smith, 'Prescribing the Rules of Health: Self-Help and Advice in Late Eighteenth-Century England' in Roy Porter (ed.), *Patients and Practitioners: Lay Perceptions of Medicine in Pre-industrial Society* (Cambridge and New York, Cambridge University Press, 1985), 249–82; *idem*, 'Cleanliness: the Development of an Idea and Practice in Britain 1770–1850' (University of London, PhD thesis, 1985).

It should be emphasized here that I am not discussing other sorts of 'popular medicine', e.g. the various kinds of 'alternative' or 'quack' medicine, or 'folk medicine', and so forth. I am not denying their existence in the late Enlightenment. Rather, this paper focuses upon works offering simplified versions of regular medicine (itself not a homogeneous entity) to a wider reading public.

2. For the radical Enlightenment, see Margaret C. Jacob, *The Radical Enlightenment: Pantheists, Freemasons and Republicans* (London: George Allen and Unwin, 1981); and for general Enlightenment faith in medicine, see P. Gay, 'The Enlightenment as Medicine and as Cure' in W.H. Barber (ed.), *The Age of the Enlightenment. Studies Presented to Theodore Besterman* (Edinburgh: St Andrews University Publications, 1967), 375–86; *idem, The Enlightenment,* 2 vols (New York: Knopf, 1967–9); for evaluation of Gay, see Roy Porter, 'Civilization and Disease: Medical Ideology and Enlightenment', in J. Black and J. Gregory (eds), *Culture, Politics and Society in Britain 1660–1800* (Manchester: Manchester University Press, 1991); *idem,* 'Was There a Medical Enlightenment in Eighteenth Century England?', *British Journal for Eighteenth Century Studies,* 5 (1982), 46–63. Paul Langford, *A Polite and Commercial People: England, 1727–1783* (Oxford: Oxford University Press, 1989) offers a convincing view of the emergence of middle class values; Peter Borsay, *The English Urban Renaissance* (Oxford: Clarendon Press, 1989) emphasizes the new importance of towns; for the uses of popular literacy at this time see David Vincent, *Literacy and Popular Culture. England 1750–1914* (Cambridge: Cambridge University Press, 1989).

3. For a strong recent statement of the 'separation' thesis, see Patrick Curry, *Prophecy and Power. Astrology in Early Modern England* (Cambridge: Polity Press, 1989). For discussion of the relations of the cultures see J.M. Golby and A.W. Purdue, *The Civilization of the Crowd: Popular Culture in England, 1750–1900* (London: Batsford, 1984); Peter Burke, *Popular Culture in Early Modern Europe* (London: Temple Smith, 1978); *idem,* 'Popular Culture between History and Ethnology', *Ethnologi Europaea,* 14 (1984), 5–13; *idem,* 'Revolution in Popular Culture', in Roy Porter and M. Teich (eds), *Revolution in History* (Cambridge, Cambridge University Press, 1986), 206–25; Bob Bushaway, *By Rite: Custom, Ceremony and Community in England, 1700–1880* (London, Junction Books, 1982). Specifically for medicine, see Mary E. Fissell, *Patients, Power and the Poor in Eighteenth Century Bristol* (Cambridge: Cambridge University Press, 1991), chap. viii, 'The Reform of Popular Medicine'.

4. On hostility to magic and the occult, see K. Thomas, *Religion and the Decline of Magic: Studies in Popular Beliefs in Sixteenth and Seventeenth-Century England* (London: Weidenfeld & Nicolson, 1971); Roy Porter, 'Medicine and the Decline of Magic', *Strawberry Fayre* (Autumn, 1986), 88–94; L.M. Beier, *Sufferers and Healers. The Experience of Illness in Seventeenth-Century England* (London: Routledge & Kegan Paul, 1987), 23–4, 161–3. For the perhaps contrasting situation in France, see J. Devlin, *The Superstitious Mind. French Peasants and the Supernatural in the Nineteenth Century* (New Haven: Yale University

Press, 1987); F. Loux, 'Presentation: langages et images du corps', *Ethnologie française*, vi (1976), 215–18; *idem, Sagesse du corps, santé et maladie dans les proverbs réginaux françaises* (Paris: Masionneuve et Larose, 1978); *idem, Practiques et savoirs populaires: le corps dans la societé traditionnelle* (Paris, Berger-Levrault, 1979); *idem*, 'Popular Culture and Knowledge of the Body: Infancy and the Medical Anthropologists', in R. Porter and A. Wear (eds), *Problems and Methods in the History of Medicine* (London: Croom Helm, 1987), 81–97; A. MacLaren, *Reproductive Rituals: The Perception of Fertility in England from the 16th Century to the 19th Century* (London & New York: Methuen, 1984).

5. For medicalization, see J.-P. Goubert, *La Médicalisation de la societé française 1770–1830* (Waterloo, Ontario: Historical Reflections Press, 1982); *idem*, 'Twenty Years On: Problems of Historical Methodology in the History of Health', in R. Porter and A. Wear (eds), *Problems and Methods in the History of Medicine* (London: Croom Helm, 1987), 40–56. R. Muchembled, *Popular Culture and Elite Culture in France, 1400–1750* (Baton Rouge: Louisiana State University Press, 1985); M. Foucault, *The Birth of the Clinic*, trans. A.M. Sheridan Smith (London: Tavistock, 1973); I. Illich, *Limits to Medicine. The Expropriation of Health* (Harmondsworth: Penguin, 1977); for a sensitive attempt to evaluate the applicability of such medicalization notions in a local context, see M.E. Fissell, 'The Physic of Charity: Health and Welfare in the West Country, 1690–1834' (Philadelphia, University of Pennsylvania PhD thesis, 1988).

6. Neil McKendrick, John Brewer and J.H. Plumb, *The Birth of a Consumer Society: The Commercialization of Eighteenth-Century England* (London: Europa, 1982); John Brewer and Roy Porter (eds), *Consumption and the World of Goods* (London: Routledge, 1991); Hohcheung and L. Mui, *Shops and Shopkeeping in Eighteenth-Century England* (London: Methuen, 1987); for the argument that medicine in the eighteenth century was heavily shaped by market concerns, see Dorothy Porter and Roy Porter, *Patient's Progress. Doctors and Doctoring in Eighteenth Century England* (Cambridge: Polity Press, 1989); Roy Porter and Dorothy Porter, *In Sickness and in Health. The British Experience, 1650–1850* (London: Fourth Estate, 1988); Roy Porter, *Health for Sale. Quackery in England 1650–1850* (Manchester: Manchester University Press, 1989).

7. Themes such as these have been examined for the nineteenth century by R. Cooter, 'The Power of the Body: the Early Nineteenth Century', in B. Barnes and S. Shapin (eds), *Natural Order: Historical Studies of Scientific Culture* (London and Beverly Hills: Sage Publications, 1979), 73–92; *idem*, 'Interpreting the Fringe: Brief Comments on a Broad Topic', *Society for the Social History of Medicine Bulletin*, xxix (1981), 32–6; *idem* (ed.), *Studies in the History of Alternative Medicine* (London: Macmillan, 1988); A. Marcovich, 'Concerning the Continuity between the Image of Society and the Image of the Human Body: An Examination of the Work of the English Physician J.C. Lettsom (1746–1815)', in P. Wright and A. Treacher (eds), *The Problem of Medical Knowledge* (Edinburgh: Edinburgh University Press, 1982), 69–87.

8. For the career of Buchan, see C. Lawrence, 'William Buchan: Medicine Laid Open', *Medical History*, xix (1975), 20–35; C. Rosenberg, 'Medical Text and Medical Context; Explaining William Buchan's *Domestic Medicine*', *Bulletin of the History of Medicine*, lvii (1983), 22–4.

9. For Beddoes's life, see J.E. Stock, *Memoirs of the Life of Thomas Beddoes MD* (London: J. Murray, 1811); D.A. Stansfield, *Thomas Beddoes M.D. 1760–1808, Chemist, Physician, Democrat* (Dordrecht: Reidel, 1984); F.F. Cartwright, 'The Association of Thomas Beddoes, M.D. with James Watt, F.R.S.', *Notes and Records of the Royal Society of London*, 22, 1 & 2, xx–xxi; F.W. Gibbs and W.A. Smeaton, 'Thomas Beddoes at Oxford', *Ambix* ix (1961), 417–19; L.S. Gottlieb, 'Thomas Beddoes M.D. and the Pneumatic Institution at Clifton 1798–1801', *Annals of Internal Medicine*, lxiii (1965), 530–33; T.H. Levere, 'Dr Thomas Beddoes and the Establishment of his Pneumatic Institution', *Notes and Records of the Royal Society of London*, xxxii (1977), 41–9; *idem*, 'Dr Thomas Beddoes at Oxford: Radical Politics in 1788–93, and the Fate of the Regius Chair in Chemistry', *Ambix*, xxviii (1981); *idem*, 'Thomas Beddoes, The Interaction of Pneumatic and Preventative Medicine with Chemistry', *Interdisciplinary Science Review* 7 (1982), 137–47; A. Miller, 'The Pneumatic Institution of Thomas Beddoes at Bristol', *Annals of Medical History* iii (1931), 253–60.

10. For Parkinson, see A.D. Morris, *James Parkinson, His Life and Times* (Boston: Birkhauser, 1989), and for the background of his radicalism see E.P. Thompson, *The Making of the English Working Class* (Harmondsworth: Penguin, 1963); S. Deane, *The French Revolution and Enlightenment in England 1789–1832* (Massachusetts and London: Harvard University Press, 1988); Albert Goodwin, *The Friends of Liberty: The English Democratic Movement in the Age of the French Revolution* (London: Hutchinson, 1979).

11. We do not yet have a definitive study of the interplay of medical and political metaphors in this period. For some suggestive writings, see S. Sontag, *Illness as Metaphor* (New York: Farrar, Straus & Giroux, 1978; London: Allen Lane, 1979); *idem, AIDS as Metaphor* (Harmondsworth: Allen Lane, 1989); C. Lawrence, 'The Nervous System and Society in the Scottish Enlightenment', in B. Barnes and S. Shapin (eds), *Natural Order* (Beverly Hills and London: Sage Publications, 1980), 19–40; R. Cooter, 'The Power of the Body: the Early Nineteenth Century', in B. Barnes and S. Shapin (eds), *Natural Order: Historical Studies of Scientific Culture* (London and Beverly Hills: Sage Publications, 1979), 73–92.

12. W. Buchan, *Domestic Medicine, or a Treatise on the Prevention and Cure of Diseases by Regimen and Simple Medicines* (Edinburgh: Balfour, Auld & Smellie, 1769); W. Buchan, *Observations Concerning the Prevention and Cure of the Venereal Disease* (London: Chapman, 1796).

13. J. Wesley, *Primitive Physick: Or, an Easy and Natural Method of Curing Most Diseases* (London: T. Trye, 1747); G.S. Rousseau, 'John Wesley's *Primitive Physick* (1747)', *Harvard Library Bulletin*, xvi (1968), 242–56.

14. Buchan, *Observations Concerning . . . Venereal Disease*, iv.
15. Buchan, *Observations Concerning . . . Venereal Disease*, iv. For Lawrence and Rosenberg, see above, note 8.
16. Buchan, *Observations Concerning . . . Venereal Disease*, iv.
17. Buchan, *Observations Concerning . . . Venereal Disease*, xvii.
18. Buchan, *Observations Concerning . . . Venereal Disease*, iv, xv.
19. Buchan, *Observations Concerning . . . Venereal Disease*, xxii.
20. Buchan, *Domestic Medicine*, xx.
21. Buchan, *Domestic Medicine*, xvii.
22. Buchan, *Observations Concerning . . . Venereal Disease*, 3. As will be evident, Buchan's characterization of the status quo – e.g. his conspiratorial vision of the medical establishment, the 'faculty' – should not be taken at face value as historically accurate. It is rather a self-serving exercise of radical rant.
23. The best source for Rush's radicalism is his letters. See L.H. Butterfield (ed.), *The Letters of Benjamin Rush*, 2 vols (Princeton: Princeton University Press, 1951).
24. Buchan, *Observations Concerning . . . Venereal Disease*, xxvi.
25. Buchan, *Observations Concerning . . . Venereal Disease*, xxvii. For political context, see John Brewer, 'Commercialization and Politics' in Neil McKendrick, John Brewer and J.H. Plumb, *The Birth of a Consumer Society: The Commercialization of Eighteenth-Century England* (London: Europa, 1982), 197–264.
26. Buchan, *Observations Concerning . . . Venereal Disease*, xxvii.
27. Buchan, *Observations Concerning . . . Venereal Disease*, xxiii.
28. Buchan, *Observations Concerning . . . Venereal Disease*, xxviii. For this theme, see Roy Porter, '"Expressing Yourself Ill": The Language of Sickness in Georgian England', in P. Burke and R. Porter (eds), *Language, Self and Society: The Social History of Language* (Cambridge: Polity Press, 1991), 276–99.
29. Buchan, *Observations Concerning . . . Venereal Disease*, xxviii.
30. Buchan, *Observations Concerning . . . Venereal Disease*, xxiii. To reiterate, it hardly needs to be said that Buchan's portrait of persecution at the hands of a united, vindictive Faculty was essentially self-serving fantasy on his part.
31. Buchan, *Domestic Medicine*, xx, xxi.
32. Buchan, *Domestic Medicine*, xxi.
33. Buchan, *Domestic Medicine*, xxix.
34. Buchan, *Domestic Medicine*, xxix.
35. Buchan, *Observations Concerning . . . Venereal Disease*, 9.
36. See Roy Porter, 'Plutus or Hygeia? Thomas Beddoes and Medical Ethics' in Robert Baker, Dorothy Porter and Roy Porter (eds), *The Codification of Medical Morality in the Eighteenth and Nineteenth Centuries*, vol. i (Dordrecht: Kluwer, 1992); *idem*, 'Reforming the Patient in the Age of Reform: Thomas Beddoes and Medical Practice' in Roger French and Andrew Wear (eds), *Medicine in the Age of Reform* (London: Routledge, 1991), 9–44 *idem*, *Doctor of Society: Thomas Beddoes and the Sick Trade in Late-Enlightenment England* (London: Routledge, 1992).
37. T. Beddoes, *Hygëia: or Essays Moral and Medical, on the Causes*

Affecting the Personal State of our Middling and Affluent Classes, 3 vols (Bristol: Phillips, 1802–3), vol. 2, Essay vi, p. 64 [henceforth references to *Hygëia* will appear thus: 2 vi 64].

38. Beddoes, *Hygëia*, 1 i 58.
39. Beddoes, *Hygëia*, 1 i 58.
40. Beddoes, *Hygëia*, 1 i 53.
41. Beddoes, *Hygëia*, xxviii.
42. Beddoes, *Hygëia*, 1 ii 30.
43. Beddoes, *Hygëia*, 1 i 54.
44. Beddoes, *Hygëia*, 2 vi 48.
45. Beddoes, *Hygëia*, 2 vi 46; D.A. Stansfield, 'Thomas Beddoes and Education', *History of Education Society Bulletin*, xxiii (Spring 1979), 7–14; D. Clarke, *The Ingenious Mr Edgeworth* (London: Oldbourne, 1965); W.A. Campbell Stewart and W.A. McCann, *The Educational Innovators, 1750–1880* (London: Macmillan, 1967).
46. Beddoes, *Hygëia*, 2 vi 47.
47. Beddoes, *Hygëia*, 2 vi 92.
48. Beddoes, *Hygëia*, 2 vi 91.
49. R. Cooter, 'The Power of the Body: the Early Nineteenth Century', in B. Barnes and S. Shapin (eds), *Natural Order: Historical Studies of Scientific Culture* (London and Beverly Hills: Sage Publications, 1979), 73–92. Obviously, such programmes were also central to nineteenth century radical alternative medicine. See R. Cooter (ed.), *Studies in the History of Alternative Medicine* (London: Macmillan, 1988); W.F. Bynum and R. Porter (eds), *Medical Fringe and Medical Orthodoxy, 1750–1850* (London: Croom Helm, 1987).
50. Beddoes, *Hygëia*, 2 viii 49.
51. Beddoes, *Hygëia*, 2 viii 6. Roy Porter, 'Reforming the Patient in the Age of Reform: Thomas Beddoes and Medical Practice', in Roger French and Andrew Wear (eds), *Medicine in the Age of Reform* (London: Routledge, 1991), 9–44.
52. Thomas Beddoes, *The History of Isaac Jenkins, and of the Sickness of Sarah his wife, and Their Three Children* (Madeley: Edmunds, 1792). I analyse this work at greater length in 'The People's Health in Georgian England', in Tim Harris (ed.) *Popular Culture in Early Modern England* (London: Macmillan, 1992).
53. A.D. Morris, *James Parkinson, His Life and Times* (Boston: Birkhauser, 1989).
54. James Parkinson, *The Villager's Friend and Physician, or a Familiar Address on the Preservation of Health and the Removal of Disease on its First Appearance, Supposed to be Delivered by a Village Apothecary, with Cursory Observations on the Treatment of Children, on Sobriety, Industry, etc. intended for the Promotion of Domestic Happiness*, 2nd edn (London: C. Whittingham, 1804), 5.
55. James Parkinson, *The Villager's Friend and Physician*, 44. Parkinson insists, 'admit no tamperings, lest you have to accuse yourself of having thereby sacrificed the child of your heart'. Parkinson was deeply hostile to quacks. 'It would undoubtedly be rendering a great benefit to society, if some medical man were to convince the ignorant, of the pernicious consequences of their reliance on advertised nos-

trums: but unfortunately, the situation in which medical men stand is such, that their best intentioned, and most disinterested exertsions for this purpose, would not only be but little regarded, but frequently would be even imputed to base and invidious motives': Parkinson, *Medical Admonitions*, 327.

56. James Parkinson, *Medical Admonitions to Families Respecting the Preservation of Health and the Treatment of the Sick, also a Table of Symptoms Serving to Point out the Degree of Danger, and to Distinguish One Disease from Another* (4th edn, London: Symonds, 1801), 5. Parkinson then emphasizes the duty of obedience to the doctor – without 'strict compliance with orders', calamities will follow.

57. James Parkinson, *The Way to Health, Extracted from the Villager's Friend and Physician* (London, 1802).

58. Parkinson, *The Villager's Friend and Physician*, 9.

59. Parkinson, *The Villager's Friend and Physician*, 10.

60. Parkinson, *The Villager's Friend and Physician*, 11.

61. Parkinson, *The Villager's Friend and Physician*, 15.

62. Parkinson, *The Villager's Friend and Physician*, 16.

63. Parkinson, *The Villager's Friend and Physician*, 16.

64. Thomas Beddoes, *Where would be the Harm of a Speedy Peace?* (Bristol: N. Biggs, 1795); idem, *An Essay on the Public Merits of Mr Pitt* (London: J. Johnson, 1796).

65. Thomas Beddoes, *A Letter to the Right Hon William Pitt, on the Means of Relieving the Present Scarcity, and Preventing the Diseases that Arise from Meagre Food* (London: J. Johnson, 1796).

66. [James Parkinson], *A Sketch by Old Hubert* (London: Burks, 1795). This one-penny, four-page pamphlet goes on in a jeering satirical way about how well the government and the rich are all eating, 'whilst the honest poor are wanting bread' – a phrase reiterated some half a dozen times.

67. Thomas Beddoes, *A Letter to the Right Honourable Sir Joseph Banks . . . on the Causes and Removal of the Prevailing Discontents, Imperfections, and Abuses, in Medicine* (London: Richard Phillips, 1808), 100.

68. Thus Beddoes discovered, on setting up his Pneumatic Institution, designed to relieve cases of tuberculosis amongst the poor, that his clients rarely came regularly for treatment. This cast him down. In order to overcome this fecklessness, he instituted systems of caution money and fines. Attendance dropped off. Thomas Beddoes, *Rules of the Medical Institution, for the Benefit of the Sick and Drooping Poor; with an Explanation of its Peculiar Design and Various Necessary Instructions* (Bristol: J. Mills, 1804). Note the foregrounding of the 'necessary instructions' in the very title.

9

'But all those authors are foreigners'

American literary nationalism and domestic medical guides

Norman Gevitz

Historians who have examined the early development of American medical literature have been concerned essentially with serious works geared towards a physician audience and have been most interested in questions regarding scientific progress and professional advancement.[1] Recently, scholars have begun to look at early publications directed at laypersons; but in this case, as with more esoteric medical genres, they have not systematically considered the relation of these works with respect to broader literary trends.[2] In the half-century following the American Revolution, many US writers placed considerable emphasis on the need to create a distinct national literature, one freed from European, primarily British, conventions. Modern attention to this literary campaign has looked at novels, poems, and essays.[3] This paper, on the other hand, will focus on the pervasiveness of nationalist themes in domestic medical books of the new republic. Especially considered will be the rhetorical assertions of American writers, their pretensions to originality, and the impact of these volumes *vis-à-vis* foreign guides in the lay medical book market in the United States over time.

Throughout the colonial period, English-speaking Americans were dependent on the mother country for their literature. Though a press had been established in Boston as early as 1639, and by the 1750s printing shops had become relatively commonplace throughout the colonies, the scarcity and quality of type, paper, and ink made the publishing of large works difficult until the dawn of the nineteenth century.[4] But the fundamental issue was not the opportunity to publish home-grown writers but whether there was much material other than religious tomes from their pens to print. Before the Revolution there was no literary class. Americans were consumed by a struggle for their continued existence. Those few who wrote verses, essays, histories or the meagre number of other secular works made their living through other means. As British subjects, the colonists considered their land an extension of England, and thus they could share pride in the accomplishments of English literature though they made no significant contribution to its advancement.

However, the books that the colonists brought with them to the new land or had imported were not so much the *belles-lettres*, but works of practical value. Reading was engaged in less for sheer enjoyment and more for the lessons in living it could provide. Religious tracts taught right conduct, and worldly books imparted useful knowledge and practical skills. In an environment where formal schooling was limited but where literacy was widespread, self-help guides constituted popular reading materials. In the absence of trained professionals, every man to survive might have to acquire the fundamentals of a number of useful trades and thus, on occasion, be prepared to become his own lawyer or doctor.

By 1620 when the Pilgrims crossed the Atlantic to settle at Plymouth Bay, there were dozens of general medical texts, surgical guides, books on regimen, recipe books, and other treatises written in the vernacular upon which they could draw.[5] As early as the 1650s, Culpeper's writings appear to have been imported into the colonies and were popular for almost a century. Indeed, Culpeper's name and works became so familiar that the first medical book published in America was a collection of recipes spuriously attributed to him and given his title, *The English Physician*.[6] The second printed medical book in the colonies was, on the other hand, his genuine *London Dispensary*.[7]

Given the costs and considerable risks associated with early American printing, it is not surprising that those medically related works that did make it to press were geared towards the broadest market. Of the first eleven publications in America up to 1720, all were designed for a general readership, and nine can be classified as domestic medical tracts, pamphlets, and books.[8] In the early 1730s, John Tennent of Virginia anonymously wrote *Every Man His Own Doctor*, the first medical bestseller in America.[9] This relatively brief work, under thirty-nine disease headings, discussed symptoms, diet, and remedies in narrative form and was more similar to later domestic medical guides and less like the typical receipt book. The latter genre, however, continued to be quite popular, especially Wesley's *Primitive Physic*, (1747) which was probably imported into the new world in considerable quantities.[10]

The reaction to William Buchan's *Domestic Medicine* (1769) was immediate and favourable. Within three years of its initial publication, it was printed in Philadelphia, and regularly reissued in America thereafter.[11] Buchan's detailed descriptions of a large number of diseases and conditions, the regimen to be followed, and their treatment constituted a comprehensive treatise which went far beyond the quality of any other previous domestic work with the exception of Tissot. The latter's translated *Advice to the People*, however, was published only once in America.[12] As other contributors of this volume have noted, within many European countries either Buchan or Tissot predominated, and it is not surprising that Americans automatically looked to their homeland for domestic advice. In succeeding decades, general and specialized guides by British physicians, most notably Thomas,[13] Reece,[14] Underwood,[15] Thomson,[16] and Wallis,[17] competed for a share of the market.

The American revolution, however, made the reception of British guides problematical. No longer were their authors 'countrymen'. Questions arose as to the relevance and appropriateness of these manuals, not only with respect to the real and imagined distinctive medical conditions that existed in the United States, but to their conformance to the political values of the new republic. In an era of intense literary nationalism, American physician–authors sought to create works that would rival and ultimately supplant their foreign competitors, at least on native soil.

In the preface to his *A Grammatical Institute* (1783), sales of which reached an estimated fifteen million copies by 1837, Noah Webster declared, 'This country must in some future time be as distinguished by the superiority of her literary improvements, as she is already by the liberality of her civil and ecclesiastical constitutions'.[18] This optimism in the nation's future literary achievements was shared in the ensuing years, not only by America's leading poets, novelists and essayists but by some of the most important lights of the American medical profession whose literary pursuits transcended the healing arts. Dr David Ramsay from Charleston, South Carolina, predicted:

Every circumstance concurs to make it probable that the arts and sciences will be cultivated, extended and improved . . . It is hoped that the free government of America will produce poets, orators, critics, and historians equal to the most celebrated of the ancient commonwealths of Greece and Italy.[19]

Dr Samuel Latham Mitchill of New York looked forward to the day 'when the proficients in benign letters and arts, doctors of philosophy, with harps and timbrels in their hands and crowns of glory on their heads, shall during their stay in this world, experience a true foretaste of the next'.[20]

American writers were urged to be original in their literary productions. Dr Benjamin Rush of Philadelphia warned young authors to stop imitating the European classics if they hoped to equal them.[21] Noah Webster exhorted his countrymen not to imitate the language, manners, and vices of foreigners.[22] During the War of 1812, which greatly intensified anti-British feelings, Washington Irving, an otherwise committed Anglophile, noted with respect to the struggle,

We would rather hear our victories celebrated in the merest doggeral that sprang from native invention, then beg, sorrow, or steal from others, the thoughts and words in which to express our exaltation. By taking our own powers, and relying entirely on ourselves, we shall gradually improve and rise to poetical independence.[23]

John Witherspoon, President of Princeton, declared that Americans should not be subject to the inhabitants of Britain, either in receiving new ways of speaking or rejecting the old. Witherspoon coined the term 'Americanism' to describe distinctive home-grown expressions.[24]

American critics tied English literature to what they believed was wrong with British social and political institutions. English literature, they declared, emphasized birth rather than merit, it tended to denigrate the common people, and put wealth above virtue. The Philadelphia novelist George Lippard, writing shortly after the accession of Victoria to the throne, noted of English novels that they are 'written very often by authors who . . . cling to the whole list of British absurdities from absurdity A no. 1 of supporting a female pope called a queen . . . to Z no. 99, of pouring all the life and blood of a people into that great funnel of degradation called the "Factory System"'.[25]

Whatever similarities the United States shared with Britain, it was the distinctive elements that nationalists now highlighted. Americans, they argued, should write about their own society, and its people's customs, habits, and values. Literature should also instruct the general public, it should teach lessons in citizenship and uplift the reader in a practical way. The American author was to be nothing less than a republican moralist, whose work should trumpet their political freedoms and extol the virtues of the common man.

Calling for an American literature and conceptualizing what it should look like was far easier than producing it. For the first fifty years of the nation, the number of works by American authors, though far greater than in the same span of time before the Revolution, was still relatively small, and the overall quality, except in the opinion of the most extreme chauvinists, rather poor. Many of the works produced were 'American' only in the sense of authorship, as British models and conventions continued to dominate. In addition, the reading habits of the American people had not substantially changed. As late as 1830, it appears that only one-third of all books purchased in the United States were written by Americans.[26] Part of the problem faced by fledgling native authors was the failure of Congress to enact a copyright law protecting the interests of foreign authors. American publishers could and did freely issue works by popular British and European writers without having to pay them any royalties. Pirating already successful works was obviously a far safer economic course than publishing an un-tested American book by a writer to whom the publisher had to pay a percentage of the proceeds.[27]

The output and quality of medical works by American authors in the first half-century after the Declaration of Independence was also disappointing. There were some significant books for the profession – treatises on the general practice of medicine, collections of papers by well-known practitioners, epidemiological studies, textbooks on basic science disciplines and clinical fields – but most of these works broke little if any new ground and were often derivative of existing British or continental works.[28] The first American medical journal, the *Medical Repository*, published out of New York City, first appeared in 1797; by 1820, seventeen periodicals had been organized, most of short duration.[29] While these journals served the useful function of disseminating the theories and practices of American physicians, and alerting readers to news of the professional societies, they offered little in the way of light. On occasion, however, they did provide heat in the form of nationalistic fervour. Overenthusiastic reviews of American works and the disparagement of British volumes, on the basis of the nationality of the author, were not uncommon. In 1820, an Anglican clergyman, Sydney Smith, reviewing the book *Statistical Annals . . . of the United States of America*, by the physician Adam Seybert, MD, acidly noted in the *Edinburgh Review*, 'In the four quarters of the globe, who reads an American book? or goes to an American play? or looks at an American picture or statue? What does the world yet owe to American Physicians and Surgeons?'[30] Dr Nathaniel Chapman, of Philadelphia, then launching his own medical journal, placed Smith's words regarding American medicine below the masthead of each issue of his periodical, undoubtedly to keep his readers ever mindful of unsympathetic foreigners and to serve as a constant spur to native medical writers to do better.[31]

The lack of American innovativeness can be explained in part by the social and medical conditions of the new republic. America was overwhelmingly rural. Though it boasted of three cities of medium size – Philadelphia, Boston, and New York – none was a medical capital in the sense that London, Edinburgh or Paris was during this period. The first medical school was established in Philadelphia in 1765 and three other continuing colleges had come into existence by 1800. The education afforded by these institutions was comparatively brief, constituting a supplement to the apprenticeship system. Graduates were encouraged to go abroad to complete their medical studies, and many of the leaders of the profession in the new nation received further training in Europe, particularly Edinburgh. Opportunities to do research upon finishing their schooling were minimal and such efforts were widely regarded as visionary and a waste of one's energies. The key to success was building a private practice.[32]

One certainly did not have to conduct research in order to write for the public, and, as opposed to the professional environment in Britain where, as Porter has shown elsewhere in this volume, significant radical figures such as Parkinson[33] and

Beddoes[34] attacked the scope of Buchan's instructions to lay-persons, there was widespread sentiment among medical leaders in America for this type of book. The necessity for domestic medical guides was self-evident; oft-cited were the comparative lack of density of population of the country and the unavailability of competent medical help – themes that find expression in British works, but which more accurately described the American situation. David A. Ramsay appears to have spoken for most of the profession in 1803 when he called domestic medical guides one of the most important medical innovations of the eighteenth century.[35] Benjamin Rush, the country's pre-eminent physician, favoured the wide diffusion of useful knowledge. During the great yellow fever epidemic of 1793, he taught clergymen, apothecaries, and Negroes how to bleed sufferers. He was active in the Philadelphia Humane Society writing directions for recovering drowned persons. He advised would-be physicians to listen to laypersons about their home remedies, and was at work on producing his own hygienic guide for the public when he died in 1813.[36] Many of the authors of early American domestic medical guides personally listened to his lecture on 'The Duties of Physicians'[37] or read it in print, and they, as well as others, including even those who diametrically opposed his heroic therapies, wrote admiringly of the man they believed inspired or directly encouraged their efforts to share medical knowledge with the people.[38]

American authors faced a seemingly formidable task in trying to compete with Buchan who, by the time of the Revolution, had established himself in America as the pre-eminent authority in the field of domestic medicine. His educational credentials, compared with those of most native writers, were superior. The scientific failings of the book, as lately noted by Lawrence, then went largely undetected.[39] In addition, Buchan had a Whiggish conception of medicine which was compatible with American values, and, most importantly, the copyright law allowed American publishers to reprint each new British edition freely and cheaply, without having to pay royalties to Buchan or his heirs. Furthermore, before the turn of the century, Rush's friend and close colleague, Samuel Griffiths, as well as another Philadelphia physician, Issac Cathrall, sought to make Buchan's work even more appealing in their separate editions of the work, by claiming to have adapted it to the climate and conditions of the United States. Both Griffiths and Cathrall saw their 'Americanized' Buchan through several subsequent printings.[40] Nevertheless, a number of American competitors did eventually step forward. As early as 1793, Henry Wilkins published *The Family Advisor*, a slim domestic medical guide, very short on narrative, which throughout its publishing life was conjoined to Wesley's *Primitive Physic*.[41] However, the first real equivalent to Buchan was James Ewell's *The Planter's and Mariner's Medical Companion*, first issued in 1807,[42] which was followed three years later by Thomas Ruble's *The American Medical Guide*.[43] In 1817, Horatio Gates Jameson wrote *The American Domestic Medicine*[44] and the next year William M. Hand anonymously issued *The House Surgeon and Physician*.[45] In the 1820s, home guides were published by Usher Parsons,[46] Thomas Ewell,[47] John Gorham Coffin,[48] Henry McMurtrie,[49] and Anthony Benezet,[50] and in 1830 there appeared the most popular manual, written by an orthodox American physician, John C. Gunn's *Domestic Medicine*.[51]

At the time they wrote their respective domestic guides, none of these authors could be considered at the forefront of the American profession. Most were reasonably well educated by American standards. Of the eleven, it appears that eight received MD degrees from American schools – four from the University of Pennsylvania. James Ewell and John Gunn did not attend a medical college and were educated solely through the apprenticeship system. The credentials of Thomas Ruble have yet to be determined. He may have been largely self-trained. Only two, Usher Parsons and John Gunn, appear to have travelled abroad to gain further medical education, but neither enrolled at a British or Continental school. In most cases, each author's domestic medical guide was their major literary work and was produced towards the beginning of their professional career. Some of these authors, however, later gained prominence by organizing medical societies or medical schools, through college teaching, or editing.[52]

From the very first page of their volumes most US writers sought to make it explicitly clear to their readers that their work was specifically designed for an American audience. Some accomplished this through dedications. James Ewell opened his volume with extended praise of the then president Thomas Jefferson and John Gunn began with lavish words in honor of President Andrew Jackson. Not all that surprisingly, patriotism was combined with Anglophobia. Among the virtues of Jefferson, Ewell included his 'exposing the misrepresentations of illiberal foreigners'[53] and Gunn observed in writing of the hero of New Orleans that 'the exemptions of [Americans] from political despotism, arose in the first instance from the knowledge of the corruptions of British power'.[54]

As in the case of American fiction, a number of US writers took on the mantle of republican moralist. They waxed rhapsodic about the form of government, the duties of citizens, the folk-ways of the populace, and the breadth and beauty of the land. They also harshly attacked the vices which threatened their vision of America, such as dogmatic religion, narrow political self-interest, and intemperance. Some promoted special causes such as education for women and, as might be expected, hygienic reform. American physicians expressly directed their works towards 'the common man'. European domestic medicine authors might declare the same purpose, but their occasional use of such disparaging terms as 'rustics' or 'peasants' to describe some of their countrymen reflected a feudal legacy and symbolized a continuing class division most Americans found antithetical to their own sense of themselves as a people – their system of slavery or their treatment of the Indians notwithstanding.

American and British writers also differed significantly in how they presented themselves to their audience. Despite 'laying medicine open', British writers maintained a social distance from their readers. In giving instructions, the layperson was always in the role of student and the patient was referred to formally in the third person. On the other hand, early American writers of domestic medical guides wrote as if their readers were their potential equals or lay colleagues, and in giving advice the familiar and informal 'you' often takes the place of 'the patient'. Both British and American authors assured their readers that they were divesting their texts of technical language and, indeed, both were largely successful, except that, in order that their audience might understand more readily what disease was under discussion, American writers were more likely to go one step further and dispense with the names of such diseases or conditions as diabetes and erysipelas, and substitute folk or more descriptive language, i.e. 'the great flow of urine' and 'St. Anthony's Fire'.[55] To whatever degree British authors sought to make the language of their texts more easily accessible to the public, their style, compared with the plainness and at times crudity of American writers, appeared positively ornamental.

In their discussion of specific diseases or conditions, Buchan and Thomas focused on general principles and only rarely dealt with particular cases. Americans, on the other hand, were great storytellers. They peppered their readers with anecdotes, generally involving themselves and how they were able successfully to bring their patients back from the jaws of death. In an American domestic medical guide no one ever dies of a curable disease brought to the physician writer in time. As a result, some of these manuals have all the appearances of an extended testimonial. Indeed, British visitors to America during this period noted the tendency of Americans to engage in self-promotion and to tell exaggerated tales.[56] The claims of domestic medical writers that they cured dozens or even hundreds of people of one disease or another with a particular remedy or regimen only provide corroborating support for this supposed national trait.

In their sometimes liberal and somewhat fanciful use of statistics, American physicians were trying extremely hard to convince their readers that they had vast experience. For in America, talking from experience was the same thing as talking with authority. A formal medical education was fine, indeed, in the opinion of many writers, essential to professional practice, but classrooms and 'college' theories were no substitute for seeing and treating patients, a view which appears to have been shared by many of their readers. Nevertheless, most American domestic medical writers also wished to convey to their audience that they had kept up with the latest medical writings and increasingly cited the works of other American physicians.

British authorities, though, continued to play an important and visible role in US works. American writers were not xenophobic to the extent of denying European contributions to the understanding of hygiene or disease. In fact, with the possible exception of Rush, prominent British practitioners were more frequently cited in American works than were Hosack, Chapman, Mitchell, Physick, and Mott. Although English domestic medical writers were also mentioned from time to time, Buchan, Thomas, Reece *et al.* had a far more significant invisible presence. American authors borrowed the format of their books and their chapter headings, were imitative in their discussions of the non-naturals and the passions, and made outright copies or at the very least paraphrases of their descriptions of diseases. Some American authors freely admitted to this in the forewords of their books and paid their intellectual debts, if not the proceeds of their royalty cheques, to British writers.[57]

However much orthodox American physicians copied the words of their British counterparts, the one area where the former were to assert their own point of view was in the realm of therapy. The American people, they maintained, not only lived in a different climate but were of a different temperament which necessitated more active intervention. This line of reasoning had the backhanded support of William Buchan, who noted in the first edition of his book that blood-letting should only be infrequently resorted to because Britons led a more sedentary existence, and that diseases were less inflammatory than in previous years.[58] American writers, both in and out of medicine, noted that the citizens of the United States were more active, spirited and hot-blooded than their English counterparts and that, unlike Britain, their country was characterized by great extremes in temperature which appeared to produce a greater severity of fevers and increased inflammation. Southern and western writers were most likely to point to regional differences as proof of the irrelevance of British guides, even if revised by Philadelphia physicians. In truth, both Griffiths and Cathrall's 'Americanized' versions of Buchan were largely cosmetic. With the primary exception of their original discussions of their experience with the great yellow fever outbreak of 1793, these volumes were word for word renderings of Buchan's British editions. As Thomas White Ruble of Kentucky observed of his competition, 'It will be remembered that all those authors are foreigners, or received their education, and whose practice have been in large maritime cities, where diseases materially differ, from those of the interior parts of a large continent . . . .'.[59]

Interestingly, in comparing the guides of Buchan and Thomas with those of American orthodox writers, there is little difference, from one disease to another, in terms of the mention of blood-letting as a primary or adjunct therapy. Where there is an apparent difference is in the emphasis and gusto many American authors gave their recommendations and the appearance with which the terms 'frequent' and 'copious' appear. Most US and British guides were not forthcoming as to the actual amounts of blood to be drawn, employing the ever ambiguous standby, 'according to the strength and age of the patient'. William E. Horner, of Philadelphia, was an exception. In his manual, first published in 1834, he noted that, in an adult of good strength, a pound of blood constituted a 'moderate bleeding', twenty-four ounces a 'full bleeding', and from thirty-two to forty ounces, a 'large one'. He then observed: 'Some inflammations are so violent, and demand such active treatment, that in one day the bleeding may require to be repeated from three to six times, the quantity in a day varying from sixty or ninety ounces, and at one bleeding from thirty to fifty ounces'.[60] Whether these numerical amounts match the descriptions of 'large' or 'moderate' in other American manuals is unclear. Whatever, it is dubious whether many readers of these guides followed these instructions. In examining a number of early nineteenth century diaries which record domestic health care management decisions, there is no evidence that venesection was commonly performed by family members.

While national differences in the recommendations regarding the letting of blood are difficult to measure, this is less the case with respect to advice regarding the use of drugs, their dosages, and the frequency of their administration. American authors urged far greater employment of purgatives and cathartics with calomel, in particular, standing out both with respect to the number of diseases in which it was seen of value, and the amount of the drug judged necessary to produce desired results. Where British authors suggested doses of from one to six grains of calomel in adults, American authors proffered a more drastic course. James Ewell observed of the drug in croup:

I have been emboldened to use it in desperate cases, in doses from thirty to sixty grains in children. On my own daughter, only four years old, and apparently in the very act of suffocation, I used it in the dose of at least sixty grains. The cure was almost instantaneous.[61]

Ewell, however, admits that such heroic doses were not always welcomed by parents. In giving one youngster a massive dose of calomel to good effect

the over-joyed parent insisted I would instruct her in the remedy . . . . On learning I had given her infant, not more than between three and four years old, forty grains of calomel, she was excessively frightened, and exclaimed, 'you have killed my child!' and indeed she could hardly be persuaded for some time though her eyes told her to the contrary, that I had not killed her child.[62]

As this case suggests, it is quite likely that lay intervention, particularly in regards to children, may not have been anywhere near as aggressive as what was recommended by American domestic authors. Indeed, while Warner has recently shown the influence of changing intellectual trends on the diminishing use of depletive therapeutics in the prescribing patterns of American physicians before the Civil War, the demands of patients, in what was very much a client-driven profession, should not be underestimated.[63]

The most nationalistic aspect of US guides, with respect to therapy, lay not in the differences in frequency and dosages of those tools shared with British manuals but in the touting of botanicals native to their own country, which were referred to as 'American remedies'. Most American writers accepted the old theological belief that God had placed in the soil all the remedies needed to treat successfully the diseases of the people of a given land. But many went further to link this therapeutic optimism with xenophobia. John C. Gunn observed:

> There is not a day, a month, a year, which does not exhibit to us the surprising cures made by roots, herbs and simples, found in our kingdom of nature, when all foreign articles have utterly failed: – and the day will come, when calomel and mercurial medicines will be used no longer, and we will be independent of foreign medicines, which are often difficult to be obtained, frequently adulterated, and always command a price which the poor are unable to pay.[64]

Some American guides listed as many as two hundred botanical items in their dispensatory sections, drawn principally from the texts of Barton,[65]Cutler,[66] Coxe,[67] and Thacher.[68] The integration of these remedies, a number of which could be found in the reader's immediate vicinity, do give American guides a distinct national caste but, unfortunately, nationalistic confidence in and recommendations of home-grown botanicals led some authors to downgrade the importance of such useful imported items as quinine, ipecacuanha, and foxglove.[69]

Therapeutic distinctiveness reached a greater extreme as self-taught botanical healers, later followed in the 1830s and 1840s by formally trained physicians from the emerging eclectic medical sect, began issuing their own domestic medical guides which not only promoted indigenous remedies but also eschewed the use of blood-letting, mercury and other mineral-based drugs.[70] On the other hand, this therapeutic nationalist theme was noticeably absent from the many contemporary homoeopathic guides written by Americans. These authors, following the materia medica of Samuel Hahnemann, did not share their competitors' beliefs in either the great differences in the manifestations of disease between the United States and Europe or the natural superiority of American drugs.[71]

How successful were the domestic guides of the early republic? Did nationalistic sentiments and characteristics bear fruit with respect to changing the reading habits of the American people? In looking at the first decade of the nine-teenth century, 1800 to 1809, American presses had produced eight domestic medical guides, six of which were by British authors. A half-century later, in the period 1850 to 1859, the total number of guides published was fifty, of which forty-one were by Americans.[72] Of orthodox foreign works, only Buchan's book proved to have had any enduring value in the American market and its apex of popularity had long passed. The best-selling British guides by Thomas and Reece issued earlier in the century did not find a wide audience in the United States.[73] On the other hand, a number of American titles proved to be large sellers over several decades. James Ewell's book, first published in 1807, went through eleven editions over six decades while the most successful American orthodox guide, John C. Gunn's *Domestic Medicine*, had 234 editions and was being printed as late as the 1920s.

The triumph of the American domestic medical guide over foreign competition may be due in part to their more accessible prose and style, their anti-British feelings or the democratic values embraced by US authors. However, the most powerful explanation is that the American people were as convinced as were the writers of American guides that national differences in terms of disease and appropriate treatment did exist and were important. British guides may have been written, they may have been more original, but they were not designed for the climate and conditions of the United States.

In this sense, lay-oriented medical guides differed from novels, poetry, and essays. Where the former were designed to be practical and therefore suited to local exigencies, and their quality judged on that basis alone, these other higher forms of literature could be read for non-utilitarian reasons and as such a wider range of criteria might be employed to explain and measure their relative success among critics and the general public. Not surprisingly, the issue of practical relevance explains why many titles of American guides were able to be published and compete successfully with British works on native soil, despite the initial pre-eminence of Buchan's work and the lack of a copyright law. In terms of the *belles-lettres*, American authors at mid-century were still struggling against foreign, mostly British, competition for recognition among their own countrymen. Cooper, Hawthorne, Emerson, Melville, and Poe each had difficulty attaining acceptance in the face of the popularity of Scott, Dickens, Carlyle, Thackeray, and the Brontës. On the other hand, unlike American writers of domestic medical guides, US novelists, essayists, and short-story writers were able to gain a readership outside the borders of the United States and some of their work would be praised by British critics. For, despite the nationalist utterings of these American authors, it was the British critics who still mattered.

Before the American Civil War, the expression of nationalist sentiments in American domestic medical guides declined. At this point, it was not because authors thought nationally based differences were unimportant, but because British guides were no longer significant competitors in the US marketplace. Domestic medical authors now battled among themselves, primarily on the issues of regional differences and sectarianism. Even in the years after the Civil War, when changing professional conceptions of disease and therapy made the idea of national or regional distinctiveness less tenable, American writers would continue to dominate the US domestic medical market, the public believing that the advice of American physicians was better suited to American conditions and American bodies.[74] At the dawn of the twentieth century, when domestic medical guides were being transformed into large multi-authored encyclopaedic works, British as well as other foreign physicians were joined by American practitioners in writing chapters, thereby internationalizing these volumes.[75] Finally, the fires of nationalistic rhetoric were reduced to mere embers, but only at a time when the traditional domestic medical guide itself was fast declining in popularity.

Notes

1. See Norman Shaftel, 'The Evolution of American Medical Literature' in F. Mart-Ibanez (ed), *History of American Medicine* (New York: MD Publications, 1959), 95–118; Henry Burnell Shafer, *The American Medical Profession, 1793–1850* (New York: Columbia University Press, 1936); Richard Shryock, *Medicine and Society in America, 1660–1860* (Ithaca: Cornell University Press, 1962).

2. See Guenter Risse, Ronald Numbers, Judith Leavitt (eds) *Medicine Without Doctors* (New York: Science History Publications, 1977; Charles Rosenberg's introduction to John C. Gunn, *Gunn's Domestic Medicine* (Knoxville: University of Tennessee Press, 1986), v–xxi; Mary Lamar Riley, '"The Family Physician": Health Advice and Domestic Medicine from the American Revolution to the Civil War' (University of Chicago, PhD thesis, 1985).

3. See Benjamin T. Spencer, *The Quest for Nationality: An American Literary Campaign* (Syracuse: Syracuse University Press, 1957); Larzer Ziff, *Literary Democracy: The Declaration of Cultural Independence in America* (New York: The Viking Press, 1981; Russel B. Nye, *The Cultural Life of the New Nation* (New York: Harper and Row, 1960).

4. Daniel J. Boorstin *The Americans: The Colonial Experience* (New York: Vintage Books, 1958), 319–24.

5. Through inventories we know that the head of their church, William Brewster, possessed a copy of Dodoen's herbal; that their military commander, Miles Standish, owned a book listed as 'The Method of Physic', quite possibly the work of the same name by Philip Barrough; and that the colony's physician and surgeon, Samuel Fuller, who appears to have been self-trained, owned an unspecified number of English titles.

6. Nicholas Culpeper [pseud.], *The English Physician* (Boston, 1708), re-printed for Nicholas Boone; see also David L. Cowan, 'The Boston Editions of Nicholas Culpeper', *Journal of the History of Medicine* 11 (1956) 156–65.

7. Nicholas Culpeper, *Pharmacopeia Londinensis, or the London Dispensatory* (Boston: Nicholas Boone, 1720).

8. This list compiled from Robert B. Austin, *Early American Medical Imprints, 1668–1820* (Washington: US Department of Health, Education, and Welfare, 1961).

9. [John Tennent], *Every Man His Own Doctor, or The Poor Planter's Physician* 4th edn (Philadelphia: B. Franklin, 1736). A further printing is recorded for 1751 and one as late as 1802.

10. The earliest American edition appears to be John Wesley, *Primitive Physic* 12th edn (Philadelphia: A. Steuart, 1764).

11. William Buchan, *Domestic Medicine* (Philadelphia: R. Aitken, 1772).

12. See S.A.A.D. Tissot, *Advice to the People* 4th edn (Philadelphia, 1771; reprinted for J. Sparhawk).

13. Robert Thomas, *A Treatise on Domestic Medicine*, revised by David Hosack (New York: Collins and Company, 1822).

14. Richard Reece, *The Medical Guide for the Use of Families and Young Practitioners* (Philadelphia: B.B. Hopkins, 1808).

15. Michael Underwood, *A Treatise on the Diseases of Children with General Directions for the Management of Infants from the Birth* (Philadelphia: T. Dobson, 1793).

16. Alexander Thomson, *The Family Physician; or Domestic Medical Friend* (New York: James Oram, 1802).

17. George Wallis, *The Art of Preventing Diseases and Restoring Health* (New York: printed by Samuel Campell, 1794).

18. Noah Webster, (1783) *A Grammatical Institute of the English Language*, Part 1 (Hartford: by the author, 1783), 14.

19. David A. Ramsay, as quoted in Spencer, op. cit. (note 3) p. 18.

20. Samuel Latham Mitchill, *Discourse on the Nature and Prospects of American Literature* (Albany: Websters and Skinners, 1821), 36.

21. Benjamin Rush, *Essays: Literary, Moral, and Philosophical* (Philadelphia: printed by Thomas and Samuel Bradford, 1798), 27.

22. See Henry Steele Commager's introduction to Noah Webster, *American Spelling Book* (New York, Columbia University Press, 1958), 1–12.

23. Washington Irving, as quoted in Spencer, op. cit. (note 3) p. 27.

24. See Varnum L. Collins, *President Witherspoon* (Princeton: Princeton University Press, 1925).

25. George Lippard, as quoted in E.P. Oberholtzer, *The Literary History of Philadelphia* (Philadelphia: G.W. Jacobs and Co., 1906), 260.

26. Nye, op. cit. (note 3) p. 249.

27. See Andrew J. Eaton, 'The American Movement for International Copyright: 1837–1860', *Library Quarterly*, 15 (1945) 95–122; Robert E. Spiller, Willard Thorp, Thomas Johnson, and Henry Canby (eds), *Literary History of the United States* (New York: The Macmillan Co., 1948).

28. See Shryock, op. cit. (note 1) pp. 34–5.

29. See Shafer, op. cit. (note 3) pp. 181–4; James H. Cassedy, 'The Flourishing and Character of Early American Journalism', *Journal of the History of Medicine*, 38 (1983) 135–50.

30. Sidney Smith, [Review of] 'Statistical Annals of the United States of America', *Edinburgh Review*, 33 (January, 1820)): 79.

31. Nathaniel Chapman, 'Prospectus to Volume 1', *Philadelphia Journal of the Medical and Physical Sciences* 1 (1820) vii–xii; see also James Eckman, 'Anglo-American Hostility in American Medical Literature of the Nineteenth Century', *Bulletin of the History of Medicine* 9 (1941) 31–71.

32. See William G. Rothstein, (1987) *American Medical Schools and the Practice of Medicine* (New York: Oxford University Press, 1987),

15–63; Martin Kaufman, (1976) *American Medical Education: The Formative Years, 1765–1910* (Westport: The Greenwood Press, 1976), 3–77.

33. James Parkinson, *Medical Admonitions Addressed to Families* 2nd edn (London: C. Dilly, 1799).

34. Thomas Beddoes, *Hygeia: or Essays Moral and Medical* . . . . 3 vols (Bristol: J. Mills, 1802–3). See Roy Porter, 'Reforming the Patient in the Age of Reform: Thomas Beddoes and Medical Practice' in Andrew Wear (ed.), *Medicine in the Age of Reform* (London: Routledge, 1991), 9–44.

35. See David A. Ramsay, *A Review of the Improvements, Progress and State of Medicine in the XVIII Century* (Charleston: printed by W.P. Young, 1801).

36. L.H. Butterfield, *Letters of Benjamin Rush*, 2 vols (Princeton: American Philosophical Society, 1951), 976, 1188. See Carl Binger, *Revolutionary Doctor, Benjamin Rush, 1746–1813* (New York: W.W. Norton and Co., 1966).

37. Benjamin Rush, 'Observations on the Duties of a Physician . . . .' in *Medical Inquiries and Observations*, 4 vols (Philadelphia: S. Kimber and S.W. Conrad, 1815), 1: 252–64.

38. Thomas Ewell quoted a letter by Rush to him stating 'Go on with your labours. In attempting to instruct others, we instruct ourselves'. Thomas Ewell, *American Family Physician* (Georgetown: J. Thomas, 1825), unpaginated frontpiece.

39. C.J. Lawrence, 'William Buchan: Medicine Laid Open', *Medical History* 19 (1975) 20–35.

40. See William Buchan, *Domestic Medicine*, Revised and Adapted to the Diseases and Climate of the United States of America by Samuel Powell Griffitts, 2nd edn (Philadelphia: printed by Thomas Dobson, 1797); William Buchan, *Domestic Medicine*, Adapted to the Climate and Diseases of America by Issac Cathrall (Philadelphia: Robert Campbell and Company, 1797).

41. Henry Wilkins, *The Family Advisor, or a Plain and Modern Practice of Physic, Calculated for the Use of Private Families, and Accommodated to the Diseases of America to which is Annexed Mr. Wesley's Primative Physic, Revised* (Philadelphia: printed by Parry Hall, 1793).

42. James Ewell, *The Medical Companion* . . . . 3rd edn (Philadelphia: For the author, 1816).

43. Thomas Ruble, *The American Medical Guide for the Use of Families* (Richmond: For the author, 1810).

44. Horatio Gates Jameson, *The American Domestick Medicine* (Baltimore: F. Lucas, 1817).

45. [Wiliam M. Hand], *The House Surgeon and Physician* . . . . (Hartford: printed by Peter B. Gleason, 1818).

46. Usher Parsons, *Sailor's Physician* . . . . (Cambridge: Hilliard and Metcalf, 1820).

47. T. Ewell, op. cit. (note 38).

48. John Gorham Coffin, *Domestic Medicine* (Boston: Phelps and Farnham, 1825).

49. Henry McMurtrie, *The Gentleman's Vade-Mecum and Travelling Companion* (Philadelphia: Poole, 1824).

50. [Anthony A. Benezet], *The Family Physician* . . . . (Cincinnati: W. Hill Woodward, 1826).

51. John C. Gunn, *Domestic Medicine, or Poor Man's Friend* (Knoxville: By the author, 1830).

52. Of these eleven American physicians, James and Thomas Ewell, Jameson, McMurtrie, Parsons, and Gunn gained sufficient prominence to have been listed in Howard Kelly and Walter Burrage, *American Medical Biographies* (Baltimore: Norman Remington, 1820): and Martin Kaufman, Stuart Galishoff and Todd Savitt (eds), *Dictionary of American Medical Biography* (Westport: Greenwood Press, 1984).

53. J. Ewell, op. cit. (note 43) p. vi.

54. J. Gunn, op. cit. (note 51) p. 10.

55. J. Gunn, op. cit (note 51) pp. 220, 224.

56. See Daniel Boorstin, *The Americans: The National Experience* (New York: Vintage, 1965), 275. The British traveller, Basil Hall, observed, 'The most striking circumstance in the American character was the constant habit of praising themselves.' See Edward Pessen, *Jacksonian America* (Urbana: University of Illinois Press, 1985) 14.

57. [Benezet], op. cit. (note 50) p. iii.

58. William Buchan, *Domestic Medicine* (Edinburgh: Balfour, Auld and Smellie, 1769), 169–70.

59. T. Ruble, op. cit. (note 42) pp. iv–v.

60. [William E. Horner], *The Family Doctor, or the Home Book of Health and Medicine* (New York: Miller, Orton, and Mulligan, 1856), 207.

61. J. Ewell, op. cit. (note 43) p. 457.

62. J. Ewell, op. cit. (note 43) pp. 457–8.

63. See John Harley Warner, *The Therapeutic Perspective* (Cambridge: Harvard University Press, 1986).

64. J. Gunn, op. cit. (note 51) p. 15.

65. Benjamin Barton Smith, *Collections for an Essay Towards a Materia Medica of the United States* 3rd edn (Philadelphia: printed for Edward Earle and Co., 1810).

66. Manasseh Cutler, *An Account of Some of the Vegetable Productions Naturally Growing in this Part of America* . . . . (Cincinnati: J.U. and C.G. Lloyd, 1903).

67. John Redman Coxe, *The American Dispensatory*, 2nd edn (Philadelphia: Thomas Dobson, 1810).

68. James Thacher, *The American New Dispensatory* (Boston: T.B. Wait, 1810).

69. Thomas Ewell was one notable exception to the general enthusiasm expressed by American domestic medical authors towards the supposedly great virtues of native plants. He noted, 'As to the cant about American Medicines, Indian Specifics, and such like baits for the vulgar, it may be observed, that there are about ten or fifteen worth preserving; the rest fill space, but give no service, and, like the obsolete words of dictionaries, should be erased from the list of medicines.' T. Ewell, op. cit. (note 38) p. xxiv.

70. See Richard Carter, *Valuable Vegetable Medical Prescriptions* Frankfurt: Gerard and Berry, 1815); Horton Howard, *An Improved*

System of Botanic Medicine (Columbus: By the author, 1832). The most important botanical manual, but not considered here a domestic medical guide due to its simplistic theory of disease and lack of description of diseases, was Samuel Thomson, *New Guide to Health; or Botanic Family Physician* (Boston: By the author, 1822). Wooster Beach's *The American Practice of Medicine*, 3 vols (New York: Betts and Anstice, 1833) was later condensed into the most popular eclectic domestic medical guide, there being 56 editions of the work through 1879.

71. See Constantin Hering, *The Homeopathic Domestic Physician* (Philadelphia: Boericke, 1835; Joseph Laurie, (1843) *Homeopathic Domestic Medicine* (New York: Radde, 1843; Egbert Guernsey, *The Gentleman's Hand-Book of Homeopathy* (Boston: Clapp, 1855).

72. A list of possible domestic medical guides was constructed from Francesco Cordasco, *American Medical Imprints, 1820–1910* (Totowa: Rowman and Littlefield, 1985)); Austin, op. cit. (note 8); and a bibliographic search of the collections of the National Library of Medicine. Each book was then examined as to format, as to whether it constituted a domestic medical guide along the general lines of the books of Tissot and Buchan.

73. Only two editions of Thomas's domestic medical guide appear to have been published in the 1820s. Reece's volume was only published once before the Civil War, and again in 1873, this latter printing based upon the 16th London edition.

74. See J. Warner, op. cit. (note 63). For a differing interpretation on changes within orthodox thinking, see William Rothstein, *American Physicians in the Nineteenth Century* (Baltimore: Johns Hopkins University Press, 1972).

75. See Carl Reissig, Smith Ely Jelliffe, William Broadbent, Sir James Crichton Browne, *The Standard Family Physician*, 3 vols (New York and London: Funk and Wagnalls, 1909).

10

'Mr Scott's case'

A view of London medicine in 1825

Stephen Jacyna

Introduction

Popularization implies a process whereby knowledge passes from an enclosed esoteric context to a more open space accessible to all. The word also suggests that a qualitative transformation occurs in the course of this transition: the knowledge becomes simplified and coarsened. Popularization is often thought synonymous with vulgarization.

One obvious way to study the applicability of this model to the transmission of medical knowledge from professional to lay contexts is to examine popular medical texts and other written manifestations of the popular understanding of medicine. This is the approach adopted by other contributors to this volume. Medicine is, however, an eminently practical form of knowledge; another measure of the extent and nature of popularization is therefore to be found in the way in which patient and doctor interacted in any particular historical period. Once medical knowledge is considered in relation to medical practice a number of further issues immediately arise. Relations of authority, dominance, and deference are manifested in the clinical encounter. These relations are determined by a variety of factors; the knowledge available to the patient and the doctor's evaluation of the layperson's medical understanding are, however, prominent among them. This paper addresses the question of how far the notion of popularization is applicable to an elucidation of the experience of one particular patient.

In the summer of 1823 James Scott, a 34-year-old Edinburgh accountant, began to notice a loss of strength in his limbs and back. There was 'a deficiency of power in the muscles – thus, for example, one day when he attempted to lift his son a boy about 7 years of age, on a poney [sic], he found his arms and back unable to perform the exertion . . . At another time when walking with some friends in the fields a small ditch about 2 or $2^1/_2$ feet broad, intercepted their progress, and when attempting to step or leap across it, he found himself totally unable'. In the ensuing months Scott tried various remedies for the complaint, some of his own devising, others prescribed by local medical practitioners. The management of his case finally devolved upon two prominent Edinburgh medical men: the surgeon John Lizars (1787?–1860) and John Thomson (1765–1846) who acted both as a consulting surgeon and a consulting physician. Despite their efforts, his condition did not improve; on the contrary, the debility of his muscles grew more pronounced until early in the summer of 1825 he was obliged to start wearing stays in order to maintain an upright posture.

We know of these events because in September 1825 Scott travelled to London to consult medical practitioners there about his illness. This visit generated a collection of documents which are now held among the Thomson papers in Glasgow University Library[1] (see Appendix 1). These include two letters: one from Lizars to Scott, undated but probably written after his return from London; and one from A. Copland Hutchinson to Lizars discussing the case. There is also an opinion of the case written by the French physician, Léon Rostan. The collection also contains a much larger document of striking appearance. Written in a fair hand on pieces of parchment sewn together with ribbon, it has a quasi-legal aspect.

This main document is a compilation apparently put together after Scott's return to Scotland for the benefit of his Edinburgh advisers and of any other practitioner whose opinion he might wish to consult. The preparation of such compilations seems to have been an established procedure among persons suffering from chronic complaints. Thomson was himself consulted in 1827 by a patient seeking 'his opinion as to the present state of a complaint with which he has been troubled for many months – the nature of which Dr T. will best be able to collect from the accompanying statement of the view entertained by different Medical men concerning it, both in London and elsewhere'.[2]

The document begins with a case history drawn up by Lizars and Thomson before Scott left Edinburgh, copies of which were circulated to the London practitioners he was to see. The details of Scott's condition quoted at the outset of this paper are drawn from this source [pp. 1–2]. The remainder of the document consists of Scott's own accounts of the consultations interspersed with the written opinions of some of the physicians and surgeons involved. Although Scott's voice predominates, the doctors also have their say. These interpolations notwithstanding, the main document consists essentially of Scott's diary of his medical encounters in London. It differs, however, from the common run of diaries from which historians have derived so much information about lay attitudes to medicine[3] in an important respect: whereas these were private documents, Scott's narrative was intended to be read by others. These intended readers were to be, moreover, not other laypeople, but members of the medical profession.

It is unusual to have both the patient's and the practitioner's accounts of a case in parallel; and much of the historiographic interest of Mr Scott's case lies in the possibility it affords of comparing the two perspectives on the same clinical event. A study of these documents permits an evaluation of many of our current presumptions about the nature of the patient–doctor relationship in the early nineteenth century. It also affords evidence of the forms of medical knowledge that mediated this relationship. The date of these documents makes them especially valuable: 1825 can be considered either as standing at the distal end of the 'long' eighteenth century or as at the outset of a new era in the history of clinical medicine. Scrutiny of these documents confirms that there is merit in both these views; Scott's case provides evidence both for the survival of what is usually considered a typically eighteenth-century absence of clear boundaries between lay and professional understandings of medicine and indications of the emergence of a more specialized and segregated distribution of medical knowledge.

Power and knowledge

In an influential article N.D. Jewson has argued that a patronage model is appropriate to an understanding of eighteenth-century clinical interactions: 'By virtue of their economic and political predominance the gentry and aristocracy held ultimate control over the consultative relationship and the course of medical innovation'.[4] The physician was thus reduced to the role of a client whose professional success depended on his ability to satisfy the demands that the patient brought to the clinical encounter.[5]

Patients were able to exert such control because they enjoyed epistemological parity with the practitioner. Medical knowledge did not constitute a discrete esoteric domain accessible only to the professional; it formed part of the common culture of gentlemen. In consequence it was possible for the polite patient to evaluate and criticize the diagnoses and prescriptions of his, or even her, medical adviser.[6]

Although an accountant, James Scott was undoubtedly a gentleman; indeed, his lifestyle, as related in the documents describing his illness, approximates more closely to that of a country squire than to that of an urban professional.[7] His clinical experiences should therefore supply some insights into how far the patron–client model of the élite patient–doctor relationship remained effective in the 1820s. Something of Scott's relationship to his Edinburgh advisers emerges from the letter addressed to him by Lizars. In response to a request from Scott for a fresh summary of his case for circulation to other practitioners, Lizars wrote: 'If I have understood you right, the accompanying is what you wish, & what in my opinion only should be sent. It appears injudicious to send the treatment you have received, as it tends to bias an opinion. The same may be considered as applicable to the incidents mentioned in your case, they in my humble opinion have no concern in your present complaint'. But he then adds, 'If you wish the treatment & these mentioned just say so and I shall approve them'. The final decision on what was to be included in the case history lay therefore with the patient, not with the practitioner. Professional judgement had to defer to the wishes of the lay patron. But, on the other hand, the fact that Scott felt obligated to ask Lizars to provide him with a case history, rather than produce his own account of the illness, implied recognition of an esoteric discourse between professionals that the layperson could not emulate.

Conversely, Scott's own account of his London experiences makes it clear that he approached each consultation with certain expectations and judged the practitioner by how far he attained these standards. In short, 'It was the patient who judged the competence of the physician and the suitability of the therapy'.[8] Above all, Scott expected his medical adviser to be assiduous – to show in an obvious manner that he had applied his mind to the problems posed by the case. This application was manifested, in the first instance, by a careful scrutiny of the precirculated case history; this was to be supplemented by putting numerous searching questions to the patient. Scott noted on several occasions the practitioner's performance in this regard: William Maton, for instance, 'appeared to have studied the written document with very great attention put many questions to me as to my habits, constitution, the effect of particular positions on my head &c &c . . . He also put questions as to the scrofula palsey &c being in the family'. [p.7]

The practitioner's skill in interrogating the patient was a matter of special moment in shaping Scott's opinion of his accomplishment. Anthony Carlisle achieved particular approval by adding new details to Scott's clinical history that his other attendants had failed to elicit. 'One of his questions,' Scott remarked, 'brought out a circumstance that it had never occurred to me to mention, that while a boy I had frequently fainting fits, and that these were sometimes caused by swallowing anything very hot, or running myself out of breath . . . .' [p.12]. 'From the questions put and the earnestness of manner with which they were accompanied, I should,' Scott declared, 'conclude Sir A to be an extremely intelligent Physician.' [ibid.]

Scott's approval of Maton and Carlisle's clinical method can in part be ascribed to the fact that they endorsed and reinforced deeply rooted perceptions of the causes of illness shared by patient and practitioner alike. Both practitioners took for granted that a long-term view of the patient's life history was necessary to an understanding of his present condition: indeed, Maton assumed that the health history of Scott's ancestors also had to be taken into account in making a diagnosis. Such concern with the 'deep' history of an individual is, as Fissell has noted, typical of patients' narratives of illness in the eighteenth century.[9]

The patient's narrative – the account he gave of his symptoms, biography, and family history – therefore remained central to the clinical encounter. Such an ability to dictate the diagnostic agenda has been identified by Jewson as one aspect of the control enjoyed by the patient under the regime of 'Bedside Medicine'.[10] Mr Scott's case suggests that at the level of élite practice, at least, this form of patient power remained largely intact in the 1820s.[11] The persistence of a primarily phenomenological definition of disease was especially evident in Scott's encounter with Robert William Bampfield who, as well as enquiring about his diet and regimen, put 'many [questions] to the nervous and muscular sensations' [p.16].

However, Scott required more from his advisers than attention to his subjective experience of disease; he also expected them to subject him to a physical examination. According to Jewson, one consequence of the concentration upon subjective symptoms under bedside medicine was a neglect of physical signs.[12] Such physical examination as did occur in the eighteenth century tended to be perfunctory and conducted chiefly with the eye.[13] The growing importance of physical examination in the nineteenth century was one aspect of the shift away from a 'subject' to an 'object' oriented medical cosmology: enquiry into the patient's subjective experiences mattered less in diagnosis than the identification of the objective causes of disease. Concomitant to this conceptual change was a transformation in the power relations between patient and doctor: 'at the same time as the sick-man found himself unequivocally subordinated to the medical investigator, the focus of medical knowledge moved away from the person of the former towards esoteric entities defined in accordance with the perceptions of the latter'.[14]

Mr Scott's case provides a different perspective on the significance of physical examination in the patient–practitioner relationship. It is seen to coexist quite amicably with a continued preoccupation with the patient's narrative. Moreover, far from being resistant to medical intrusion upon his body or finding such investigation demeaning, Scott demanded such an examination from his advisers. When a practitioner failed to provide a physical examination, the patient regarded the doctor as remiss: thus Scott remarked with clear disappointment that William Lawrence 'did not put many questions, and did not examine my spine' [p.4].

Where physical examination did occur Scott applied epithets such as 'careful' and 'minute' to characterize the scrutiny he had received. Sometimes he detailed the nature of the examination. As well as the verbal investigation already noted, Maton 'examined the strength of the different muscles particularly those of the fingers, and the effect of strong and sudden light on the pupils of the eyes' [p.7]. A readiness to undertake a hands-on investigation of Scott's ailment was thus one criterion by which the practitioner's assiduity was judged. While the norms of polite behaviour were on the whole strictly observed, the clinical consultation was already emerging as a site where conventional restrictions on physical contact might with all propriety be systematically violated.

As well as evidence of technical competence and genuine application, Scott sought some token of a practitioner's personal concern with and involvement in his predicament. Thus he notes on several occasions that the doctor asked to be kept informed of the future progress of the case; Maton, once again, achieved a high approval rating in this respect. At the end of his account of their meeting Scott noted that 'He will be particularly anxious to have a report from Dr Thomson or Dr [sic] Lizars or me within six or eight weeks after I return, and particularly in case an issue is tried, and it will give him great pleasure to correspond further with them as to my case.' [p.8] Likewise, A. Copland Hutchinson, who had seen Scott some time before in Edinburgh, asked Lizars to 'assure Mr Scott that I feel a very deep interest in his Case, and I shall trust to your kindness in acquainting me how he proceeds'. [Hutchinson to Lizars]

A picture of the ideal physician begins to emerge: he is conscientious, skilful, courteous, and concerned. Most of the practitioners Scott saw in London attempted to conform to this ideal; Maton and Carlisle perhaps came closest to satisfying their patient's expectations. William Lawrence was less successful. Scott's first consultation with him on 29 September seems to have been perfunctory and unsatisfactory. Lawrence managed, however, to emerge with more credit from a second meeting on 9 October. He showed his genuine application to the matter by insisting that he had 'again and again considered my case and that it was an extremely anomalous one'. He also showed his concern for the patient by asking to hear from Scott's Edinburgh advisers upon his return [p.4].

But there is a much more egregious exception to the conventional pattern of behaviour expected of the medical practitioner; the treatment Scott received from John Abernethy was *sui generis*. Scott was accompanied on his visit to Abernethy by Goldsworthy Gurney, a surgeon whom he had previously consulted. Gurney,

> having made some observations in regard to the peculiarity of my way of walking, Dr [sic] Abernethy stopped him

with a 'D-n you sir have I not read the statement, and read it with attention. I have not time to hear you speak, but wish to tell this gentleman what I think of his case.'

Then addressing me he delivered a lecture of twenty minutes on disease in general, on his own case in particular as affected with rheumatism, and on some other cases which had come under his observation, but without any particular reference to the peculiarities of mine. [pp.8–9]

Leaving aside the gratuitous rudeness to a colleague in the presence of a patient, Abernethy's performance apparently violated the standards of behaviour Scott expected and on the whole received from his advisers. Abernethy had, it is true, read the case history 'with attention'; but he neglected to complement this with a careful interrogation of the patient. Instead of dealing with Scott's case in particular, he chose to deliver a monologue on disease in general; instead of making Scott the centre of attention, he presumed to speak about his own condition and about that of other patients; instead of stressing the individuality of Scott's condition, he sought to subsume it in a wider scheme:

Sir, [he declared] nothing is of so vast importance as attention to the proper regulation of the bowels. Imperfect and irregular action in them is the root of all other disease. Even disorders or weakness of the spine I have successfully treated by tracing them to the bowels – One patient applied to me having the lower part of his spine much disordered, and was in consequence unable to walk without assistance. I saw at once that the bowels acted irregularly, I referred him confidently to my book and he followed the advice contained in it – Two years afterwards he again called upon me strutting and stamping as if in the heyday of health – I have a knack at recollecting cases, and egad I at once knew him – He thanked me for having compleatly cured him – No no friend, I answered, you are not cured, you cannot stand with your knees bent. He tried, and down he fell upon that table before you. The disease was fast leaving him – It had left his loins, but his thighs remained still to be cured – I recommended the continuance of the same treatment of the bowels, and I have no doubt that he is now what he thought himself when he last called upon me, perfectly and completely cured.

This, Abernethy declared, was his 'practical theory of disease'. For further education in this theory Scott was referred to 'the 1st part of my surgical Observations page 72'. [p.9] He evidently saw no incongruity in referring a layman to a professional text. Otherwise, Abernethy had little in the way of specific advice to offer his patient.

He had, moreover, come to his opinion of Scott's case without any physical examination. When Gurney ventured to ask where Abernethy thought the disease to be seated, the retort was: 'Good God Sir, how can you expect that I am to form a more specific opinion without an accurate examination of the patient's body, and minute study of the history which you see is impossible here'. But he added, 'I do not know that were I to give this examination I should at all recommend any thing more than I have done'. [p.10] Not only did Abernethy regard physical examination as of secondary importance, he apparently had no facilities to perform it in his consulting room. He did, however, visit Scott at his residence five days after their first encounter and performed an examination there. As predicted this did nothing to alter his original diagnosis: 'He stated that it was just as he had supposed – There is evidently no disease in the spinal column itself . . . He pressed upon my stomach and made me feel considerable pain where upon he at once observed that there the cause of the weakness was to be sought for'. [pp.9–10] The belated hands-on examination served, therefore, only to confirm Abernethy's prior diagnosis.

From other sources we know that Scott's treatment at the hands of Abernethy was by no means untypical. Indeed, he probably escaped relatively lightly: Abernethy seemed to have confined his customary rudeness during these consultations to the unfortunate Gurney; he was, however, quite capable of being offensive even to aristocratic patients.[15]

Abernethy therefore seemingly violated the basic premises of the doctor–patient relationship – yet he prospered. Although some patients did flee his consulting-room in terror (part of Astley Cooper's vast practice was said to consist of these refugees[16]), Abernethy remained a fashionable practitioner; indeed, according to Macilwain, he 'had . . . an amount of practice to which neither he nor any other man could do full justice'.[17] This paradox can, in part, be explained in terms of the contrast Abernethy offered to the more conventional practitioner; in a normally sycophantic society a reputation for bluntness could work in a practitioner's favour.[18] This was the view taken by an obituarist who maintained that Abernethy's 'roughness of manner' was cultivated 'from inclination – habit – or perhaps DESIGN'. This claim might surprise those who thought that Abernethy had 'lost many thousands annually by his MANNER of treating patients', but

> we never participated in this opinion, nor do we believe that the individual himself did so. We firmly believe that this same rudeness drew more visitors than it deterred from fear of insult. Let it be remembered that it caused the man to be talked of everywhere – and this very circumstance, leaving all ability out of the question, was sufficient to make his fortune.[19]

In short, Abernethy's outrageous behaviour could be seen as a shrewd form of self-publicity.

There are, however, hints in Scott's account that Abernethy's departure from the conventions of patient–practitioner interaction was not as complete as might at first sight appear. Scott's opinion of Abernethy seems to have materially improved between the first and second consultation. After the bruising physical examination Abernethy persisted in his earlier egotism: he proceeded to regale Scott with an account of a joint consultation in which his opinion had been vindicated against that of Matthew Baillie; he also regretted that Scott had still not read his book. But at the same time Abernethy showed greater concern for Scott's own condition, its likely outcome, and the most efficacious mode of treatment. He also demonstrated his solicitude by stating that 'he would be much gratified to hear from me as to the progress I made'. As a result of this second consultation Scott revised his previous assessment of Abernethy: 'although I had formerly conceived that he had not much attended to my case – I felt now convinced from the deliberate way in which he referred to it that he had given it every consideration in his power'. [p.11] One is tempted to conclude that Abernethy played something of the role of a licensed jester in the court of élite medicine: he tacitly upheld the structures that he overtly subverted. Apparent lapses from the norms of accepted behaviour, such as Abernethy's digressions about his marvellous memory for past cases, might, for example, be viewed not as mere conceit but as an attempt to demonstrate his abiding long-term interest in his patients.

Mr Scott's case thus shows that the kind of power relations between patient and doctor that Jewson and others have seen as characteristic of eighteenth-century 'bedside' medicine were still evident in the 1820s. Just as a patron who commissioned a portrait would expect the painter to conform to certain conventions, so Scott required his medical advisers to observe certain patterns of behaviour. The medical men, for their part, by and large accepted this framework and sought to comply with their patron's demands. There is, however, an apparent difference in what was demanded by the patient: by the 1820s physical examination, far from being *infra dig.*, was *de rigueur*.[20]

The transition from a reliance on the patient's narrative in diagnosis to a preference for what can be derived by physical examination is usually considered as marking a fundamental shift in the epistemological basis of the clinical encounter. The initiative had passed from patient to doctor; the latter, moreover, now based his assessment of the case upon arcane knowledge accessible only to him using his special professional skills. Obviously, on this reading, a major shift in power from layman to professional had also occurred. Scott's lay understanding of medicine, however, encompassed and endorsed physical diagnosis; and one way in which he manifested his continued strength in the clinical encounter was by requiring that his advisers employ these techniques.

There is evidence also that, early nineteenth-century developments in medical concepts and technique notwithstanding, the epistemological parity between doctor and patient remained intact. Scott felt competent to discuss his case on a basis of equality with his advisers, and they acquiesced. Thus the practitioners he saw accepted the need to explain and justify, rather than merely state and dictate, their diagnoses and treatments; Scott for his part felt free to question them and to make his own suggestions. Thus he questioned Maton about the possible role of the digestion in his complaint; entered into a discussion with Carlisle about the therapeutic efficacy of mercury; and listened to a pathological discourse from Armstrong on the processes of chronic inflammation [pp.8,12,15]. Later

Scott questioned one aspect of Armstrong's diagnosis, noting that 'Dr Armstrong founded a great deal upon the circumstance of my feeling pain in the lower part of the back in case of a sudden jerk – But I find that that pain is below the spine in the *os sacrum*'. [p.16] Scott's use of the technical anatomical term is noteworthy.

Nor did Scott scruple to check the diagnosis of one practitioner against that of another: Armstrong was of the view that – *pace* Abernethy – 'the pain felt on pressing my stomach is not more than he thinks would be felt by most people in my state of health. He does not therefore think that there is any derangement of the action of the stomach and bowels'. [p.14]

The fact that Abernethy advised Scott, as he did many of his private patients, to 'read his book' also indicates the extent to which medical knowledge remained the common property of all educated persons. The book in question – *Surgical Observations on the Constitutional Origins and Treatment of Local Diseases* – was not a 'popular' guide to medicine comparable to Buchan's *Domestice Medicine*. It was a work written for the profession, but which also had a considerable lay readership. Its circulation among the educated classes 'served to give the *public* some notion of those principles which [Abernethy] was so beautifully unfolding to the younger portions of the profession in his lectures'.[21] The 'public' in question was presumably the polite educated class of person who might consider consulting a practitioner like Abernethy in times of illness. Popularizing medical ideas could serve as a method of self-advertisement. The boundary between the esoteric knowledge imparted to medical students and colleagues and what was suitable for public dissemination was virtually invisible.

This view of an equality between lay and professional knowledge needs, however, to be qualified. Even for the eighteenth century it is easy to exaggerate the degree to which doctors and patients shared a common discourse. William Cullen cast doubt on the extent to which even

the acutest genius or the soundest judgment will avail in judging of a particular science in regard to which they have not been exercised. I have been obliged to please my patients with reasons, and I have found that any will pass even with able divines and acute lawyers; the same will pass with the husbands as with the wives. No person is qualified to judge of the soundness of a theory, unless he has been much exercised in reasoning upon the same subject.[22]

In other words, while educated laypeople might be able to comprehend medical doctrines, they were incapable of discriminating between them or of appreciating their application in a particular case. In order to gratify a patient's vanity or curiosity, the practitioner might discuss matters of medical theory with him; but this did not imply a concession of intellectual parity. There remained a 'higher' level of discourse in which only medical men could participate.

Cullen was not, of course, an impartial observer of the doctor–patient relationship. But his remarks do indicate that Jewson's notion of the practitioner's enforced deference to his patron is simplistic. A more subtle process of negotiation between lay and professional pretensions structured the clinical encounter.

The operation of the two-tier system of discourse at which Cullen hinted is apparent in Mr Scott's case. Although Carlisle had discussed matters of diagnosis and therapy at length with Scott, he proposed to send a written opinion to his Edinburgh physician because 'he feels it necessary to explain himself technically . . . in place of putting into my hands a formal written opinion'. [p.13] This implied that there were limits to what could be communicated about a case directly to the patient. The definition of this boundary gave the practitioner a useful tool in negotiating his relations with the patient.

Closely related to the question of what a patient could understand was the question of what it was fit for him to be told. Although Scott had direct access to much of what was said about his case, private consultations between practitioners did occur. The surgeon Gurney who accompanied Scott to some of the consultations occasionally acted as a sieve, deciding what information should be passed on to the patient. Thus he withheld Carlisle's written opinion from Scott for a while 'from its being unfavorable'; only when later consultations produced a more optimistic prognosis did Gurney let Scott see the document [p.13]. Gurney and Astley Cooper also held 'a long conversation' about Scott's condition after the patient had left the room [p.19]. Scott apparently accepted the propriety of such confidential conversations between his advisers.

Despite the obvious power enjoyed by the patient, the practitioners were not, therefore, entirely without resources. They could occasionally invoke a 'technical' discourse intelligible only to colleagues. Moreover, Abernethy's indiscretions notwithstanding, they could rely upon a certain professional *esprit de corps* which allowed them to structure their relations with members of the public. This solidarity, moreover, allowed doctors to exercise a degree of control over the patient's access to information about his case.

A genteel, affluent patient such as James Scott enjoyed, however, ultimate control in his relations with the medical profession because he was in a position to choose which practitioner to consult. If the treatment he received in one consulting-room failed to give satisfaction, he could go elsewhere. Such freedom to choose between a selection of potential clients is a definitive feature of the role of patron. But this freedom was not absolute; the patron's choice was itself regulated by certain conventions. 'Fashion' is one obvious constraint acting on patrons: it does much to define what is a 'good' service or product in any given context. Those who ostensibly served the patron's needs were, however, able to structure these demands by disseminating notions of what constituted a desirable medical adviser. It is sometimes forgotten that, in the case of medicine, knowledge of individuals as well as of ideas is popularized. Scott's choice of consultants provides some indication of what was the fashion in medical practitioners at the time of his visit to London in 1825.

The patient's choice

Many of the practitioners Scott consulted were fashionable in the usual sense of the word. They were society doctors who waited on aristocracy and royalty; they were, in short, the lineal successors of such eighteenth-century figures as William Heberden and Richard Warren. The reputation of such men rested less upon their attainments in medical science than on their tact, sensibility, manner, and connections.[23] Of the practitioners who figure in Mr Scott's case, Anthony Carlisle and William George Maton fit this stereotype most closely.

Carlisle published on a variety of clinical and physiological topics. Some of these works may have been known to lay readers, but they were chiefly aimed at the profession. While these publications may have enhanced Carlisle's reputation as a 'scientific' surgeon in the Hunterian mould, they did not impinge directly upon his standing as a clinician; his close connections with the Prince Regent, the future George IV, were much more important in that respect. He gained further valuable exposure through holding the post of Professor of Anatomy at the Royal Academy; this provided the opportunity for Carlisle to develop the persona of a learned and cultured gentleman, who happened also to be a medical practitioner.

Maton could also claim to be a 'learned' and possibly ornate practitioner; but his erudition had still less direct bearing on his professional activity. Even the DNB concedes that this published papers 'do not show much depth of medical attainment'. *The Lancet* was less tactful in its language, dismissing Maton as one 'celebrated for the degree of fame he had managed to acquire without enlarging the bounds of medical science'.[24]

During his days as an undergraduate Maton had, however, developed an interest in botany, which was to be of service to him in his subsequent career:

> During the Weymouth season Maton used to practice in that town. One day as he was walking there an equerry summoned him to Queen Charlotte, who asked him to name a [botanical] specimen . . . . He named the plant and acquired the confidence of the royal family.[25]

In 1816 Maton became Physician Extraordinary to the Queen; his practice was soon exceeded only by that of Henry Halford.

The anecdote about Maton and the Queen may be apocryphal. But it does illustrate the fact that general learning and deportment rather than any professional expertise could be crucial in assuring a practitioner's fame and fortune in Georgian England. The fact that Scott consulted doctors of this ilk can be seen as an acquiescence in a traditional conception of what made a 'good' doctor: he was one that had the confidence of and aped the manners of the social élite who, it was assumed, were capable of discerning quality in this as in other departments.

But all of Scott's choices cannot be explained on such premises. On 30 September he consulted John Shaw, a relatively young surgeon, who possessed no credentials as a 'quality' practitioner. What Shaw did possess was some claim to particular expertise in the kind of complaint from which Scott suffered: he had in 1823 published a work *On the Nature and Treatment of the Distortions to which the Spine, and the Bones of the Chest, are Subject*. In short, Shaw was something of a back specialist. An examination of this work reveals, moreover, that he claimed to derive his special competence in these matters not from clinical experience alone, but from his profound acquaintance with the anatomy and pathology of the subject. The knowledge needed to distinguish between the different forms of distortion of the spine and to decide what remedy was appropriate in a given case could not be gained by clinical experience alone: 'This power can only be acquired by a careful examination of the different organs of the body, both in a natural and diseased condition.' Shaw realised that such an assertion might not go unchallenged, 'when we find it argued, that a person unacquainted with anatomy or pathology, is sometimes successful in the treatment of distortions, where surgeons of eminence have failed'.[26] Nonetheless, it was on this explicitly scientific basis that Shaw based his claim to special skill in the treatment of affections of the spine.

Shaw was well-placed to carry out the kind of researches that he considered essential to a rational practice. As assistant to Charles Bell (whom he consulted before giving an opinion of Scott's case) at the Great Windmill Street Anatomy School he enjoyed extensive opportunities for dissection. He had, in addition, performed many of the experiments on the nervous system of animals on which Bell's fame rested. These research opportunities were complemented by access to patients at the Middlesex Hospital.

Shaw was therefore clearly a different kind of practitioner to a gentleman–physician like Maton or (putative) gentleman–surgeon like Carlisle. His credentials rested upon scientific attainments rather than cultural refinement. Moreover, while most of the practitioners Scott encountered were generalists, Shaw had cultivated an interest in the disorders of a particular organ system. Scott was drawn to him because of the specialist knowledge to which he laid claim. We do not know how Scott came to know of Shaw's reputation. He may as a sufferer from a chronic back complaint have read his book. More likely, however, there was a lively oral culture which disseminated medical reputations among potential patients.

R.W. Bampfield, whom Scott consulted on 8 October, possessed similar credentials. One feature of Scott's condition was a lateral curvature of the spine. Bampfield had taken a particular interest in cases of curvature of the spine since settling in London as a civilian surgeon after the end of the

Napoleonic wars; in 1824 he published a monograph on the subject. In his book, Bampfield outlined the social conditions that enabled and encouraged such specialization among London practitioners: 'The immense population of the British metropolis,' he wrote,

> favors this research into particular and rare diseases, and facilitates the acquisition of experience and practical facts, whilst an impulse and encouragement to such useful and exclusive investigations are given, by the prospect of obtaining from so large a population, a compensation for the most fatiguing labours, such as the attendance on those diseases has occasioned me. Rome, in the zenith of her greatness and during her most numerous population, had separate practitioners for many diseases, and such will probably be the case in London, if the increase of its population proceeds at its present ratio.[27]

Bampfield thus anticipated with remarkable precision George Rosen's emphasis upon the role of the 'city' as a social precondition for medical specialization.[28]

That claims to specialist knowledge were among the considerations governing Scott's choice of practitioner is made explicit in the preamble to one of his later consultations. He remarked that 'Dr Armstrong has been stated by several of my acquaintances to have paid more attention to, and to have more opportunity of experience in diseases of the brain, spine, and nerves, than any other medical man in London'. [p.14] It is not clear whether these acquaintances were lay, medical, or both; what is evident is that by the mid-1820s a reputation for specialization had become one way in which a practitioner could attract patients.

John Armstrong is better known for his writings on fever than as a specialist in nervous complaints.[29] His biographer maintains that Armstrong's success as a practitioner depended largely on his reputation as an authority on febrile disorders.[30] But he had early in his career published papers on brain fever and caries of the spine based upon his clinical work in Sunderland.[31] An examination of Armstrong's published lectures shows, moreover, that he continued to take an interest in nervous complaints after his removal to London.[32] Armstrong also displayed an interest in insanity, which he regarded as invariably the result of disorder of the brain.[33]

Armstrong, like Shaw, maintained that clinical experience alone could not supply the basis of a rational practice. In order to diagnose disorders of particular nerves he stressed that 'you must make out their natural functions; and those have been very much illustrated lately by the French physiologists'.[34] Elsewhere he insisted that:

> The investigation of chronic affections requires to be preceded by physiological anatomy; physiology and anatomy being taken in conjunction to explain the natural structure and healthy functions of the various parts . . . . By cultivating pathological anatomy we arrive at a condition or conditions which explain the symptoms as well in chronic as in acute or sub-acute diseases; and to this condition or these conditions I would apply the term pathological cause or causes of disorder or disease.[35]

Only if he possessed these conceptual resources could the practitioner at the bedside hope to diagnose conditions accurately and to treat them successfully.

In his emphasis on the direct clinical utility of the medical sciences, Armstrong diverged from the type of conventional élite physician. He made his disdain for such practitioners explicit through a critique of their doyen, William Heberden. 'No man,' he claimed, 'can read the works of Heberden without perceiving he was a very superficial observer of nature. He was one of those who referred almost exclusively to symptoms, without reference to conditions; and his opinions, however popular he might have been in his day, are of little use.' Moreover, Armstrong coupled this critique of the epistemological foundations of Heberden's practice with an attack upon the social role of the 'popular' physician:

> When a man becomes a popular physician he soon ceases to be useful; he is called in generally in the advanced stages, when the patient is moribund, just to give a sanction to the measures which have been previously adopted. This is the common routine of popular physicians in London. Heberden was a very popular physician; but his

literary productions will soon be forgotten – they will be
swept away by time, as wrecks from the shore by a spring
tide.[36]

Armstrong represented a dissident element in the London
medical community – one which placed greater emphasis upon
scientific attainment than on social deportment and which was
openly critical of certain aspects of the old order. He was, in
effect, a medical radical who was not afraid to denounce such
totems of learned physic as Cullen's nosology.[37] Indeed, he
numbered medicine, as at present practised, among the causes
of disease: 'Physic in this country,' he declared, 'is as fatal as the
plague in Asia: its operation is often less speedy, but its baneful
and fatal effects are no less certain.'[38]

These views can be attributed to Armstrong's background
and his early experience of London medicine. He was very
much an outsider who had not trained at one of the London
hospitals and who consequently lacked the personal connections that facilitated entry to the medical élite; indeed, it was
alleged by some that Armstrong 'had severe and constant opposition from his professional brethren in the metropolis'.[39]
Armstrong was, moreover, a teacher in a private medical school
and therefore subject to the harassment those institutions
suffered from the medical establishment. He became associated
with the reformist party centred upon Thomas Wakley which
was critical of all aspects of the activity of the consultant hierarchy that dominated London medicine.[40] Conversely, Armstrong was supported by London general practitioners, who
formed the chief constituency of the reformist group.[41] After
Armstrong's death, *The Lancet* approved the vehemence with
which 'this honest child of nature [breathed] forth his contempt against the empty, impertinent and conceited frippery of
the upstart wearers of 'gowns' and 'wigs'!'[42]

Wakley had commended Armstrong's course on the practice
of medicine, laying special stress upon its pathological content.[43] But in these lectures Armstrong's substantive views on
medicine were conjoined to an ethic of medical practice that
differed in important respects from those he ascribed to the
professional élite. In particular, Armstrong expounded his own
principles of correct conduct towards patients.

He took for granted the ability of all but a minority of
patients to understand medical matters: the dissemination of

such knowledge throughout society – and not merely among
the better sort – was a condition of the efficiency and honesty of
medical practice. 'The general state of intellect,' he argued,
'influences that of particular professions; and this is so especially the case with physic, that it is now the furthest advanced
where most general information prevails among the people at
large.'[44] It was incumbent on the practitioner to respect the
intelligence of the layman; but Armstrong decried all attempts
to impress or deceive patients by the use of medical theory:

> A physician should appeal to the common sense and not
> the ignorance of his patient. If he have a direct reason to
> give why he uses certain remedies, there is no reason why
> he should not explain it. If a patient ask of you the nature
> of his disease, it is your bounden duty to point it out, and
> the effects which you expect from the remedies. I would
> not employ a physician unless he explained his opinions
> thus. It may be that a man, although he had paid attention
> to diseases, has no reason to give; and then let him confess
> his ignorance, and not be ashamed of it, for he can at least
> abstain from doing mischief. Why should he deceive his
> patient, when his want of honesty may destroy his patient's
> comfort and even his life? I would rather not practice
> physic at all than practice it as a system of deception.
> Patients have a right to know, and ought to know these
> things; and if a physician attempt to cover his ignorance
> with the flimsy texture of sounding names, common sense
> will detect it; and it is humiliating to think that any man
> can so far descend from the dignity of his profession as to
> affect information which he does not possess. Candour is
> absolutely necessary in order that a physician should prac-
> tice successfully.[45]

Armstrong would therefore have condemned as dishonest
Cullen's patronizing readiness to give theoretical justifications
of his practice to his polite patients simply to gratify their
curiosity. His polemic insinuated that such disingenuousness
was too prevalent in contemporary practice: Cullen's nosology
provided a convenient vocabulary of obfuscation with which
'popular' physicians deceived their patients.[46] The mark of the
ideologically correct medical radical was, in contrast, an
eschewal of all such subterfuge. Elsewhere, however, Armstrong

qualified this unambiguous commitment to an equal and open relationship between practitioner and patient. While he advised his students on most occasions to abandon meaningless technicalities and to 'address yourselves to the common sense and understanding of the persons to whom you speak', when dealing with 'persons so ignorant that all you could do would not make them understand the real nature of the case, then the best mode is to announce the disorder in some Greek or Latin word, with which they are perfectly satisfied, and will not ask you another question. (A laugh.)' When treating such patients even Cullen's nosology had its uses.[47]

James Scott, however, did not belong to the latter category of patient. In his consultation with him, Armstrong seems to have remained faithful to his professed principles. He sought to attribute Scott's symptoms to an underlying pathological condition. He answered his patient's queries about the possibility of the complaint being rheumatic. And he explained to Scott the nature and likely outcome of chronic inflammation of the spinal cord [pp.14–15].

Armstrong did not, however, consider his own opinion of the case as definitive. He referred Scott to a yet higher source of specialist knowledge: 'he strenuously urged me to consult Dr [Léon] Rostan of Paris who has long had charge of the Infirmary established there entirely for diseases of the nervous system [i.e. the Salpêtrière], and who in the course of this practice sees more cases of that description than he, Dr Armstrong, or any medical man in London can possibly see in a life-time'. [p.15] Armstrong referred to Rostan's researches on the pathology of the nervous system in his lectures;[48] and from the manuscript it appears that the two were personally acquainted. Such deference to French achievements in medical science was another mark of medical radicalism in this period.

Armstrong suggested only that Scott should consult Rostan 'by letter'; it is apparent, however, from the written opinion Rostan gave of the case that he saw and examined the patient. Presumably, Scott went on from London to seek further assistance in Paris.[49] He was prepared to go to considerable trouble and expense to secure the best specialist advice available to him.

It has been argued that a hostility to specialization, together with a disdain for the scientific knowledge which was employed to justify this form of practice, was a leading feature of London élite practice throughout the nineteenth century. The kind of values embodied by Maton, rather than the skills and knowledge professed by Armstrong, remained the qualities demanded of consultants.[50] Mr Scott's case shows, however, that at a relatively early date rival notions of medical excellence were to be found in the London medical scene. These attached much greater importance to the scientific foundations of practice and favoured a degree of specialization. From other sources we know that these attitudes were sometimes coupled to a disenchantment with the existing medical establishment and with wider programmes of reform. Alternative codes of medical behaviour sometimes accompanied a particular stance on the epistemological foundations of rational practice.

Scott's case shows also that patients were aware of the existence of these specialist, scientific practitioners and appreciated the kinds of knowledge and insight to which they laid claim. Even observers hostile to the growth of specialization were forced to acknowledge this fact. Thus Johnson in 1829 demanded why if 'physic and surgery be indivisible in themselves, or from each other, . . . is it that we see them split and splitting in all directions?' He went on to lament:

> The Profession appears like a congregation of various wild animals around a carrion. One pecks out the *eyes*; and another the *teeth*; a third tugs at the *ears*; a fourth shews its predilection for the *skin*; a fifth of the true vulture species) gorges on the *liver* . . .:- in short, there is scarcely an organ or structure of the human body, which does not furnish a PROFESSORSHIP in physic and surgery – down even to the SPINE, and the more crooked or carious this is, the more to the taste of the professor of spinalogy!

But, whatever 'are the opinions as to the utility or inutility of these divisions and sub-divisions in practice; . . . it is evident that the PUBLIC has already decided the question in their favour'.[51]

The public, moreover, also valued the scientific attainments of a practitioner *per se*. Benjamin Brodie explained much of Matthew Baillie's outstanding success in practice early in the nineteenth century in these terms:

> Being the only physician of that time who had been engaged in teaching anatomy, the public naturally, and very justly, considered that he must have some knowledge

of disease which others, in his department of the profession, did not possess. But this was not all. Bred up in W. Hunter's museum, of which the anatomy of diseased structures formed an important part, and having had ample opportunities of investigating disease by dissection at St. George's Hospital, he had become, after his uncles, William and John Hunter, the most distinguished pathologist of the day.[52]

Scott's choice of medical advisers reveals something of the diversity of forms of medical expertise and reputation available at the time of his visit to the capital. He visited the consulting-rooms both of practitioners who derived their standing from their aristocratic manners and connections and of others whose claims rested on possession of scientific knowledge and specialist expertise. In Jewson's terms Bedside Medicine coexisted in the London of the 1820s with a form of practice that possessed at least some of the characteristics of 'Hospital' Medicine.[53] The same patient's complaint could, in consequence, be viewed by different practitioners in radically divergent ways.

Conceptualizing Mr Scott's case

Jewson argues that the particular forms of social interaction constituting Bedside Medicine had as a concomitant a certain type of pathology. There was a tendency to produce monistic schema which sought to encompass all disease by a single principle. Although these systems differed in detail, they had structural features in common; in particular, they tended to conform to a holistic or constitutional notion of disease.[54]

Among the practitioners Scott saw Abernethy's concept of disease conforms most closely to this type: indeed, it is almost a caricature of the Jewson scheme. The fact that he sought to reduce all ailments to a single root – namely, disorder of the digestive organs – has already been noted. Moreover, his approach was resolutely constitutional: he declared that 'Though the disorder of particular organs thus gives a character and denomination to the disease, it is sufficiently evident, in the instances adduced, that the whole constitution is disturbed . . .'[55] In consequence, 'It is a principal object of medicine to give strength and tranquillity to the system at large, which must have a beneficial influence on all its parts, and greatly promote the well-doing of every local disease'.[56]

The most effective method of achieving tranquillity of the system was by regulating the digestion. In Abernethy's view, bad diet and in particular overeating was at the root of most contemporary disease:

> Nature seems to have formed animals to live and enjoy health upon a scanty and precarious supply of food; but man in civilized society, having food always at command, and finding gratification from its taste, and temporary hilarity and energy result from excitement of his stomach, which he can at pleasure procure, eats and drinks an enormous deal more than is necessary for his wants or welfare . . .[57]

This was clearly a class-specific pathology; only a narrow section of society would have found Abernethy's diagnosis of their ills plausible, or his prescription of greater dietary restraint at all beneficial. His was, in short, a concept of disease adapted to the wealthy patient. We have seen how Abernethy sought (by force if necessary) to make Scott's case conform to his 'practical theory' of disease.

Although patients were apparently tolerant of Abernethy's style of practice and adherence to a single theory, some of his professional brethren regarded such 'routinism' as 'generally ludicrous, but sometimes tragical'.[58] The same journal had in 1828 stigmatized a case where an 'eccentric surgeon' had summarily diagnosed a case as a disorder of the digestive organs, which terminated in the patient's death, as an example of 'positive error arising from a preposterous adherence to a preconceived doctrine that blinds the eye to every object'. Abernethy's was a 'monstrous mode of prescribing for diseases of the most dangerous and fatal nature, without giving one's self the least trouble to investigate the history, symptoms, or seat of the complaint'.[59]

At the opposite extreme is Rostan's approach to Scott's case. His whole enterprise was, from the outset, to localize the complaint; to find as precisely as possible the anatomical site of the lesion to which the symptoms were attributable. Again, this conforms well with Jewson's claim that a new form of medical cosmology came out of the Parisian hospitals in the early decades of the nineteenth century, one that attributed disease to local rather than systemic causes.[60]

The other British doctors that Scott saw tended to fall somewhere between these two extremes. Most took the view that there was a disease of the nervous system. Bampfield agreed, however, with Abernethy that the digestion was primarily affected [p.16]. Shaw also thought the disease constitutional; it proceeded not from any of the injuries Scott had suffered in the past, but was the result of 'exhaustion consequent upon over exertion of mind or body'. [p.5] (Thomson and Lizars in their case history noted that Scott had in the winter of 1822–23 been 'induced greatly to over-exert himself at his desk'. [p.3]) Among those who considered the case as nervous in origin, there was general agreement that the origin of Scott's symptoms was to be found in a fall from a horse in 1819.

Of the London practitioners, Armstrong and Brodie came closest to the localizationist pathology exemplified by Rostan. But Brodie also displayed a certain scepticism about the degree of precision with which the site and character of a lesion could be identified. In a letter to Lizars he maintained that there was 'abundance of evidence that symptoms such as those described by Mr Scott may be produced by disease in the lower part of the brain or upper part of the cervical marrow; but no knowledge which I possess will enable me to give any thing like a positive opinion as to the exact nature of the disease, or its *precise* situation'. Because the exact nature of the lesion had not been specified, the treatment could only be formulated 'on general principles'. In his remarks Brodie alluded to contemporary French pathological thought on chronic inflammation [p.22].

Conclusion

James Scott came to London at what can be seen as a pivotal point in the history of medicine. Aspects of the medical world he encountered would have been perfectly familiar to an eighteenth-century patient. But at the same time his experiences reflected something of the profound transformations in medical theory and practice that had occurred in the aftermath of the French Revolution.

Jewson is among the few to attempt to provide a framework for understanding how this transformation became manifest in the clinical encounter. Mr Scott's case gives general support to Jewson's characterization of the definitive features of both 'Bedside' and 'Hospital' medicine. A concrete instance like this can, however, help to refine our notions of what significance can be attached to these categories. Clearly they cannot be seen as mutually exclusive moments in the history of medicine. To a remarkable extent the two medical cosmologies were able to coexist within a community of practitioners and even within the same consulting-room.

What is perhaps the most valuable aspect of Jewson's thesis is less his demarcation of different epochs in medical history than his recognition of the importance of the form of social interaction between patient and practitioner in determining the form and content of the clinical event. The role of patron enjoyed by a patient like James Scott imposed a particular structure upon his encounters with medical men. This, rather than the fact that his tour of London occurred in 1825, and not in 1775 or in 1875, is crucial to understanding his experience.

But we need to appreciate that the demands patrons made on doctors were themselves subject to change. While such requirements as courtesy and concern from the practitioner may have remained constant, there was scope for new items to enter into the definition of what constituted a satisfactory clinical encounter. The influence of such novel demands from a powerful class of consumers of medical services upon the development of styles of medical practice deserves further attention. Conversely, it is necessary to ask how far practitioners were able to influence the development of patient demand through a judicious use of the channels of communication and means of publicity available to them. In particular, the role of publications as a form of self-advertisement needs to be reconsidered. Too often it is assumed that technical works were produced solely for professional consumption – that the author's medical peers were the only relevant 'patron group'. The simple antithesis between professional and 'popularizing' publications must be abandoned; it was possible for a work to address simultaneously both these audiences. Judicious publication on technical topics could enhance a practitioner's standing with prospective patients as well as impressing his peers. Brodie revealed that his income in 1819 increased by more than £1,000; he attributed this rise in part 'to the publication of my work on 'Diseases of the Joints,' which had taken place in the previous year'.[61] While Armstrong 'came to London . . . on the sole faith of the reception which his work on TYPHUS had experienced from the periodical press'.[62]

Finally, a sense of the wider context in which clinical medicine proceeded is necessary. Although he restricts himself to a micro-sociological perspective, Jewson does make certain presuppositions about this larger setting; the predominance of the aristocratic patient under 'Bedside' medicine presupposes a society in which the mores of this class enjoyed widespread authority. From the 1780s there was, however, a concerted challenge to the political and cultural hegemony of the landed classes. Medicine was not aloof from this movement. Armstrong's case demonstrates how such radicalism could be represented in concepts of the proper form of the patient–doctor relationship. The equality of discourse, which Jewson regards as a fact of aristocratic eighteenth-century medicine, becomes in Armstrong's writings a democratic ideal which polite medicine notably failed to achieve. Only a practitioner imbued with correct principles could overcome this hypocrisy and treat his patients as true equals. Armstrong's notion of the community of medically cogniscent laymen was more extensive than the 'gentlemen' who act as patrons in Jewson's scheme of eighteenth-century medicine; only the lowest classes of society were excluded. They remained proper objects for medical condescension and deception. Armstrong coupled his critique of the ethics of élite practice with an attack upon its epistemological basis; a modern, ostentatiously 'scientific' approach to medicine thus formed an integral part of his programme.

Armstrong's radicalism can, as we have seen, be ascribed to his marginal position within the London medical community. However, similar strands can be discerned in the writings of Benjamin Brodie who was much more part of the medical establishment. Brodie made his career at St George's, the 'most *Aristocratic*'[63] of the London hospitals. He moved in aristocratic circles; was 'employed by the Court of three successive Sovereigns'; and was 'consulted by the élite of the nobility and gentry of the land'.[64] Nonetheless, he did not acquiesce in the values of those whom he thus served; on the contrary, Brodie displayed a disdain for the mores and pretensions of the aristocracy. He decried their ignorance and gullibility about medical matters.[65]

Brodie urged his students to behave as 'gentlemen'; but his definition of gentlemanly conduct was in many ways constructed to exclude the manners and predilections of the upper classes. A gentleman was not 'he who is fashionable in his dress, expensive in his habits, fond of fine equipages, pushing himself into the society of those who are above him in their worldly station'.[66] This could be seen as an attack upon the polite practitioners who set such store upon mimicking aristocratic habits. Brodie also criticized the intellectual foundations of this sect's practice: Sir William Knighton, for instance, possessed much 'practical knowledge', but 'had no scientific attainments. He pursued [medicine] in the first instance with no other object than obtaining a livelihood, and afterwards with a too great anxiety to amass a fortune'.[67] Love of pelf and a devotion to medical science were mutually exclusive.

Sir Henry Halford, probably the most successful London physician of his day, was subject to similar strictures: he 'was a clever and sagacious physician, with a great deal of practical information, but without any of that scientific knowledge which is necessary for a right diagnosis of disease'. In fact, 'his views of disease were very limited, and he was too apt to be contented with relieving the present symptoms, instead of tracing them to their origin, and making it his object to remove the cause which produced them'.[68] The fact that Halford adhered to the epistemological norms of 'Bedside' medicine was, therefore, grounds for censure. But Brodie was also contemptuous of Halford's cultural and social pretensions. He mocked the fact that Halford 'prided himself rather over-much on his skill in composing Latin verses'; further, 'From being in frequent attendance on the Royal Family, with whom he was a favourite, he had acquired too much of the habits and feelings of a courtier'.[69]

Brodie's critique of Halford was more measured than Armstrong's of Heberden; despite his shortcomings, Halford was still 'in many respects an ornament to his profession'.[70] It, nonetheless, reveals how unfavourably even a member of the medical establishment could perceive the values and achievements of a previous generation of his peers. Moreover, the intellectual achievements and the social persona of the likes of Knightley and Halford were coupled together by Brodie and Armstrong alike as grounds for censure.

When he came to define his own professional identity, Brodie identified his work as a hospital doctor as central to his endeavours: for thirty-two years of his career 'the hospital as far as my profession was concerned, was the greatest object of interest that I possessed'. It was there that he acquired 'the best part of the knowledge which I had been able to attain. It had rendered my professional life one of agreeable study, instead of one of mechanical and irksome drudgery'. Brodie also stressed the significance of the teaching role he had performed at St George's.[71] He published the materials gleaned from his hospital experience in numerous contributions to pathology.

Brodie, in short, obligingly satisfies many of Jewson's criteria for characterizing a practitioner wedded to the cosmology of Hospital Medicine. But whereas Jewson stresses the social conditions within which this system of medical knowledge and practice emerged and flourished, this study suggests an alternative way of viewing the notion of medical cosmology: namely, as a normative structure, a medical morality, which established certain norms and values which practitioners could invoke and manipulate. Even in a setting like early nineteenth-century London where some of the conditions that Jewson regards as necessary to Hospital Medicine were absent, these values were still available to a rising surgeon like Brodie; they assisted him in defining his own priorities, and supplied him with criteria by which to judge the achievements of others.

Most of the practitioners Scott visited in London were 'hospital' doctors in the straightforward sense that they held hospital posts; some were, however, more inclined than others to carry aspects of hospital medicine over into their private practice. Moreover, Armstrong who had no connection with a major teaching hospital, was among those who did approach Scott's case with some of the assumptions and methods of 'hospital' medicine. The link between medical cultures and their institutional bases is more problematic than Jewson suggests.

The overt political element present in Armstrong's attack on the 'polite' medicine of a previous era and on its surviving adherents is lacking in Brodie's case; he was more a whig than a radical. It is, however, possible to discern a shift of sensibility in his writings on the duties and goals of the medical practitioner. There is something distinctly Victorian in his emphasis upon diligence, obligation, and disinterested exertion; his definition of a 'gentleman', in particular, owes much more to evangelical than to aristocratic models. The history of medical values must, therefore, be considered in relation to those of society at large. Hospital Medicine, no less than its predecessor, possessed an extra-professional 'client' group whose characteristic rhetoric and biases were embodied in the cosmology of its adherents.

Acknowledgements

I am grateful to Roger Cooter, Mary Fissell, Chris Lawrence, John Pickstone, and Roy Porter for their comments on an earlier version of this paper.

Appendix 1

Documents in Glasgow University Library contained in envelope marked 'Mr Scott's Case Spinal Cord &c'.
Letter from John Lizars to James Scott, Queen St [Edinburgh], undated.
Letter from A. Copland Hutchinson, His Majesty's Dockyard Sheerness, to John Lizars, 33 York Place, Edinburgh, 19 March 1827.
Léon Rostan's opinion of the case, Paris, May 1826.

Main document comprising the following items:
1. 'Case drawn up by Dr Thomson and Mr Lizars.'
2. Account of James Scott's consultations in London, September to October 1825 together with written opinions subsequently received from the physicians and surgeons he saw.
i. 'Note of Mr Lawrence's verbal opinion 29 September.'
   Report of further meeting with Lawrence, 9 October.
ii. 'Note of Mr Shaw's verbal opinion 30 September.'
   Account of further meeting with Shaw 6 October.
iii. 'Note of Dr Maton's verbal opinion – 1st October.'
   Dr Maton's prescription.
iv. 'Note of Mr Abernethy's verbal opinion 1st October.'
   Account of further meeting with Abernethy, 6 October.
   'Mr Gurney's note of Mr Abernethys opinion.'
v. 'Note of Sir Anthony Carlisle's verbal opinion 1 October.'
   Note of communication from Carlisle via Gurney that the former has altered his opinion of the case. Scott receives Carlisle's verbal opinion from Gurney, 11 October.
   'Sir Anthony Carlisle's written opinion 1st Octor 1825 –'
vi. 'Note of Dr Armstrong's verbal opinion 8 October –'
vii. 'Note of Mr Bampfield's verbal opinion 8 October –'

Description of demonstration of Bampfield's couch, 11 October.

'Mr Bampfield's written opinion –'

'Mr Bampfield's regimen or diet –'

viii. 'Note of Sir Astley Cooper's verbal opinion 10 October –'

'Mr Gurney's note of Sir Astley Coopers opinion.'

ix. 'Note of Mr Brodies verbal opinion 10th October.'

'Mr Brodie's letter to Mr Lizars –'

x. 'Note as to Mr Gurney.'

'Mr Gurney's written observations –'

Appendix 2

Medical practitioners figuring in Mr Scott's case

Edinburgh

John Lizars (1787?–1860) surgeon and extramural lecturer in anatomy and surgery.

John Thomson (1765–1846) former Professor of Military Surgery in Edinburgh University; by 1825 consulting physician and surgeon and extramural lecturer on practice of medicine.

London

John Abernethy (1764–1831) surgeon at St Bartholomew's Hospital and lecturer on anatomy, physiology, and surgery. Address: 14 Bedford Row.

John Armstrong (1784–1829) physician to London Fever Hospital and Lecturer in Medicine at the Webb St Medical School. Address: 48 Russell Square.

Robert Western Bampfield (?–?) surgeon to Royal Metropolitan Infirmary for Diseases of Children. Address: 37 Bedford Street, Covent Garden.

Benjamin Collins Brodie (1783–1862) surgeon at St George's Hospital. Address: 16 Savile Row.

Sir Anthony Carlisle (1768–1840) surgeon to Westminster Hospital. Address: 6 Langham Place.

Sir Astley Cooper (1768–1841) surgeon at Guy's Hospital. Address: 2 New Street, Spring Gardens.

Goldsworthy Gurney (1793–1875) surgeon and lecturer in chemistry at the Surrey Institution. Address: 7 Argyle Street, Oxford Street.

William Lawrence (1783–1867) surgeon to St Bartholomew's Hospital. Address: 14 Chatham Place, Blackfriars.

William George Maton (1774–1835) physician and botanist. Address: Spring Gardens.

John Shaw (1792–1827) surgeon to Middlesex Hospital and lecturer at Great Windmill Street School. Address: 65 Berner's Street, Oxford Street.

Paris

Léon Rostan (1791–1866) physician at the Salpêtrière.

Notes

1. Thomson Collection, Glasgow University Library, Gen. 1476, Box 18.
2. Moncrieff Threipland to John Thomson, 25 March 1827, ibid.
3. On the uses of this source see J. Lane, '"The Doctor Scolds Me": the Diaries and Correspondence of Patients in Eighteenth Century England' in R. Porter (ed.), *Patients and Practitioners: Lay Perceptions of Medicine in Pre-industrial Society* (Cambridge, 1985), 205–48.
4. N.D. Jewson, 'Medical Knowledge and the Patronage System in Eighteenth-Century England', *Sociology* (1974), 382–3.
5. ibid., p. 378.
6. This aspect of the Jewson model has been developed and confirmed in R. Porter, 'Laymen, Doctors and Medical Knowledge in the Eighteenth Century: The Evidence of the *Gentleman's Magazine*', in Porter, *Patients and Practitioners*, pp. 283–314; see also D. Porter and R. Porter, *Patient's Progress: Doctors and Doctoring in Eighteenth-century England* (Cambridge, 1989), 78–9, 85–8.
7. This is typical of the tendency of the professions in Edinburgh, especially lawyers, to maintain close links with the land. See S. Nenadic, 'The Rise of the Urban Middle Class', in T.M. Devine and R. Mitchinson (eds), *People and Society in Scotland: Volume I, 1760–1830* (Edinburgh, 1988), 117.
8. Jewson, 'Medical Knowledge', 375.
9. M.E. Fissell, 'The Disappearance of the Patient's Narrative and the Invention of Hospital Medicine', in R. French and A. Wear (eds), *The Origins of Modern British Medicine* (Cambridge, 1991), 92–109.
10. Jewson, 'Medical Knowledge', 376–7.
11. Fissell, 'Patient's Narrative', argues that the central role of the patient's narrative had by this period been considerably eroded among practitioners treating the lower orders of society.
12. ibid., 377.
13. Porter and Porter, *Patient's Progress*, 74.
14. D. Jewson, 'The Disappearance of the Sick Man from Medical Cosmology, 1770–1870', *Sociology* (1976), 234.
15. See the anecdotes listed in T.J. Pettigrew, *Biographical Memoirs*

of the most Celebrated Physicians, Surgeons, etc. etc., Who Have Contributed to the Advancement of Medical Science 3 vols (London, 1840), vol. 1, 3–4. On Abernethy's fearsome reputation, see Porter and Porter, *Patient's Progress*, 57.

16. ibid., 4.

17. G. Macilwain, *Memoirs of John Abernethy, with a View of his Lectures, his Writings, and Character; with Additional Extracts from Original Documents, now first Published* 3rd edn (London, 1856), 161.

18. Porter and Porter, *Patient's Progress*, 88.

19. 'Mr Abernethy', *Medico-Chirurgical Review* (1831), 286.

20. Manual examination of even as accessible a site as the scalp could, however, give rise to patient resistance. While John Armstrong advised his students always to examine the scalp when there was a suspicion of injury to the head, he admitted that 'in some cases this examination of the hairy scalp cannot be made; for some old maiden lady, with a flaxen-coloured wig, may call out, and prevent any such investigation'. J. Armstrong, *Lectures on the Morbid Anatomy, Nature, and Treatment, of Acute and Chronic Diseases; Delivered in the Theatre of Anatomy, Webb Street* (London, 1834), 56. Elsewhere, however, Armstrong hinted that female modesty could inhibit the discovery of serious conditions by physical investigation: *idem, The Morbid Anatomy of the Stomach, Bowels, and Liver* (London, 1838), 98.

21. Macilwain, *Memoirs*, 158–60.

22. Quoted in J. Thomson, *An Account of the Life, Lectures, and Writings of William Cullen, M.D., Professor of the Practice of Physic in the University of Edinburgh* 2 vols (Edinburgh, 1859), vol. 1, 503.

23. See M.J. Peterson, *The Medical Profession in mid-Victorian London* (Berkeley, 1978), 155–6; Porter and Porter, *Patient's Progress*, 123.

24. 'Dr Maton and Sir George Tuthill', *Lancet* (1834–5), 63.

25. DNB.

26. J. Shaw, *On the Nature and Treatment of the Distortions to which the Spine, and the Bones of the Chest, are subject. With an Enquiry into the Merits of the Several Modes of Practice which have hitherto been followed in the Treatment of Distortions* (London, 1823), ix–x.

27. R.W. Bampfield, *An Essay on Curvatures and Diseases of the Spine, including all the Forms of Spinal Distortion* (London, 1824), ii.

28. G. Rosen, *The Specialization of Medicine: With Particular Reference to Ophthalmology* (New York, undated), 34–6.

29. See J.V. Pickstone, 'Dearth or Dirt: Notes on the Theory and Practice of "Fever" in British Towns, 1780–1850', unpublished, 16.

30. F. Boott, *Memoir of the Life and Medical Opinions of John Armstrong, M.D.* (London, 1833), 32–3.

31. J. Armstrong, 'On the Brain Fever Produced by Intoxication', *Edinburgh Medical and Surgical Journal* (1813), 58–61; 'Case of Brain Fever Following Intoxication; with Some Observations', ibid., 146–53; 'Cases of Diseased Cervical Vertebrae Terminated by Anchylosis. With Observations on the Treatment of Caries of the Spine; and an Outline of a Carriage, Partly upon a New Construction, for the Use of Patients Labouring under that Disease', ibid., 385–98; 'Brief Hints, Relative to

the Improvement of the Pathology and Treatment of the Chronic Diseases usually Termed Nervous', ibid., (1815) 416–18.

32. See: J. Armstrong, *Lectures*, 55.

33. ibid., 58–9.

34. ibid., 64.

35. ibid., 657.

36. ibid., 654.

37. ibid., 655. Armstrong thought Cullen's contribution to medicine grossly overrated; his system was 'a mere metaphysical' "thing of shreds and patches"'. He thought that 'Brown, whom Cullen seemed to despise, had the ascendant in talent'. 'Lectures on the Principles and Practice of Physic, by Dr Armstrong', *Lancet* (1824–5), 355.

38. Armstrong, *Lectures*, 662.

39. 'The Late Dr Armstrong', *Med. Chir. Rev.* (1831), 243. See also Boot, *Memoir*, 30–1.

40. On the background to medical radicalism, see A. Desmond, *The Politics of Evolution: Morphology, Medicine, and Reform in Radical London* (Chicago, 1990) 26–33; on the position of teachers in the private medical schools, pp. 154–65.

41. 'The Life of Dr John Armstrong', *Med. Chir. Rev.* (1829), 284.

42. [Editorial], *Lancet* (1830–1), 401.

43. [Review of Thomas Alcock, *An Essay on the Education and Duties of the General Practitioner in Medicine and Surgery*], *Lancet* (1823), 271.

44. Armstrong, 'Lectures', 357.

45. Armstrong, *Lectures*, 655–6.

46. ibid., 655.

47. Armstrong, 'Lectures', 112.

48. Armstrong, *Lectures*, 665.

49. Such resort to continental authorities for medical advice was not unique: James Johnson mentions the case of 'Mr Charters, an eminent coach-builder in this metropolis, who has consulted almost every physician and surgeon, of any reputation, both in this country and the Continent'. Among them were the Parisian practitioners, Antoine Portal and François Magendie. 'Empyema and Pneumothorax', *Med. Chir. Rev.* (1828), 132.

50. C.J. Lawrence, 'Incommunicable Knowledge, Science, Technology, and the Clinical Art in Britain, 1850–1914', *Journal of Contemporary History* (1985), 503–20.

51. 'The Anatomy, Physiology, and Diseases of the Teeth. By Thomas Bell', *Med. Chir. Rev.* (1829), 328–9.

52. B.C. Brodie, 'Autobiography', in C. Hawkins (ed.), *The Works of Sir Benjamin Collins Brodie Bart. D.C.L. Serjeant-Surgeon to the Queen, President of the Royal Society, etc. With an Autobiography* 3 vols (London, 1865), vol. 1, 86.

53. Bampfield maintained that his special knowledge of diseases of the spine could not have been acquired in private practice; it derived from his experience as a surgeon at the Royal Metropolitan Infirmary for Diseases of Children. Bampfield, *An Essay*, iii–iv.

54. Jewson, 'Medical Knowledge', 370–3.

55. J. Abernethy, *Surgical Observations on the Constitutional Origins and Treatment of Local Diseases; and on Aneurisms*, 3rd edn (London, 1814), 2–3.

56. ibid., 65.

57. ibid., 67.

58. 'Mr Abernethy', 286.

59. 'Fatal Disease of the Brain Mistaken', *Med. Chir. Rev.* (1828), 454–5.

60. Jewson, 'The Disappearance', 228–9.

61. Brodie, 'Autobiography', 80.

62. 'The Life of Dr John Armstrong', *Med. Chir. Rev.* (1829), 282.

63. 'Medical Seed-time. Professional Omnibuses', *Med. Chir. Rev.* (1831), 146.

64. 'In Memoriam', in Hawkins, *The Works*, xiii.

65. Brodie, 'Autobiography', 479, 528.

66. ibid., 502.

67. ibid., 78.

68. ibid., 110.

69. ibid.

70. ibid.

71. ibid., 115.

Index